The
Holistic Nursing Approach to Chronic Disease

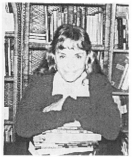**Carolyn Chambers Clark, ARNP, EdD, FAAN, AHNC,** founded The Wellness Institute and is now Director, Wellness Resources (http://home.earthlink.net/~cccwellness), providing continuing-education materials, newsletters, seminars, and practice management consultation. She also is host of http://HolisticHealth.bellaonline.com and http://Menopause.bellaonline.com. As a certified advanced holistic nurse and mental health nurse practitioner, she has maintained a private practice with clients for more than 30 years, focusing on whole person wellness.

She was elected a Fellow of the American Academy of Nursing in 1980 and is an award-winning author who has conducted research and published widely on wellness, holistic, and self-care topics, including *Wellness Practitioner, Integrating Complementary Procedures into Practice, Health Promotion in Communities: Holistic and Wellness Approaches,* and *The Encyclopedia of Complementary Health Practice.* She was also founding editor of the *Alternative Health Practitioner: The Journal of Complementary and Natural Care* and is the author of *Group Leadership Skills,* now in its fourth edition.

The
Holistic Nursing Approach
to Chronic Disease

Carolyn Chambers Clark
ARNP, EdD, FAAN, AHNC

 Springer Publishing Company

Springer Publishing Company, Inc.
536 Broadway
New York, NY 10012-3955

Acquisitions Editor: Ruth Chasek
Production Editor: Pamela Lankas
Cover design by Joanne Honigman

04 05 06 07 08 / 5 4 3 2 1

Library of Congress Cataloging-in-Publication Data

Clark, Carolyn Chambers.
  The holistic nursing approach to chronic disease / by Carolyn Chambers Clark.
       p. ; cm.
  Includes bibliographical references.
  ISBN 0-8261-2504-2
  1. Chronic diseases—Nursing. 2. Holistic nursing.
  [DNLM: 1. Chronic Disease—nursing. 2. Holistic Nursing.
WY 152 C592h 2004] I. Title.

RT120.C45C537 2004
610.73'6—dc22

                                                      2004014929

Printed in the United States of America by Maple-Vail Book Manufacturing Group.

*In grateful thanks for your support and colleagueship,
I dedicate this book to four holistic nurses who nominated
me for the Holistic Nurse of the Year, Charlotte Eliopolous, PhD,
MPH, RN, who spear-headed the effort; Nancy Oliver, PhD, RN;
Rorry Zahourek, PhD, RN; and Mary Anne Bright, RN, CS, EdD.*

CONTENTS

ACKNOWLEDGMENTS

Thank you to all the clients, students, and nurses who, over the years, have provided me with important questions and enthusiasm for my answers.

Special thanks to Dr. Ursula Springer, who has supported my writing efforts since 1977; and to Ruth Chasek, my editor, a true diplomat and organizational genius; to Pamela Lankas, an editorial professional; to Joanne Honigman, a delight to work with and a creative book cover designer; and to all the others at Springer Publishing Company who have assisted with this book.

CHAPTER 1

Introduction to the Holistic Nursing Approach

Florence Nightingale recognized the importance of whole-person approaches. She integrated the healing arts with conventional treatments, including touch, light, aromatics, empathetic listening, music, and quiet reflection (American Holistic Nurses' Association, 2001). Her *theory of natural healing* defined the nurse as the provider of an environment conducive to the reparative process, and the client as having vital, natural, reparative power that can be accessed within the appropriate environment (Selanders, 1993).

To achieve this reparative state, holistic nursing combines traditional and complementary modalities (American Holistic Nurses' Association, 1997). It is up to you, as a holistic nurse, to collaborate with clients to create a plan of care based on their unique health beliefs, cultural background, sexual orientation, values, and preferences. This plan focuses on health promotion, disease prevention, recovery or restoration, or peaceful dying, all the while assisting the client to be as independent as possible (American Holistic Nurses' Association, 2001).

A holistic nursing approach embraces interventions focused on client responses that heal the whole person and help bring balance, realizing that modalities, therapies, and healing arts by themselves are not the essence of holism and wellness. Holistic nurses also assist clients to assume personal responsibility for wellness by serving as wellness role models who integrate self-care procedures into their own lives. Be sure to build wellness self-care procedures into your daily regime. It will help you ward off stress and give you plenty of energy to help clients by establishing a balance between what you give to yourself and what you give to others (American Holistic Nurses' Association, 1997).

Holistic nursing includes assessment, intervention, and evaluation phases, although the process rarely works in a linear fashion. As you gather more information and begin to intervene, you may have to double back and collect more assessment information. Likewise, after beginning an intervention, you may find that a specific approach is not useful for a particular client. This finding should make you pause, gather more information from the client, reassess, and collaborate to find a more useful intervention or combination of approaches. Despite the interactive nurse–client process in holistic nursing, for the purposes of discussion, the phases will be discussed separately, but bear in mind that they are most often circular and fed by the verbal and nonverbal feedback you receive from clients.

COMMUNICATION IN HOLISTIC NURSING

Throughout the holistic nursing process, the importance of two-way communication is emphasized. Holistic nursing approaches are not driven by an "expert" who chooses an intervention and applies it. Holistic nursing approaches occur while communicating respect for clients' uniqueness and the integrity of their mind-body-spirit, and by fully listening to and checking out the meaning of client statements.

USE REAL, NOT "PSEUDO" LISTENING

Holistic nursing interventions are collaborations based on real listening. *Real listening* means that you have the intention to understand, enjoy, learn, and/or give help or solace (McKay, Davis, & Fanning, 1995). Some needs and intentions that may get in the way of real listening include being concerned with whether the client likes you, worrying about being rejected, ignoring all but one piece of information the client presents, preparing for your next comment, sifting through information to find vulnerabilities, and checking to make sure your comment produced the desired effect. Other situations that may result in less than real listening involve only half-listening because you're waiting for your turn to talk or because you know you should listen but feel the pressure to get away and complete other tasks.

ELIMINATE BLOCKS TO LISTENING

Take heart. Everyone is a pseudo-listener at times. You may only half-listen because you're pushed by time pressures or other types of stress. Even if you are feeling the strain, keep in mind that half-listening can harm your communication process with clients.

One important step you can take to enhance the amount of real listening you do is to consciously affirm to yourself that your intent is to really listen. Do this before entering the room. When you are with the client, make a conscious effort to focus on really listening. Consider letting clients know when you are under time pressures (e.g., "Sorry if it seems I'm only half-listening today, but I'm under some work pressures. Let's make an appointment to talk later today when I'll be able to give you my full attention.").

This kind of comment is useful because clients are smart; they know when someone isn't really listening, and they may conclude it's because of something they're doing. If you state the real problem, it is much less likely that clients will continue to think they are at fault. Another important step you can take to enhance real listening in your practice is to identify any blocks to listening that may crop up in your conversations. These include comparing, mind reading, rehearsing, filtering, judging, dreaming, identifying, sparring, being right, derailing, and placating (McKay et al., 1995).

Comparing makes it hard to listen to clients because you're assessing if you know the right answer or are competent or how you stack up against clients. Some thoughts that show this kind of listening block are, "Boy, this person's really had it bad," or "I've had it harder than she has," or "I know just what this person needs to do." The best defense against this kind of pseudo-listening is to catch yourself doing it and bring your focus back to what the client is saying at the moment.

Mind reading happens when you doubt what you hear and observe and try to figure out what clients are *really* thinking and feeling. This can lead to making assumptions about clients that aren't backed up with clinical data (e.g., "He says he doesn't drink, but yet he has bruises consistent with being drunk," and "She says she's ready to try to walk, but she must be tired after not sleeping all night"). Instead of mind reading the best response is to state your observations and ask if they are correct, not assume you know. Of course, clients always have the right to deny their actions, feelings, or thoughts, and that's okay because it means they aren't completely comfortable sharing their thoughts and feelings. As well, a denial provides a starting point for making encouraging comments, such as, "Only tell me what you feel comfortable saying." This kind of statement lets clients know that they set the level of disclosure. Most often, once you give them that power, they will feel more comfortable and will more readily disclose.

Rehearsing occurs when you're thinking about what to say next after the client stops talking. When you put your attention on rehearsing, you can't be really listening. Try to catch yourself rehearsing, then focus on listening to the client fully, prior to thinking about how to respond.

Filtering occurs when you listen to some client statements and not to others. There is an old saying in mental health circles: "You can only help clients up to and as far as you've resolved your own problems." What this means is our own internal roadblocks prevent us from hearing and exploring client issues that set off anxiety in us. No one has resolved all of life's issues, and we're all struggling to understand ourselves and each other. To reduce filtering, it would be wise to study what happens when you filter conversations. Otherwise, you may find yourself filtering or totally denying, having no memory of upsetting topics, and not hearing someone's anger, unhappiness, or other upsetting feelings.

Judging occurs when you place labels on clients. If you find yourself thinking about a client as an "alcoholic," "drug addict," or "immoral," "not Christian," "crazy," or some other judging statement, you've ceased to really listen and instead are using a knee-jerk response. Avoid making judgments at all, although it is useful to come to conclusions and then validate them with clients (e.g., "If I understand you correctly, you're saying that _____.").

Dreaming can happen when a client says or does something that triggers a chain of your private associations. Suppose a client says her husband left her and you're newly divorced. In a flash, you're back to your divorce and not really listening to what is being said. When you're dreaming, you will miss a lot of really important information. If you've been through a traumatic situation or are currently in one, be sure to get professional counseling from someone you trust and who is a good listener. That way, you'll be less apt to dream while working with clients.

Identifying can happen when you take what the client says and actually bring in your own experience. Suppose a client tells you about his recent surgery and you begin to tell her about your surgery or another client's surgery. This will cut off communication with the client, so be very careful about sharing private information unless you are totally sure it can help. The best thing to do in this instance is to discuss what you plan to share with a more experienced communicator, perhaps a psychiatric/mental health clinical specialist, prior to sharing your personal information with a client.

Sparring occurs when you disagree, put down, or discount what a client says. Nurses are probably most apt to discount their own worth and to refuse to accept compliments from a client. This leaves the client feeling unsatisfied that you really heard the compliment. And the client is probably right because you didn't, not in a real sense. A simple "thank you" when a compliment is given could solve this block.

Being right means going to any lengths to avoid being wrong. As a professional, it may be hard to admit that you made a mistake, that you didn't listen fully, or even that you misunderstood a client's statement. There is nothing wrong with making a mistake, just acknowledge it (e.g., "You're right, I did misunderstand you," or "You're right, I didn't take your suggestion for change"), and then refocus on the topic that was being discussed.

Derailing occurs when you change the subject. Let's suppose a client is talking about masturbating or having sex with his wife. If you're uncomfortable with these topics (or others), you're more apt to derail and change the subject. Another way to derail is to make a joke or quip to take the tension out of a situation. This can result in clients' concluding that situations that are important to them can't be discussed with you.

Placating means you verbally agree with everything clients say. Some clues that you might be placating are finding yourself saying, "I know what you mean," or "Of course you are" or "Right, right." Placating often has to do with wanting clients to like you. When the focus becomes you and not the client, you are the roadblock to communication. Try to catch yourself placating others. If you can't, ask for feedback from colleagues, friends, and even clients, until you can identify your placating statements.

Now that you're familiar with the blocks, you probably have a pretty good idea which ones you use. Use the steps in Table 1.1 to help you stop blocking. Consider the steps as an experiment in objectively observing yourself and evaluating the results.

At first, you may feel uncomfortable trying to change your communication patterns, but in time, you will begin to use more real listening. You will also reap the following gigantic rewards when you change the way you relate: clients will deeply appreciate it, crises will cool down, miscommunication will stop, you will learn to remember what was said, and blocking will stop.

TABLE 1.1   Steps to Stop Blocking Communication and Start Listening

1. Identify a communication block you use often and keep a count of how many times a day you use it.

2. Identify what subjects or situations usually trigger the block.

3. Identify what you were feeling (bored, anxious, irritated, hurt, frustrated, rushed, down, tired, preoccupied, etc.) when you started to block.

4. The next day, consciously avoid using your blocking comments and use paraphrasing instead, choosing one of the following, and fill in what you heard the client saying, "Let me see if I understand: you're saying _____." "I want to understand your feelings; is this the way you feel? _____." "Do you mean _____?" "If I heard you right, what happened was _____." "From what you said, you're very angry (frustrated, upset, fearful, etc.) about what's happened to you."

Pay attention to your reactions and your efforts to resist blocking. If you are able to cut back at all, consider this experiment a success. If you don't learn as fast as you'd like, find a colleague who agrees to help. Ask that person to tell you the details of an important but upsetting event. At intervals, paraphrase what's been said and then ask your colleague if you really understood. As you work together, ask questions until you understand. Use *clarifying* to let the other person know that you're interested (e.g., "What do you mean by that?" or "Give me an example of that."). If you didn't really understand what was said, re-paraphrase until your colleague is satisfied. Keep at it until you don't use the block anymore.

If you find none of these suggestions works for you, consider obtaining counseling. Remember that the more healed and whole you become, the more you will have to offer to clients (Quinn, 1997).

HOLISTIC NURSING ASSESSMENT

As with any other type of nursing intervention, a client assessment is completed. Whatever approach is used, teaching and learning are paramount. Clients must be informed consumers who know the cause of their condition and the rationale for suggested treatment so they can participate as fully as possible. Even a client who is dying can make simple decisions. Does he want a massage first or a nap? Does she want to try eating her lunch as a juice drink or soup? Does she want to hold your hand or not? Use the information below to sharpen your holistic nursing skills.

KNOWLEDGE

You may teach clients information, provide handouts, or assist them in their search for information so that they can become informed consumers. To assess client learning needs, ask them to tell you what they know about their dis-ease and treatment. (The word "dis-ease" is used throughout this book because from a metaphysical view of things, a great many physical symptoms are believed to be caused by negative thoughts and attitudes that can be correlated with a lack of balance and increased stress. This stress can weaken body organs and body functions, leading to distress, and if it becomes chronic, to body malfunctioning.)

The good news is that dis-ease can be often be reversed by reversing mental patterns (Hay, 2000). Louise Hay is an example of someone who, when given the diagnosis of vaginal cancer, began to examine the cause. As a five-year-old, she had been raped and battered. Aware that cancer could come from a pattern of deep resentment that is held for a long time until it eats away the body, she knew she had work to do. She worked hard to clear the mental pattern that had created the dis-ease. After three months of mental and physical cleansing, she was pronounced free of cancer (Hay, 2000).

Clients are often not aware of how their mental patterns may be creating their dis-ease. As you talk with them, information they lack will become readily apparent and you can provide needed knowledge or assist clients to find their own sources. Some may be aware of how their behavior is affecting their dis-ease, but may not be ready to strike out on a wellness path. A sample list of holistic nursing assessment questions is provided in Table 1.2.

MEANING

When you use a holistic nursing approach, keep in mind that you will be working with an autonomous individual who is your therapeutic partner in the journey to healing and wholeness. Make sure you use a holistic framework that encompasses bodymindspirit, one that views the client as a dynamic interacting system of complex energy existing in a complex energy environment. This will help you to better understand the underlying causes of dis-ease or dis-ability.

TABLE 1.2   Holistic Nursing Assessment Questions

Below you will find a list of suggested questions to ask clients about their dis-ease. Revise or add to them depending on your style of speaking and your experience.

1. What would you like to tell me about your dis-ease?
2. What is your usual diet?
3. What kind of exercise do you do and how often?
4. What kinds of things do you usually think about or worry about?
5. What do you think led up to your dis-ease?
6. How do you feel about being diagnosed with _____?
7. Who is the one person you can talk things over with and feel understood?
8. How has this person helped or hindered you in getting well?
9. What would be a sign to you that you're getting better?
10. What is your goal(s) in relation to your condition?
11. What goal(s) do you have that you need help to achieve?
12. What do you need to learn to achieve your goal(s)?
13. How can I help you feel better?
14. What story can you tell me about your life journey and struggle?
15. From the list below, what kinds of self-help approaches have/haven't worked for you?
    Put a yes if they've worked; no if they haven't.

    ____ acupressure   ____ affirmations   ____ aromatherapy
    ____ energy therapy   ____ guided imagery   ____ hypnosis
    ____ massage   ____ prayer   ____ relaxation therapy
    ____ touch therapies ____ other: explain
    ____ other: explain
    ____ other: explain

Of the totality of bodymindspirit, perhaps the least well understood is spirit or soul. *Soul* is the individualized form of spirit, and is roughly the equivalent of the Jungian unconscious, creative and full of inspiration and spiritual connection. *Spirituality* is the process of developing a relationship with the hidden, transcendental realm of existence, the grounded being—God, if this is personified, or the Universal Energy or Universal Power if it isn't. Spirituality also encompasses life purpose, reverence for the earth and each other.

Think of spirituality as a process, not a state or a place to get to, but a relationship. Re-storying helps give meaning to earlier experiences and provides a format for discussion.

How is this accomplished with clients? See Table 1.3 for some ideas (Blatner, 2003).

For best results, complete the work in Table 1.3 yourself prior to using it with clients. When using the questions with clients, change the words to fit with your speech patterns and what you feel comfortable saying. Just remember to keep to the main idea for each task.

As you work with this process for yourself and with clients, remember that spiritual individuals tend to be more hopeful and to experience more meaning or purpose in life than their nonspiritual peers. Themes most strongly associated with spirituality are community or connectedness, charity, hope, forgiveness, meaning, and morality (Mahoney & Graci, 1999).

As with any nursing intervention, client readiness is an important factor. Whether clients are ready to change their dis-ease-related patterns or not, they all have strengths you can build upon. Some clients may verbalize or demonstrate feelings of hopelessness and powerlessness. Often these are the individuals who have lost (or have never found) a life purpose or spiritual path, or who have been disappointed so often they have given up.

Keep in focus that the mind is the primary or at least a coequal factor in all conditions. Use the information in Table 1.4 as a guide.

By using the information in Table 1.4, you can begin to evaluate the whole client, including finding out the meaning attached to the person's symptoms. There are perhaps as many meanings for dis-ease or the disharmony in the individual as there are clients. Be sure to check out your hunches with clients. Not only will this procedure validate that you're reading meanings, but it can also provide helpful feedback for them.

To begin a holistic nursing assessment, gather data about client symptoms and how they are perceived. Table 1.5 provides examples of meaning clients could ascribe to their dis-ease process. Keep in mind that these are only examples. Clients are unique in the meaning they ascribe to their dis-ease process.

As you work with clients, become aware of patterns that may have led to the chronic condition and that could lead out of it. Begin to understand what the process of this condition is and how it can be accepted, modified, or even prevented. Notice the attitudes clients hold that make it difficult for them to get past the

TABLE 1.3   A Spiritual Journey: Re-storying with Clients

Directions: To help clients reframe or re-story their spiritual journey, ask them to

1. tell a story about their lives

2. use the words "my journey," "my struggle"

3. tell how their soul got a little lost, a little diminished, a little suppressed in the course of time, and how they began to find it again, and restore its wholeness

4. identify personal symbols, such as an animal, a design, a poem or song, a piece of music or art, a talisman, a treasure, or any other valued object

5. tell how they chose their symbol or if it was thrust upon them

6. describe what the symbol means to them

7. tell how the symbol can be used in their healing journey

8. draw the symbol

9. let the drawn symbol speak to them about how it was formed and what the symbol says about them.

condition and back to health and wellness, and begin to get a handle on their ability to participate in care as well as some hunches about how to engage them in a wellness process.

RELATIONSHIPS

When completing a holistic assessment, evaluate the relationships between the client and significant others and explore how these relationships affect the client's dis-ease. For example, do family members act as enablers, buying fatty and sugary foods for clients who want to lose weight and then chiding them if they don't eat those forbidden foods? Other family members may denigrate clients, keeping them at a low level of self-esteem so that they will perform in ways the family deems is correct. In some cases, family members may be willing and ready to provide additional support, but the client lags behind. In other cases, family members may need educational experiences or support from you so they can provide what is needed for clients.

The client's relationship with you is another piece of the puzzle. Assess what role the client tries to cast you in. It will often mirror

TABLE 1.4   The Mind as Coequal Factor in All Conditions

Directions: As you listen to clients speak, search for patterns. Use the ideas below to guide you.

1. What verbalized thought or value patterns are involved in this dis-ease?
2. What gut feelings or intuitions do I get about this client?
3. What does the client report or demonstrate about the basis of this dis-ease?
4. What valuable signals of internal conflict do the client's pain and dis-ease portray?
5. How can I explore these conflicts in a helpful, nonintrusive way?

the roles clients play in relation to other family members. Identify any ethical dilemmas that may be trapping the client (or you) and retarding the growth process.

HOLISTIC NURSING TREATMENT PLANNING

When using a holistic model, be sure to include caring approaches as a component of healing. Whenever possible, encourage minimally invasive wellness approaches. Emphasize the prevention of illness and the achievement of maximum bodymindspirit wellness. The word could just as well be written mindbodyspirit or spiritbodymind because in a dynamic, holistic sense, it is not a linear concept, but a fully interactive one.

Despite the type of approaches you and the client choose, keep in the forefront of your mind various ways to communicate respect for clients' uniqueness, integrity of mindbodyspirit, personal power, and self-healing processes. The first step in moving in this direction, as mentioned earlier, is to learn to listen fully to clients. If you find yourself talking a lot about yourself or introducing topics of conversation, these behaviors may be clues that you need to obtain training in listening skills. Socializing with clients and talking about yourself or your problems will only dilute the help you can give to them.

APPROACHES

To facilitate healing, holistic nurses use many methods of knowing and being (Quinn, 1997). *Process-oriented approaches* focus not so

TABLE 1.5   Examples of Meaning and Potential Action for Client Dis-Ease

Dis-ease process	Client meaning	Client action
AIDS	a punishment	periods of fighting to survive, followed by giving up
cancer	challenge	rise to the occasion, take positive self-care action
overweight or obesity	the enemy, something outside them that takes over, leaving them powerless	eating more to forget
heart conditions	a weakness, belief that if only they were stronger perhaps they could have avoided becoming ill	frantic searching alternating with wellness self-care
arthritis	Seeking loving care missed while growing up	escape to the bed or to complaining
fibromyalgia	damaged goods	unworthiness; nursing hurts
diabetes	deep sorrow	grieving for what might have been

much on the outcome or even on what is said, but on the process that occurs between you and a client or between clients and their conditions. A *nurturing/caring approach* may be of the most use for clients who are feeling helpless and who lack energy to collaborate. Until they recover their self-esteem, strength, or goal direction, this may be the best approach. Other clients who are ready to function at a higher level and who have found a way to meet their basic needs may profit from a *collaborative approach*. In this intervention, you share power with clients and collaborate with them to find the best way to deal with their condition. An *intuitive approach* may work well when you feel especially in tune with some clients. With them, following your intuition about what may help them may be the best approach. An *analytic approach* may work with clients who are interested in talking about details and specifics. They like to keep diaries and write in journals, hoping to understand what their condition is about and how they can influence it. Clients functioning at this level of development are ready to view themselves as a case study or as their own one-person experiment, trying new activities and self-evaluating the result.

INFORMATION

Throughout the treatment phase, it is helpful to go to the literature and look up studies that provide information to assist you in your work. PubMed.com is a good place to start this exploration. This effort will provide the *empirical knowledge* that puts your approaches in a scientific perspective. When possible, share the findings with the client. If you have suffered the same symptoms or worked with clients or family members who have, you can share your *personal knowledge* base and use it as a support for current planning. This kind of approach can inspire confidence in you and in your clients because you know the pathway back to wellness. *Ethical knowledge* sources and approaches may be critical when working with clients. For example, when working with a depressed client who threatens suicide, sharing lifesaving information with family members or others may create an ethical dilemma after pledging privacy and confidentiality. *Aesthetic knowledge,* including pictures and other art objects produced by clients, can provide important information and insight about thoughts, feelings, and needs. Any artistic production by clients deserves mention, and if possible, discussion. Because the right brain is used in this kind of work, more holistic and free expression may be evoked. Aesthetic approaches may be the treatment of choice with clients who cannot verbally express themselves or whose thoughts are blocked from verbal expression but released during drawing or other artistic actions.

It is expected that the holistic nursing process will be used with each condition. See Table 1.6 for questions to ask yourself when planning nursing approaches.

HOLISTIC NURSING INTERVENTIONS

There are many ways to promote healing in clients. For example, you can assist clients in the physical realm by using measures that help cells and tissues to grow and bond. You can assist clients in

TABLE 1.6   Planning Nursing Approaches

1. According to the client, what is the relationship between the condition and nutrition, exercise, stress, environmental concerns, social support, spiritual and/or cultural beliefs?
2. What additional information about the relationship between the condition and nutrition, exercise, stress, environmental concerns, social support, and spiritual and/or cultural beliefs have I identified and shared with the client?
3. What patterns has the client identified as leading to the condition?
4. What additional patterns or knowledge have I identified and shared with the client?
5. What is the client's understanding of the process of this condition?
6. What additional clarity can I bring to the client to help in the understanding of the process of this condition?
7. What is the client's level of acceptance of the condition?
8. What strategies can I use and teach the client that could enhance acceptance of the condition?
9. What is the client's understanding of how to modify the condition?
10. What attitudes must change in order for the client to heal?
11. What will assist in integrating or balancing the client's body, mind, and spirit so this condition recesses or resolves?
12. How can I strengthen the client's responses to facilitate the healing process and wholeness?
13. How can I integrate self-care into my life so as to serve as a role model for this client?
14. What actions can I use and teach the client to use to avoid absorbing others' negative energy patterns?
15. How can I use the interconnectedness of individuals and their relationships to each other and the global community to facilitate healing?
16. What is the best mix of mind, body, and spirit approaches (especially those that are evidence based) to assist the client toward wholeness and well-being?

the mind/emotion aspect by helping to potentiate the shift from resentment to forgiveness, and finding ways to release energy for new growth and expanded consciousness. You can assist clients in the spiritual realm by helping them to experience unconditional love and transcend separateness from the source of universal energy (or whatever are their spiritual beliefs) and all creation. Specific interventions can range from guided imagery to therapeutic or healing touch, journal writing, artistic creations, and rituals to many other holistic approaches that can meet agreed-upon goals.

To achieve these outcomes, you must be well grounded in the difference between curing and healing. It may not be possible to cure all clients, but they all can be healed if they agree to be and if they put forth the effort or consciousness that is required. Realize that each healing process is unique and cannot be coerced, manipulated, or controlled. Because this is true, it is necessary to assess what the healing process is for each client, and then to respect it.

Important questions to ask yourself in this regard are:

- How can I help this client to formulate a healing intention?
- How can I teach this client to support this intention through the healing process with this condition?
- How can I use a meditative state to maximize the healing environment of the client in this condition (e.g., by centering myself)?
- How can I use nonverbal communication methods to enhance healing (e.g., using a caring and calm tone of voice and facial expression; using touch to convey care, support, nurture, and confidence; conveying safety and sufficient time through tone of voice, expression, and touch)?
- How can I shift consciousness, or assist the client to shift consciousness, to enhance the healing state for this condition (e.g., tuning into and modifying my own state of consciousness and well-being)?
- How can I use my own healing process with similar symptoms to understand and be a courageous companion on the healing journey for clients?
- How do I help create a sacred healing space to assist the healing process for this condition?
- How do I use the following processes to enhance healing of clients with this condition: being open to self-discovery, modeling self-care, offering clients methods for working on life issues, guiding clients in the discovery of creative options, and recognizing that clients know the best life choices for themselves so that they can cope with life processes?

TREATMENT EVALUATION

Healing outcomes reflect a change in client awareness, perception, behavior, and relationships. Outcomes could include decreased pain, enhanced wound healing, increased energy, enhanced ability to express or name feelings, perceptual reframing of an upsetting situation, healing of a painful memory, improved relationships, improved self-concept, enhanced understanding of reciprocity in relationships, forgiveness, deeper sense of connection to life or self, alignment of life's purpose and path of expression in work, greater excitement and creativity in work, recognition of the meaning and healing rhythms of the environment, enhanced ability to cope with stress, verbalized sense of well-being/quality of life, increased ability to perform self-care tasks, establishment of healthy boundaries, and willingness to change (McKivergin, 1997).

Unlike traditional models of treatment in which the professional conducts the evaluation, in the holistic nursing model, the client is a partner in evaluating the effects of treatment. There are many ways to do this. Some suggestions appear below.

1. Ask the client to evaluate the effect of a treatment by giving you specific examples of observed changes.
2. Teach the client how to chart observations in a journal or diary and discuss the findings at the next meeting.
3. Use an agreed-upon rating scale.

THE CHRONIC DISEASES

Chronic conditions discussed in this book include AIDS, allergies/asthma, Alzheimer's, arthritis, cancer, carpal tunnel syndrome, chronic fatigue syndrome, depression, diabetes, digestive problems, fibromyalgia, heart and blood vessel disorders, kidney disease, liver and gallbladder disease, multiple sclerosis, osteoporosis, overweight/obesity, pain, Parkinson's disease, and sleep disorders.

I've chosen to cover these conditions because they're chronic and because a lot can be done beyond standard medical treatment to help clients strengthen themselves and reduce or prevent symptoms. Self-care advice in this book is backed by research. Studies that support the validity of each self-care approach can be found at the back of each chapter.

Each condition section includes specific examples of a holistic nursing assessment with a sample client, collaborative treatment plan/interventions, and their possible effects. Use the assessment/evaluation presented for each condition as a starting point, remembering that each client is unique and that the assessment/plan/evaluation was developed for the client presented.

REFERENCES

American Holistic Nurses' Association. (1997). *AHNA standards of holistic nursing practice.* Flagstaff, AZ: Author.

American Holistic Nurses' Association. (2001). *Position on the role of nurses in the practice of complementary and alternative therapies.* Flagstaff, AZ: Author.

Hay, L. (2000). *Heal your body.* Carlsbad, CA: Hay House.

Mahoney, M. J., & Graci, G. M. (1999). The meaning and correlates of spirituality: Suggestions from an exploratory survey of experts. *Death Studies, 23*(6), 521–528.

McKay, M., Davis, M., & Fanning, P. (1995). *Messages: The communication book.* Oakland, CA: New Harbinger.

McKivergin, M. (1997). The nurse as an instrument of healing. In B. Dossey (Ed.), *Core curriculum for holistic nursing* (pp. 17–25). Gaithersburg, MD: Aspen.

Nightingale, F. (1860). *Notes on nursing.* London: Harrison.

Quinn, J. F. (1997). Transpersonal human caring and healing. In B. Dossey (Ed.), *Core curriculum for holistic nursing* (pp. 13–16). Gaithersburg, MD: Aspen.

Selanders, L. C. (1993). *Florence Nightingale: An environmental adaptation theory.* Newbury Park, CA: Sage.

Chapter 2

AIDS/HIV

It is believed that a virus called HIV causes AIDS, but only 50%–60% of those exposed to HIV actually develop AIDS. There is much that can be done to strengthen the immune system so that AIDS does not develop (Perdue, 2000) and to reduce or eliminate complications (Nicholas et al., 2002). AZT is not a cure for the HIV infection, but it is commonly prescribed, as are 3TC and Combivir. There are many other drugs used and new medications are being developed. They are toxic drugs. The side effects of AZT include blood disorders, nausea, vomiting, muscle pain, headaches, liver abnormalities, anxiety, tremors, and confusion. The long-term toxicity of this drug is not known, but the risk for children born to HIV-infected women who take AZT is nearly three times greater than in the general population.

HOLISTIC NURSING ASSESSMENT

Study the holistic nursing assessment that follows. The nurse devised this nursing assessment after working with Mr. H., a 35-year-old man diagnosed with AIDS. Use the format and information as an exemplar for your holistic work with clients who suffer from HIV/AIDS.

Client learning needs: "I'm trying to figure out how I got AIDS."

Indicants of readiness to learn: "Can you help me? I read somewhere there was a nutritional connection. Do you know anything about that?"

Soul/spirituality symbol(s): Draws inspiration from a seascape by his bedside.

Meaning of the condition to client: "This is a punishment for having sex, isn't it?"

Relationship needs/effects as perceived by the client: "My father thinks he's being helpful, but he's really very critical. Always has been. I want to work things out with him before I die, but I'm too angry."

Patterns/attitudes that may create dis-ease for this client: Client uses negative affirmations often (e.g., "I'm never going to get well," and "This thing has a strangle hold on me."). Client reports eating "junk foods" and "taking drugs for years." Unresolved feelings toward his father may be adding stress. Client reports no stress reduction tools except "not thinking about this."

Life purpose: Client indicates no life purpose and facial expression indicates hopelessness.

Client strengths: Client is able to verbalize feelings and willing to discuss a plan of care.

Ability to participate in care: Client has periods of weakness, but expresses interest in learning and changing nutritional patterns.

Ethical dilemmas: Should the client be given "comfort only" measures even though the physician in charge wants to continue medication? The client has asked for assisted suicide information—what is the nurse's role?

Nurse–client process: The client talks in an angry tone to the nurse. With discussion, the client reveals the nurse reminds him of his mother.

TREATMENT PLANNING: SETTING JOINTLY AGREED-UPON GOALS

A good way to focus treatment planning is to develop goals in collaboration with a client. Assume clients know the best life choices for themselves and will reveal their wishes if you listen closely and observe.

In the case of the client discussed above, the following goals were agreed upon:

1. Reduce anxiety/stress level.
2. Reduce angry feelings toward father.
3. Reduce guilt feelings.
4. Enhance healing.

Goals can be individualized, but for clients in advanced stages of HIV-AIDS, comfort and rest may rank high. Inquire what goals the client has for treatment and state your intention to help meet them. If the client is unable to state a goal, you can state two or three goals you think might be helpful and ask the client for verbal or nonverbal agreement. Examine the treatment plan that follows and use it as a starting point for your work with clients diagnosed with AIDS.

TREATMENT

Acceptance of condition/attitude change: The client chose the following affirmation to use to replace the guilt he feels: "I do not accept any energy that is contrary to the unlimited positive power that lies within me." Client agreed to write or say the affirmation at least 20 times each day.

Facilitating the healing process/healing intention formulation: From a list of meditative statements, client chose the following one to assist in the healing process: "I love and appreciate all of myself." Nurse asked client to write this statement as an affirmation on 3 x 5 cards, put them in prominent places around the room, and meditate on the words while in a relaxed state. Nurse will use caring nonverbal communication, centering, and a meditative state to enhance client healing, and will verbalize observed patterns that may be holding the client back and offer alternate approaches.

Creating a sacred space: Client requested natural light, Mozart, and removal of papers and unnecessary materials from his bedside. Agreed to use prayer to cleanse the energy of the working space.

Encouraging re-storying: Client has begun to tell stories about his life path and agreed to write in a journal about elements of his struggle and journey.

Integrative practices planned: Client stated he felt tense and wanted to learn relaxation procedures and how to ask his friends to stop bringing in junk foods. Nurse made an appointment to work out a relaxation script for developing an audio tape and suggested ways of asking his friends not to bring him junk food.

Role model strategies: Showed client some of the affirmation cards she used to heal herself.

Protection plan: Agreed to teach client centering procedures and picture a white light around nurse and client to protect against negative influences in the environment.

Family strategies: Client agreed to write a letter to his father about how he feels, but not to mail it. Instead client will discuss the content and the pros and cons of mailing the letter vs. calling and asking him to visit. Client chose an anger release ritual to reduce additional anger toward his father.

Life issues/life purpose work: Will encourage client to be open to self-discovery and offer client methods for working on life issues. Client has agreed to begin journal writing and drawing, focusing on forgiveness of himself and others.

Treatment possibilities/considerations: AIDS treatment is very expensive and the new drugs aren't working as well as once thought. Prevention remains the best hope against AIDS, including condoms, providing needle exchange programs for drug addicts, and education about how unprotected sexual intercourse and intravenous drug injections can lead to AIDS. Even after being diagnosed with AIDS, clients can take actions to enhance the immune system. Suggested treatments appear below. Most are evidence-based.

ADDITIONAL INFORMATION AND TREATMENTS TO SHARE WITH CLIENTS

NUTRITION

Encourage clients to:

1. *Eat foods high in vitamins C (1,000 IU/day) and E (800 mg/day)* to reduce stress and infectious organisms (Allard et al., 1998). Foods high in vitamin C include green peppers, honeydew melon, cooked broccoli or Brussels sprouts, cooked kale, cantaloupes, strawberries, papaya, cooked cauliflower, oranges, watercress, raspberries, parsley, raw cabbage, grapefruit, blackberries, lemons, onions, sprouts, spinach, and tomatoes. Foods high in vitamin E include wheat germ, peanuts, outer leaves of cabbage, leafy portions of broccoli and cauliflower, raw spinach, asparagus, whole grains (rice, wheat or oats), cold pressed wheat germ or safflower oil, cornmeal, eggs, and sweet potatoes.

2. *Take a selenium supplement.* Selenium is an essential trace element that is important in the optimum function of the immune system. Many soils have been depleted of the nutrient (Hori, Hatfield, Maldarelli, Lee, & Clouse, 1997), so a supplement is often needed. Selenium supplements can suppress the human immunodeficiency virus type 1 (Hori et al., 1997), increase the immune defense of HIV-infected clients, and reduce death due to AIDS (Patrick, 1999).

3. *Eat foods high in Vitamin B12 or take a supplement* (Patrick, 2000). Foods high in cyanocobalamin include mackerel, seafood, soybeans, tofu, tempeh, kelp, soy cheese, nori, and eggs. Try to obtain the organic versions of these foods. Combine with calcium foods (soy cheese, broccoli, kale) for better assimilation.

4. *Eat foods rich in sulfur.* Sulfur-containing amino acids (SAAs) such as methionine, cysteine, homocysteine, and taurine provide protection. Dietary SSA and supplementation may be indicated for clients with HIV because of their increased risk for SAA deficiency (Parcell, 2002). Sulfur compounds have a low level of toxicity and the element is found in many common foods including cabbage, peas, beans, cauliflower, Brussels sprouts, eggs, horseradish, shrimp, chestnuts, mustard greens, onions, and asparagus. MSM, a volatile component in the sulfur cycle, can also be taken as a supplement (Parcell, 2002).

5. *Increase intake of foods high in vitamin A, zinc, and magnesium* (Patrick, 2000). Foods high in vitamin A include carrots, broccoli, kale, turnip greens, watercress, beets, dandelion greens, spinach, eggs, papaya, parsley, red peppers, pumpkin, yellow squash, apricots, and cantaloupes. Some foods rich in zinc are pumpkin seeds, whole grains, oysters, herring, liver, eggs, nuts, and wheat germ. Magnesium can be found in whole grain breads and cereals, fresh peas, brown rice, soy flour, wheat germ, nuts, Swiss chard, figs, green leafy vegetables, and citrus fruits (Clark, 1996).

6. *Cleanse the liver.* It's important to keep the liver and immune system as healthy as possible when the body is being stressed by medications or by fighting off infection. To assist with liver and lymphatic cleansing, clients can drink a combination of olive oil and lemon juice. Blend the following: 1 washed whole lemon (pulp, rind, seeds, and all), 1 tablespoon of extra virgin olive oil, and 1½ cups of distilled water. Strain the blend through a wire strainer to remove the pulp, which is discarded. Divide the juice into four equal portions and consume one with each of the three daily meals and the last one before bedtime. This will stimulate lymphatic flow, increase the flow of bile from the liver and gallbladder, and digest essential fatty acids in the intestine (Williams, 1995a).

7. *Drink distilled water.* Recent tests have shown that cryptosporidium, a waterborne parasite, is commonly found in lakes, rivers, and some reservoirs across the country, according to the Centers for Disease Control and Prevention. Because of this danger, cryptosporidium experts at the University of California Medical School, in San Francisco suggest that anyone with AIDS should definitely not drink tap water (Aragon et al., 2003). Two federal agencies have also warned that drinking tap water could be fatal to Americans with weakened immune systems and that they should take precautions such as boiling water before consuming it, or better yet, drink *distilled water.* Another reason to drink distilled water is that traces of pharmaceuticals, hormones, and other organic contaminants (from disinfectants to fire retardants) have been found in drinking water. Although the levels are low, not all are tested at drinking water facilities and their interactive or synergistic effects are unknown (Boyd et al., 2003; Kolpin et al., 2002; Ternes et al., 2002).

8. *Have a green drink daily.* For clients having difficulty digesting their food or if they want their minerals and vitamins to get right into the bloodstream, they can "drink" their vitamins and minerals. To make a *"green drink,"* put a cup or two of a green lettuce (except iceberg) in a blender. Add a handful of parsley and another of fresh spinach or kale. Fill the blender with pineapple juice and blend until frothy. Drink it slowly, chewing each mouthful (to get the digestive juices in your mouth flowing). Also suggest making carrot juice 1–3 times a day. A juicer can be obtained at a local health food store. Counsel clients to wash carrots and cut their ends off. Put a glass measuring cup (enough to hold 2 cups) under the spout. Put 5 to 6 or enough carrots in the top of the juicer to make at least 8 ounces. Add a handful of fresh spinach or parsley to the juicer and then another carrot or two. Juice. Drink slowly, chewing.

9. *Eat foods rich in vitamin A, especially when pregnant.* Infants born to women with vitamin A deficiency consistently have lower weight and height for their ages (Newschaffer et al., 2000). When HIV-infected pregnant women took vitamin A and beta-carotene, their newborn infants had an improved digestive system (Filteau et al., 2001). Vitamin A supplements for children of HIV-infected women kept babies alive and reduced their diarrhea (Coutsoudis et al., 1995). Taking large doses of vitamin A is not a good idea because it is oil soluble and the vitamin will stay in the body and could do harm. The best approach is to eat more carrots, broccoli, kale, turnip greens, watercress, beets, dandelion greens, spinach,

eggs, papaya, parsley, red peppers, fish, sweet potatoes, pumpkin, yellow squash, apricots, cantaloupes, and organ meats (liver, sweetbreads, etc.).

HERBS/ESSENTIAL OILS

Share the following information with clients.

1. *Take echinacea and ginseng.* These herbs have been shown to stimulate the immune system (See, Broumand, Sahl, & Tilles, 1997). Extracts of *Echinacea purpurea* and *Panax ginseng* were shown to enhance cellular immunity both in healthy individuals and patients with AIDS. (Counsel clients not to use Siberian ginseng if they have low blood sugar, high blood pressure, or a heart condition.)

2. *Use blue-green algae* (DeClercq, 2000).

3. *Take glycyrrhizin* (extracted from the licorice root *Glycyrrhiza radix*). Avoid taking this herb for more than 7 days in a row and advise clients with high blood pressure to avoid it (DeClercq, 2000).

4. *Use the spice curcumin.* It has proved helpful with AIDS (DeClercq, 2000).

5. *Take Astragalus for AIDS-related infections* (Yao, Wainberg, & Parniak, 1992). Caution clients not to use Astragalus if they have a fever.

6. *St. John's Wort* has also shown promise for AIDS (Barnes, Anderson, & Phillipson, 2001; Collins, Ng, Fong, Wan, & Yeung, 1997). All studies concluded that St. John's Wort was safe and effective.

7. *Drink 3 ounces of aloe vera juice after each meal.* The juice contains ingredients that can boost the immune system (Pugh, Ross, El Sohly, & Pasco, 2001). Caution clients never to try to make their own aloe vera juice because they might get too much of the laxative portion right next to the leaf that is removed before making the juice. Explain the importance of using the commercially prepared aloe juice available in half-gallon and gallon jugs in the health food store. It contains the healing portion of aloe. **WARNING:** Encourage clients to consult with an herbologist or obtain an herb reference book and make sure they look up (alone or in your presence) the feasibility of combining any prescribed medications with herbs.

CASTOR OIL PACKS

Clients with AIDS may need to prevent liver overload. Large amounts of toxic AIDS medications can tax the liver. Conditions that tax or compromise the immune system may benefit from castor oil packs. The skin is a living organ that absorbs external substances, so remind clients to make sure that any oil used on the body is cold-pressed and of the highest quality. It is not exactly known how castor oil packs work but they may affect the lymphatic system that filters toxins out of the body. Advise clients to check with their local health food store for cold-pressed castor oil. Share the following directions with clients: Warm the oil and dip a clean piece of natural cotton or flannel in it. Place the castor oil packs on sores, leave them there for an hour, then dispose of the packs (Williams, 1995b).

GENTLE ACUPRESSURE

Sit at top of client's head, teach client to hold on each spot with 2nd, 3rd, and 4th fingers until all three fingers pulsate, then move up the spinal cord to next spot: (a) either side of the spinal cord at waist, (b) bottom of scapula, (c) middle of scapula, (d) top of scapula, (e) top of shoulder, (f) bottom of neck, (g) bony prominence that runs across back of head. Finish with 3rd, 4th, and 5th fingers on bony hinge of jaw and index fingers first at cheeks (either side of nose) then above eyebrows, then right hand on top of head while placing left fingers between eyebrows. To enhance peace, hold spot on bony prominence on either sides of spinal column and then bottom of big toes (Dayton, 1994).

STRESS MANAGEMENT

A study that took place at the University of Florida's College of Medicine and the UF Brain Institute showed that for every severe stress reported in a 6-month period, the risk of early disease progression doubled. This study provided evidence that stress is a powerful influence on the development and severity of HIV-AIDS. Encourage clients to:

1. *Join a cognitive-behavioral stress management group.* A program for HIV-positive gay men using cognitive-behavioral techniques in a group setting decreased anxiety and depression about symptoms and enhanced some immunological measures (Lutgendorf et al., 1997).
2. *Play a relaxation tape upon awakening and prior to sleep.* You may decide to devise a relaxation tape based on the client's fears and wishes about treatment and the dis-ease process. A sample

relaxation script appears on pages 97–98 that you can revise to use for AIDS. Advise clients that they can also purchase relaxation/guided imagery self-help tapes at many bookstores.

EXERCISE

Wasting and abnormal distribution of body fat occurs with AIDS, which is why exercise is so important. *Try a progressive resistance training program.* Roubenoff (1999) described an 8-week intensive progressive resistance training program for people with AIDS. The 24 people who completed the study had significant increases in strength and lean body mass, and reduced fat. Those participants suffering from wasting were also able to gain weight, mostly in lean body mass. If body wasting is a problem for clients, consider finding a similar program or encouraging them to hire a personal trainer to help develop an intensive resistance training program. Encourage clients to engage in exercise at whatever level possible.

MASSAGE

Dr. Tiffany Field showed that massage helped HIV-exposed infants to gain weight and stay calm. Massage therapy also helped HIV-positive adolescents improve their immune function (Diego et al., 2001). Either provide massage or refer clients to a nurse massage therapist.

DISTANCE HEALING

AIDS patients paired with distance healers, who prayed for healing, acquired significantly fewer new AIDS-related illnesses, had lower illness severity, and required significantly fewer doctor visits, fewer hospitalizations, and fewer days of hospitalization (Sicher, Targ, Moore, & Smith, 1998). They also had a significantly improved mood compared to a group of controls who did not receive *distance healing.* Talk to clients about using distance healing.

SELF-HYPNOSIS

Self-hypnosis can significantly influence immunity (Gruzelier, Smith, Nagy, & Henderson, 2001). If you don't have self-hypnosis skills, you can either learn them or you might want to find a psychologist or psychiatric/mental health nurse practitioner with hypnosis skills to whom you can refer clients.

AFFIRMATIONS

Optimism and positive thinking have been shown to affect disease progression. Being chronically hostile, depressed, and apathetic can lead to dis-ease. Friedman (1991) found that hardy people have self-healing personalities that make them resilient and healthy.

Consider using one or more of the following *affirmations*. Adapt them if necessary and ask clients to write or speak the affirmations at least 20 times a day to replace the negative thoughts that may be holding back self-healing capabilities: I am powerful and capable. I am loved. I love and appreciate myself.

EVALUATING TREATMENT ACTIONS

Assess the effect of holistic nursing treatments by asking the client to provide specific examples of observed changes. If you've collaborated to set treatment goals and indicants of meeting them early on, you can simply refer back to these goals and ask the client to evaluate movement toward them. For example, if the client decided that comfort was an important goal, indicants could be number of nights of restful sleep per week and avoiding the use of pain medication. The client can be assessed prior to, during, and after treatment, by providing feedback on the number of restful nights of sleep per week and the number of pain medications used. Clients who choose to heal a painful memory, align their life's purpose and path of expression, or even achieve harmony with nature can rank themselves on their movement toward achieving these goals, too.

Another evaluation method involves teaching the client how to chart observations related to goals in a journal or diary and discuss the findings at the next meeting. You could ask the client who indicated guilt and anger to write about his level of guilt and anger now, preferably in separate paragraphs, and to write about them in his journal or diary at weekly intervals.

You can also develop a rating scale or choose an agreed-upon rating scale. It can be used as a pretreatment and posttreatment evaluation. Simply ask the client to rate his or her pain on a scale of 1 (no pain, anger, guilt, etc.) to 10 (extreme pain) and then compare ratings pre- and post-treatment. Separate scales can be devised for each feeling or goal (e.g., the one for anger would read "On a scale of 1 [no anger toward father] to 10 [extreme anger toward father], rate your current feelings."). Asking clients to rate their own feelings helps them feel more involved in their care and also provides a written and permanent record of progress.

REFERENCES

Allard, J. P., Aghdassi, E., Chau, J., Tam, C., Kovacs, C. M., Salit, I. E., & Walmsley, S. L. (1998). Effects of vitamin E and C supplementation on oxidative stress and viral load in HIV-infected subjects. *AIDS, 12,* 1652–1659.

Aragon, T. J., Novotny, S., Enahoria, W., Virgin, D. J., Khalakdina, A., & Katz, M. H. (2003). Endemic cryptosporidiosis and exposure to municipal tap water in persons with acquired immunodeficiency syndrome (AIDS). *BMC Public Health, 3*(1), 2.

Barnes, J., Anderson, L. A., & Phillipson, J. D. (2001). St. John's wort: A review of its chemistry, pharmacology and clinical properties. *Journal of Pharmacy and Pharmacology, 53,* 583–600.

Boyd, G. R., Reemtsma, H., Grimm, D. A., & Mitra, S. (2003). Pharmaceuticals and personal care products (PPCPs) in surface and treated waters of Louisiana, USA and Ontario, Canada. *Science of the Total Environment, 311*(1–3), 135–149.

Clark, C. C. (1996). *Wellness practitioner: Concepts, research and strategies.* New York: Springer Publishing Co.

Collins, R. A., Ng, T. B., Fong, W. P., Wan, C. C., & Yeung, H. W. (1997). A comparison of human immunodeficiency virus type 1 inhibition by partially purified aqueous extracts of Chinese medicinal herbs. *Life Sciences, 60,* PL345–PL351.

Coutsoudis, A., Bobat, R. A., Coovadia, H. M., Kuhn, L., Tsai, W. Y., & Stein, Z. A. (1995). The effects of vitamin A supplementation on the morbidity of children born to HIV-infected women. *American Journal of Public Health, 85*(8, pt.1), 1076–1081.

Dayton, B. R. (1994). *An introduction to a gentle acupressure for caregivers.* Friday Harbor, WA: High Touch Network.

De Clercq, E. (2000). Current lead natural products for the chemotherapy of human immunodeficiency virus (HIV) infection. *Medical Research Review, 20,* 323–349.

Diego, M. A., Field, T., Hernandez-Reif, M., Shaw, K., Friedman, L., & Ironson, G. (2001). HIV adolescents show improved immune function following massage therapy. *International Journal of Neuroscience, 106*(1–2), 35–45.

Filteau, S. M., Rollins, N. C., Coutsoudis, A., Sullivan, K. R., Willumsen, J. F., & Tomkins, A. M. (2001). The effect of antenatal vitamin A and beta-carotene supplementation on gut integrity of infants of HIV-infected South African women. *Journal of Pediatric Gastroenterology and Nutrition, 32,* 464–470.

Friedman, H. S. (1991). *The self-healing personality.* New York: Henry Holt.

Gruzelier, J., Smith, F., Nagy, A., & Henderson, D. (2001). Cellular and humoral immunity, mood and exam stress: The influences of self-hypnosis and personality predictors. *International Journal of Psychophysiology, 42*(1), 55–57.

Hori, K., Hatfield, D., Maldarelli, F., Lee, B. J., & Clouse, K. A. (1997). Selenium supplementation suppresses tumor necrosis factor alpha-induced human immunodeficiency virus type 1 replication in vitro. *AIDS Research in Human Retroviruses, 13,* 1325–1332.

Kolpin, D. W., Furlong, E. T., Meyer, M. T., Thurman, E. M., Zaugg, S. D., Barber, L. B., & Buxton, H. T. Pharmaceuticals, hormones and other organic wastewater contaminants in U.S. streams, 1999–2000. *Environmental Science and Technology, 36,* 1202–1211.

Lutgendorf, S. K., Antoni, M. H., Ironson, G., Klimas, N., Kumar, M., Starr, K., & McCabe, P. (1997). Cognitive-behavioral stress management decreases dysphoric mood and herpes simplex virus-type 2 antibody titers in symptomatic HIV-seropositive gay men. *Journal of Consulting and Clinical Psychology, 65*(1), 31–43.

Newschaffer, C. J., Cocroft, J., Anderson, C. E., Hauck, W. W., & Turner, B. J. (2000). Prenatal zidovudine use and congenital abnormalities in a Medicaid population. *Journal of Acquired Immune Deficiency Syndrome, 24*(3), 249–256.

Nicholas, P. K., Kemppainen, J. K., Holzemer, W. L., Nokes, K. M., Eller, L. S., Corless, I. B., Bunch, E. H., Bain, C. A., Kirksey, K. M., Davis, S. M., & Goodroad, B. K. (2002). Self-care management for neuropathy in HIV disease. *AIDS Care, 14,* 763–771.

Parcell, S. (2002). Sulfur in human nutrition and applications in medicine. *Alternative Medicine Review, 7*(1), 22–44.

Patrick, L. (1999). Nutrients and HIV: Part one—beta carotene and selenium. *Alternative Medicine Review, 4,* 403–413.

Patrick, L. (2000). Nutrients and HIV: Part two—vitamins A and E, zinc, B-vitamins, and magnesium. *Alternative Medicine Review, 5*(1), 39–51.

Perdue, S. (2000). *NIAID researchers discover why some HIV-infected people don't develop AIDS.* News release. Washington, DC: National Institutes of Health, National Institute of Allergy and Infectious Diseases, U.S. Department of Health and Human Services.

Pugh, N., Ross, S. A., El Sohly, M. A., & Pasco, D. S. (2001). Characterization of Aloeride, a new high-molecular-weight polysaccharide from Aloe vera with potent immunostimulatory activity. *Journal of Agricultural Food Chemistry, 49,* 1020–1024.

Roubenoff, R. (1999, Spring). Exercise: A major component in treating HIV. *Tufts Nutrition,* p. 3.

See, D. M., Broumand, N., Sahl, L., & Tilles, J. G. (1997). In vitro effects of echinacea and ginseng on natural killer and antibody-dependent cell cytotoxicity in healthy subjects and chronic fatigue syndrome or acquired immunodeficiency syndrome patients. *Immunopharmacology, 35,* 229–235.

Sicher, F., Targ, E., Moore, D., & Smith, H. S. (1998). A randomized double-blind study of the effect of distant healing on a population with advanced AIDS. *Western Journal of Medicine, 169*(6), 356–363.

Ternes, T. A., Meisenheimer, McDowell, D., Sacher, F., Brauch, H. J., Haist-

Gulde, B., Dreuss, G., Wilme, U., & Zulei-Silvert, N. (2002). Removal of pharmaceuticals during drinking water treatment. *Environmental Science and Technology, 36,* 3855–3863.

Williams, D. G. (1995a). AIDS. *Alternatives, 6*(1), 8.

Williams, D. G. (1995b). AIDS and castor oil. *Alternatives, 6*(1), 7.

Yao, X. J., Wainberg, M. A., & Parniak, M. A. (1992). Mechanism of inhibition of HIB-1 infection in vitro by purified extract of *Prunella vulgaris. Virology,* 187(1), 56–62.

CHAPTER 3

Allergies/Asthma

Allergies, including asthma, are often marked by obstructed breathing, chest constriction, and coughing. Histamine release is one of the factors responsible. Medical treatment includes antihistamines and steroids. Complementary holistic nursing interventions may be especially needed by clients with allergies/asthma because (1) inhaled corticosteroids have failed to halt the progression of the asthma epidemic (Leonard & Sur, 2002); (2) long-term steroid use even if only inhaled, poses a cataract risk (Smeeth et al., 2003); (3) NSAID use may trigger a fatal asthma attack (National Asthma Education and Prevention Program Expert Panel Report 2, 1997); (4) children who receive a minimum of both antibiotics and early childhood vaccinations have a 60% higher risk of developing allergies (Alm, 1999); and (5) children who are overweight or obese are significantly more likely to receive a diagnosis of asthma (Gilliland, 2001).

HOLISTIC NURSING ASSESSMENT

Study the assessment that follows. The nurse devised this holistic nursing assessment after working with Ms. H., a 50-year-old woman who works as a clerk in a yard goods store. The answers may give you ideas when completing holistic nursing assessments with clients diagnosed with allergies/asthma.

Client learning needs: "I don't understand why I have so many allergies."

Indicants of readiness to learn: "Where did these allergies all come from?"

Soul/spiritual symbol(s): None identified.

Meaning of the condition: "When I start coughing and sneezing, I feel that I'm being taken over by my allergies."

Relationship needs/effects as perceived by client: "My father told me big girls don't cry. He used to slap me if I did. My mother and I don't get along. I wish we did."

Patterns/attitudes that may create dis-ease for this client: "My mother told me I'm never going to get over this." "The doctor told me I should get rid of my dog and cat because I'm allergic to them, but I won't give them up." "I get very worked up every time I start sneezing or coughing."

Life purpose: "I just want to feel better."

Client strengths: Client is intelligent, well-nourished, and interested in learning about her dis-ease.

Ability to participate in care: Client works part-time and is mobile and energetic.

Ethical dilemmas: The clerk in the ER reported to the nurse that the client's friend, not the client, signed the consent for treatment form. No one else knows this fact.

Nurse–client process: The client is dependent on the nurse, asking what to do, what to decide, and how to handle her family and work situation.

TREATMENT

Acceptance of condition/attitude change: To counter negative thoughts and feelings, ask the client to say or write an affirmation daily, such as, "The world is safe and friendly." "I am at peace." "I choose to be free." Client agreed to write an affirmation on 3 x 5 cards, put them in prominent places around her home and office, and read them 20 times a day.

Facilitating the healing process/healing intention formulation: From a list of meditation statements, client chose the following one to say 20 times a day to assist in the healing process: "I am at peace with others and with my life."

Creating a sacred space: Client requested using prayer and a tape of Beethoven.

Integrative practices planned: Client requested a guided imagery/self-hypnosis tape to help her be less reactive to allergens.

Re-storying: Client started telling segments of her life story and drawing cartoons to explain her feelings.

Role model strategies: Showed client information about a HEPA filter she had used to help her husband reduce his allergic reactions.

Protection plan: Client is learning centering procedures and plans to use them to protect herself from allergens. Has started to question whether working in a fabric store may be adding to her allergic responses.

Family strategies: Teaching client assertive and empathic communication skills that she plans to use to mend relationships with her family.

Life issues/life purpose work: Will encourage client to get in touch with her life purpose by writing on the topic in her journal.

Treatment possibilities/considerations: Suggestions for client use appear below. Most are evidence-based.

ADDITIONAL INFORMATION AND TREATMENTS TO SHARE WITH CLIENTS

ENVIRONMENT

Environmental actions can reduce asthma symptoms, need for medication, and airway hyperresponsiveness (Bush, 2002). The following approaches are recommended. Ask clients to:

1. *Buy a high-efficiency particular air cleaner (HEPA filter).* It can remove the pollen and mold spores that may be setting off your allergic responses.

2. *Use a vacuum cleaner with a HEPA filter* to eliminate many airborne allergens.

3. *Stay out of the dampness.* Turn on the air conditioner in your car and at home, clean damp areas with bleach or a citrus cleaner, use a dehumidifier for damp spaces, or leave a fan on.

4. *Avoid household pets* and/or give them frequent baths to reduce noxious dander that creates allergic responses. Also, keep pets outside as much as possible. Avoid birds as pets. Bird antigens linger in a house for as long as 18 months. The best action to take for lung irritations (hypersensitivity pneumonitis) is to avoid the room in which a bird was kept.

5. *Remove carpets and install tile or wood floors* because you may be allergic to the glues and content of carpets. Wall-to-wall carpeting also invites roaches and their waste products. Carpeting plus increased insulation and sealed windows can lead to symptoms of "sick building syndrome," including eye, nose, throat, and skin irritation; headache; fatigue; and breathing problems. Chronic colds and dull headaches have also been associated with sick building syndrome.

6. *Make bedrooms allergy-proof.* Encase pillows, mattress, box springs, and furniture in allergen-proof plastic to protect against dust mites; wash sheets, blankets, pillowcases, and mattress pads every week in water that is at least 140°F to kill dust mites; and use hypoallergenic bedding materials. Use of house dust mite–impermeable encasings results in a significant decrease in atopic dermatitis (Oosting et al., 2002) and in a reduced need for inhaled steroids in children with asthma and house dust mite allergy (Halken et al., 2003).

7. *Keep windows shut* to ensure that outdoor allergens stay outside.

8. *Avoid wood-burning stoves and fireplaces.* They release irritating particles.

9. *Avoid strong chemicals,* carbonless paper, toners (from laser printers and copy machines), adhesive floor coverings, smoking or being around those who do, permanent-press clothes (containing formaldehyde), baby powder, talcum powder, perfume, moth balls, air fresheners, spray deodorants, and hair spray. Avoid nail cosmetics, including enamels and hardeners. They contain up to 5% formaldehyde fixative (Baran, 2002). Stay away from any strong chemicals, including exposure to air pollution and cigarette smoke (Bowler & Crapo, 2002).

10. *Wear natural fiber clothing* such as cotton, silk, and wool.

11. *Use chamomile preparations* to reduce the itching and inflammation of eczema. It has been shown to relieve symptoms without the long-term side effects of corticosteroid therapy (Ross, 2003).

12. *Use a salt water solution to clear sinuses.* Combine 1 quart of boiled water, 1½ to 3 heaping teaspoons of table salt, and 1 rounded teaspoon of baking soda. For a dry nose, add 1 tablespoon of white Karo syrup or glycerine. Mix the ingredients in a 1-quart glass jar with a lid. Warm the solution in a microwave or on the stove in a pot. Make sure it isn't too hot, then place a small amount in a baby bulb syringe. Bend over the sink and squirt the solution into one nostril and then into the other one. Repeat two or three times. Discard the unused solution and clean the syringe in warm soapy water.

13. *Take a rice bath for dermatitis.* Rice starch added to bath water can repair damaged skin, particularly in the case of atopic dermatitis (De Paepe, Hachem, Vanpee, Roseeuw, & Rogiers, 2002).

14. *Apply tea tree oil for skin inflammations* (Koh, Pearce, Marshman, Finlay-Jones, & Hart, 2002).

15. *Avoid unnecessary medication.* In one study, more than 91% of college seniors used over-the-counter medications for allergies (Howland, Weinberg, Smith, Laramie, & Kupka, 2002). In another study, the overdiagnosis of asthma and the overuse of asthma treatments with significant side effects was a common occurrence in children with persistent cough referred to a tertiary respiratory clinic. The authors suggest that children with persistent cough deserve careful evaluation to minimize the use of unnecessary medications and if medication is used, adequate follow-up is important (Thomson, Masters, & Chang, 2002).

NUTRITIONAL ACTIONS

1. *Start a food diary to eliminate offending foods.* Record all the foods, beverages, medications/drugs taken. Also record the time of day, mood, and symptoms for 6 hours afterward. Any of the following symptoms could suggest a food allergy: warmth, itchiness, head stuffiness, headache, fatigue, stomach upset, canker sores, chronic diarrhea or gas, ulcers, bladder infections, bedwetting, kidney disease, chronic infections, frequent ear infections, anxiety, depression, insomnia, irritability, mental confusion, joint pain, low back pain, asthma, chronic bronchitis, wheezing, acne, hives, rashes, itching, sinusitis, watery swelling from edema, fainting, fatigue, headache, hypoglycemia, itchy nose or throat, or migraines. The most common allergens are cow's milk, eggs, fish, wheat, soy, nuts, and citrus fruits (Nelsen, 2002; Stögmann & Kurz, 1996). Follow the same procedure with children. Forty percent of children with atopic dermatitis have food allergies (Miraglia del Giudice, De Luca, & Capristo, 2002), often to cow's milk. In young children, bedwetting, sleep disorders, excessive coughing, bad breath, "growing pains," abdominal pains, constant runny nose, nausea, recurring middle ear infections, ringing in the ears, or hyperactivity could mean a food allergy. Food additives such as yellow dye no. 5 (tetrazine) and benzoates can increase the production of mast cells, elevating the possibility of an allergy. The following food additives have also been associated with allergies and/or asthma: azo dyes and food colorings, salicylates, aspartame, benzoates, nitrites,

sorbic acid, hydoxytoluene, sulfites, gallates, polysorbates, and vegetable gums.

2. *Reduce allergic symptoms in infants and children up to two years of age by breast feeding them* (Kull, Wickman, Lilja, Nordvall, & Pershagen, 2002). If breast feeding is impossible, a hypoallergenic formula of pork and soya proteins, hydrolysate of casein or amino acid substitute may also work (Moneret-Vautrin, 2002).

3. *Avoid processed foods.* They often contain allergy-producing preservatives such as BHA, BHT, and MSG.

4. *Avoid salt.* Sodium chloride has been implicated as an asthma aggravator for some men. A low-salt diet can lead to less wheezing and easier breathing (Carey, Locke, & Cookson, 1996).

5. *Drink at least 10 glasses of water every day.* Acute asthma attacks often occur during periods of dehydration (Tanner, 2001). Atopic eczema/dermatitis has been shown to decrease in clients drinking deep-sea water as opposed to distilled water (Kimata et al., 2002).

6. *Avoid ice-cold drinks and wheat* (bread, pasta, pie crust, cake, rolls, cookies, etc.). Ice-cold drinks have been implicated in physical urticariä, and exercise-induced anaphylaxis is frequently food dependent, with wheat being an important allergen (Chong, Worm, & Zuberbier, 2002).

7. *Take a selenium supplement.* It can improve cellular oxidative defense, counteracting the inflammation and disordered respiration associated with asthma (Hasselmark, Malmgren, & Zetterstrom, 1993). Due to the poor quality of soil in the northeast, Florida, parts of Washington and Oregon, and parts of the Midwest, selenium may have to be taken as a supplement (do not exceed 50–70 micrograms a day), although seafoods, whole-grain breads and cereals, asparagus, garlic, and mushrooms contain selenium.

8. *Eat foods that contain fatty acids.* Fatty acids protect against the inflammation of allergies by forming prostaglandins, substances that control many body actions such as blood pressure, muscle contraction, kidney function, stomach secretion, intestinal absorption, and contractions of the uterus (Das, 2002). Eat cold-water fish (mackerel, herring, sardines, and salmon) and use flaxseed oil to reduce inflammatory/allergic responses. Consumption of oily fish can protect against asthma in childhood (Hodge et al., 1996) and mussels may also protect against asthma (Emelyanov et al., 2002).

9. *Avoid animal foods* (meat and dairy products). They irritate because they contain saturated fats and arachidonic acid, both of which can increase an allergic response.

10. *Cook with olive, macadamia nut, and cold-pressed canola oil.* They are high in omega-9 fatty acids. Avoid all other cooking oils and margarine. Use only salad dressing made with olive oil, which reduces the activity of "adhesion molecules" that can promote inflammation (Challem, 2003).

11. *Choose organic foods.* Buy organically produced foods from a health food store or grocery store. The label will indicate if the food is organically grown, confirming that it does not contain toxic pesticide residues or genetically engineered properties, both of which could increase allergic responses. ("Bt-treated Crops May Induce Allergies," 1999).

12. *Try honey.* Although there is no research evidence, anecdotal reports have shown that eating a daily teaspoon of honey obtained from local bees can improve allergies ("Bee Wise about Allergy," 1998).

13. *Rotate foods.* Eat a food only once every 5 days to reduce allergies. The most common food allergens include milk, cheese, yeast, wheat, rye, corn, soybeans, eggs, oranges, white potatoes, peanuts, chocolate, various spices, beef, coffee, tomatoes, malt, and pork. Before purchasing food, examine container labels of ingredients for corn or malt syrup, cheese or beef flavorings, peanut oil, malt, and other common food allergens. Because it may not be easy to identify what substances in processed foods may be causing the allergic reaction, eat whole, unprocessed foods, and reach for the fresh form of whatever food is being considered.

14. *Eliminate sugar, caffeinated and decaffeinated beverages, and foods with a high glycemic load.* Sugars, potatoes, breakfast cereals, muffins, white rice, and pasta raise insulin levels and may lead to high levels of pro-inflammation C-reactive protein (Liu et al., 2002).

15. *Eat fruits, vegetables, grains, and seeds every day.* Salad greens, broccoli, and green beans enhance the anti-inflammatory effect of fish and its omega-3 fatty acids. In one study, children who ate an Indian diet (more vegetables, less meat, and fewer additives and packaged and processed foods) had fewer symptoms of allergy and asthma than Indian youngsters eating a mostly Western diet (Carey et al., 1996). The children with fewer symptoms avoided meat, fish, eggs, green peas, soybeans, salt, sugar, coffee, ordinary tea, chocolate, potatoes, grains, apples, citrus fruits, or dairy products. They maintained a vegetarian diet and drank only nonchlorinated tap water. Ellwood and colleagues (2001) came to the same conclusions in their study of children and teenagers in 56 countries. Even

drinking tomato juice can help. It worked as well as a high dose of vitamin E to decrease C-reactive protein (Upritchard, Sutherland, & Mann, 2000).

16. *Eat foods high in zinc, magnesium, manganese, and vitamin C* (Romieu et al., 2002; Souter, Seaton, & Brown, 1997). Some foods that are high in zinc include herring, nuts, oysters, liver, and wheat germ. Green leafy vegetables, whole grain bread and cereals, wheat germ, brown rice, nuts, figs, and Swiss chard are high in magnesium. Whole grains, seeds, nuts, fruits and vegetables, oatmeal, and dry beans and peas are high in manganese. Honeydew melon, cooked broccoli or Brussels sprouts, kale, cantaloupe, strawberries, papaya, cooked cauliflower, green pepper, oranges, raspberries, watercress, parsley, raw cabbage, onions, blackberries, spinach, tomatoes, and rose hip tea or powder contain vitamin C.

17. *Increase intake of bioflavonoids.* Antioxidants, such as bioflavonoids, can protect against asthma (Knekt et al., 2002). Drink 1–2 cup of green tea daily or eat grapes (the seeds and skins have the most bioflavonoids). Every day drink 3 glasses of freshly squeezed orange juice followed by a glass of water (Davis, 1980).

18. *Increase intake of vitamin E.* This vitamin decreases the production and release of inflammatory mediators in mast cells (C2), suggesting it might have a role in controlling inflammatory diseases (Gueck, Aschenbach, & Fuhrmann, 2002). Eating foods high in vitamin E (olive oil, wheat germ, whole grain cereals, fruits, green vegetables, and fish) may protect against asthma, as the condition is related to increased levels of oxidants. Vitamin E is an antioxidant that reduces levels of these harmful compounds (Fogarty, Lewis, Weiss, & Britton, 2000).

19. *Eat more berries.* Berries can produce anti-asthmatic effects (Seeram, Momin, Nair, & Bourquin, 2001; Sellappan, Akoh, & Krewer, 2002).

20. *Drink more fresh juices.* Buy a juicer from a health food store. Wash seven or eight carrots, cut off the tops and stems, and put the cleaned carrots through the juicer. This will remove the indigestible fiber and many of the toxins from pesticides while providing an easy-to-digest, energizing drink. Add 1 or 2 radishes to the juicer and mix them into the carrot juice. Drink several glasses a day. This juice will reduce mucus, especially if fewer mucous-forming foods such as dairy products, white bread, cookies, pies, cakes, and sugary cereals are eaten.

21. *Eat asparagus for congested lungs* (Davis, 1980). Four tablespoons daily of pureed fresh, cooked, or canned asparagus may help.

22. *Lose weight.* A high prevalence of obesity exists in clients diagnosed with asthma. It is not known whether the increased prevalence of obesity reflects a true increase in asthma in obese individuals or whether asthma-like symptoms occur because of obesity. Weight reduction and weight maintenance should be important aspects of treatment (Nathell, Jensen, & Larsson, 2002).

Children who are overweight or obese are significantly more likely to be diagnosed with asthma (Gilliland et al., 2003), as are women who take postmenopausal hormones (Barr et al., 2004). To prevent allergies, feed children fewer processed sweet and fatty foods, and give them more whole fruits and vegetables.

23. *Try capsicum.* Made from cayenne or hot chilies, capsicum may be helpful because it can boost the immune system and circulation, clean the blood, thin bronchial secretions, and reduce the itch of contact dermatitis (Wallengren, 2002). The substance can be found in capsules, in salves, or can be sprinkled on food. Coupled with garlic, it may dry up the sinuses.

24. *Eat horseradish.* Try eating 1/4 to 1/2 teaspoon of fresh ground horseradish pulp (without the juice) mixed with lemon juice between meals to clear the sinuses.

25. *Take pantothenic acid.* One of the B-vitamins, this nutritional supplement can clear the head of congestion, but it also acts as a heart protector, may improve circulation, helps the body store sugar, eliminates waste by-products (ketones), and plays an important role in various body processes, especially the production and breakdown of fatty acids. Because it is water soluble, unneeded amounts of the ingested vitamin are eliminated in the urine and do not accumulate in the body. There are no known side effects (Shimizu, 1999: Smith, Narrow, Kendrick, & Steffen, 1987).

26. *Use probiotics.* These friendly bacteria are available in health food stores. They can help manage atopic eczema and cow's milk allergy (Kirjavainen, Salminen, & Isolauri, 2003) and other food allergies (Montalto et al., 2002).

27. *Eat onions and other sulfur-rich foods.* The sulfur compounds in onions, called thiosulfinates, provide anti-asthmatic and anti-inflammatory properties (Dorsch et al., 1988). Onions can also build the immune system and help heal lung tissue (Griffths, Trueman, Crowther, Thomas, & Smith, 2002). Other foods high in sulfur include cabbage, peas, beans, cauliflower, Brussels sprouts, eggs, horseradish, shrimp, chestnuts, mustard greens, and asparagus. MSM is a sulfur supplement that may be effective for the treament of allergies (Parcell, 2002).

28. *Try alfalfa to halt sneezing attacks and clear sinuses, and fenugreek in capsules or as a tea to ease sinus headaches.*

REPLACEMENT HORMONES

Women nearing menopause should think carefully about taking replacement hormones. One study found that women who never used replacement hormones had a significantly lower risk of asthma than those women who take HRT (Carey et al., 1996).

EVENING PRIMROSE OIL

Individuals suffering from itchy, dry, scaly skin (atopic dermatitis) benefited from taking evening primrose oil (Yoon, Lee, & Lee, 2002). The researchers concluded that those using the oil showed a significant decrease in serum IFN-gamma levels, demonstrating its effectiveness as an anti-inflammatory agent.

HERBS

Some herbs have anti-inflammatory, immune system-building, respiratory-soothing and anti-mucus effects. Consult a herbalist about using fenugreek, rose hips, saw palmetto, boswellia, chamomile, eyebright, garlic, gingko, licorice, sage, fennel, thyme, or pau d'arco teas or capsules. Eucalyptus oil used in a mister or nebulizer can also help, as can drinking two to four ounces of aloe juice a day. Ginger tea has also been used successfully to reduce sinus inflammation. The steam from grated ginger is simmered in water and then breathed in for 5 to 7 minutes, 2–3 times a day until symptoms subside. Unlike drugs that treat symptoms, herbs may strengthen the immune system. Once it has been strengthened, it may be possible to gradually reintroduce an allergen and get no allergic response. Astragalus, licorice, pau d'arco, ginseng, ginger, and garlic may tone the immune system so that it doesn't react to unsafe substances with an allergic response. Consult a herbologist or herb book and ask clients to share the results of any herb taken with their primary care provider.

HOMEOPATHY

Reilly and colleagues (1986) used homeopathically prepared dilutions of grass pollens or dust mites in the treatment of nasal allergies.

The treatment group that received the highly diluted preparations improved considerably more than those treated with a placebo that did not contain the allergens. Runny noses, itchy throats, and sneezing may be helped by the homeopathic remedies Arsenicum album or sabadilla. Homeopathic remedies for temporary relief of allergies include eyebright, monkshood, phosphate of iron, wind-flower, red onion, trioxide of arsenic, iodide of potassium, quicksilver, and poison-nut. Since most allergies are long-term problems, they require consultation with a trained homeopathic practitioner. Because most homeopathic remedies are so highly diluted that little, if any, of the original substance remains in the treatment, and so it is unlikely that there will be a reaction with prescribed or over-the-counter drugs. To be sure, caution clients to share information about any homeopathic remedies used.

EXERCISE

Physical activity, especially walking and more vigorous activity, can enhance quality and length of life, especially for those having difficulty breathing (Rockhill et al., 2001). It's important to start slowly and to carefully supervise clients, but urge them to move, even if it's only a walk or two around the house at the start. Heavy exercise in polluted air with high concentrations of ozone is to be avoided for children as it may contribute to the development of asthma, as does scuba diving for individuals with asthma (Lecomte, 2002).

Use the lung exercise. Stand with feet shoulder-width apart and parallel. Keep back straight and chin slightly toward chest, with back of neck stretching up. Exhale all air from lungs while clasping hands behind the back. Inhale slowly, keeping chin tucked into the chest, expanding the lungs, and pushing the hands away from the back. Exhale and drop the hands while bringing arms out in front, then raising them up to the head and then around behind the back, keeping fingers pointed out while making a full circle. Lace the fingers behind the back and repeat the exercise (Chang, 1986).

YOGA

A study of the effect of a yoga therapy program on chronic bronchial asthma found that yoga had beneficial effects on some objective and subjective measures of the impact of asthma (Manocha, Marks, Kenchington, Peters, & Salome, 2002). Encourage clients to look into local yoga programs.

STRESS REDUCTION

Strong emotions such as anxiety, anger, depression, and even happiness can trigger an asthma attack (Ritz & Steptoe, 2000). Finding a way to reduce stress, be it positive or negative stress, will help. The first step is to identify what triggers asthma attacks. Once that is achieved, clients can take steps to reduce the effects of these triggers. Strategies that may work include practicing yoga or guided imagery or taking B-vitamins.

WRITING

Writing about the most stressful life events could reduce asthma symptoms. Ask clients to spend at least 20 minutes a day on three consecutive days writing about the most stressful event they've encountered. It could reduce asthma symptoms for 4 months or longer (Smith, Stone, Hurewitz, & Kaell, 1999).

ACUPUNCTURE

Stress and allergies can play havoc with energy flow. Although a meta-analysis of published data from 11 randomized controlled trials did not find an effect of acupuncture in reducing asthma, it may reduce brochoconstriction (Martin et al., 2002).

Two acupuncture points, K-27 (Kidney 27) are located on the front of the body, where the first rib, collar bone, and breast bone come together. To find the location:

1. Place several fingers on one collar bone and several fingers of your other hand on the other collar bone and slowly flow them toward the center of your chest. The small depression or hole between them is where the three bones come together and K-27 is located.
2. Put the index and middle finger of one hand on either side of the belly button. Place the index finger of the other hand on K-27 on the right side of the body.
3. At the same time, apply gentle pressure to both areas and rub in a rotary fashion for 15–20 seconds.
4. Move top index finger over to the left K-27 point and rub both places again for 15–20 seconds.

ACUPRESSURE

Lung flow. Hold the 2nd, 3rd, and 4th fingers of each hand on the bottom rib approximately 2 inches to the side from midline, then move the hand to the middle back of the arm, and end with holding separately, first one thumb and then the other in the fleshy part before the wrist. Hold each spot until pulses are felt in all three fingers of a hand (Dayton, 1994).

Liver flow. Hold three fingers of each hand until pulsation is felt first on bony prominence that runs across the bottom of the skull, two inches from the spine, then on the coccyx, then on the outside of the heel, and then on the bottom rib (Dayton, 1994).

MASSAGE

Histamine production is affected by the sphenoid sinus located in the center of the head. The suboccipital muscles have a powerful impact on the sphenoid sinus and may be key to treating allergies (Griner & Nunes, 1996). Massage the muscles just below the bony ridge running across the back of the head. Use only the index and middle fingers, using a 30-degree angle of the palm to the area being massaged. Stroke quickly (so as not to activate the stretch reflex) and stroke across the muscle, working up, over, and down, using about six long strokes. Alternately stroke and percuss the muscle (tapping) short and very fast. Avoid smashing, grinding, pummeling, rubbing, stretching, or massaging the length of the muscle because these will activate the stretch-reflex response and increase spasms (Griner & Nunes, 1996).

AROMATHERAPY MASSAGE

An aromatherapy massage can be calming for adults or children, thereby helping to open up constricted breathing passages. Dilute 5 drops of essential lavender oil in 2 tablespoons of vegetable oil and massage the back in long sweeping movements. Start at the base of the spine, with your hands on either side of the vertebrae. Move up the back slowly in upward strokes, coming over the shoulder and down the sides of the body.

WARM SOAKS AND TEA

For an asthma attack, lie down and place a cloth dipped in hot water and vinegar as warm as can be borne on the chest. When the cloth cools, replace with another. If attack returns or client cannot lie down, place the cloth on the stomach. Next, place a warm soak on the legs and feet. Sip milk with fennel boiled in it, or chamomile and mint tea (Davis, 1980).

GUIDED IMAGERY

A physician, William Mundy, M.D. (1993), utilized guided imagery to treat allergies (as well as depression and unhappiness), and reduce the need for allergy medication. It used to be thought that body chemistry dictates behavior and symptoms and that feelings and thoughts were separate entities, but due to Candace Pert (Pert, Dreher, & Ruff, 1998) and her work with psychoneuroimmunology, it is now agreed that body chemistry interacts with symptoms and feelings. Mind and body chatter back and forth, using the language of biochemicals.

Pert's work at the National Institutes of Mental Health showed that certain white blood cells are equipped with the molecular equivalent of antennas that are tuned in to receive messages from the brain. A mosaic of evidence suggests that human body systems communicate with one another through messengers carried back and forth on tiny molecules. These biochemical messengers, called neurotransmitters, neuropeptides, lymphokines, and other tongue-twisting terms, are informational substances that have a powerful effect on moods and emotions. Based on these ideas, it is possible that by changing thoughts and feelings, body responses, including immune response, can also be changed (Pert, Dreher, & Ruff, 1998).

A combination of relaxation, guided imagery, and self-esteem workshops reduced the number of asthmatic episodes and the use of bronchodilator medication in asthmatic children, compared to 6 months prior to the intervention (Castes et al., 1999). Consider using the following script to teach an immune system not to react to allergens. Record the directions into a recorder, pausing often, especially at the . . . and speak in a slow monotone. When you've made the tape that sounds right for you, play it back to yourself when you're in a quiet, safe place. Remember to play it several times a day so it will be firmly planted in your mind and body, and follow its directions.

1. Loosen your clothes . . . slip off your shoes . . . close your eyes and relax into a comfortable chair.

2. Allow a relaxing warmth to spread from the tips of your toes throughout your body . . . Take your time . . . breathing in relaxation . . . and comfort.

3. Picture little particles of allergens that have plagued you in the past. Make them colored or polka-dotted or however you wish to see them . . . Take your time . . . making sure you have them looking exactly as you wish to see them . . .

4. Imagine a thick plexiglass wall separating you completely from those allergen particles . . .

5. Sit safely behind that thick plexiglass . . . imagine yourself on the other side of that wall, having an allergy attack. You are separated from that person on the other side of the wall, but can clearly see what's happening. Allergic molecules circulate around the you on the other side of that plexiglass shield, while the you on this side remains safe and protected, behind your plexiglass shield . . .

6. Once you have the picture of you on the other side of the plexiglass having an attack, shift your attention to some peaceful, quiet, and soothing place . . . Smell the smells you associate with that spot . . . Hear the sounds you associate with that spot . . . Feel the sensations you associate with that place . . . See the sights you associate with that spot . . .

7. Notice that there are certain particles in that air . . . particles that come in through your lungs and into your mouth . . . They smell and taste good and healthy . . .

8. Picture those healthy particles becoming part of you, filling every cell of your body with peace and relaxation . . . calm and serene . . . totally relaxed and healthy . . . totally surrounded by the healthy molecules, keeping you safe from harm.

9. Look through that plexiglass protective shield and see yourself over there, behind it, having that allergic attack . . . You remain behind your shield, safe and healthy.

10. In your mind's eye, reach through that plexiglass shield and get a handful of those allergic particles . . . see how calm and safe you remain, even though you're holding those allergic molecules in your hand. If at any time you lose that feeling of calm safety, just dissolve those allergic molecules and take yourself in your mind's eye to that safe and comfortable spot you pictured before . . . Stay there until you feel safe and comfortable again, then come back and reach through that plexiglass shield and get another handful of allergic particles.

11. See how those allergic molecules just disappear . . . swallowed up by the healthy molecules surrounding every part of you . . . keeping you healthy, calm, safe . . .

12. Reach through that plexiglass shield and grab another handful of allergic particles . . . Notice how they can't touch you . . . you are totally protected by your healthy molecules . . . staying safe, healthy, and comfortable . . .

13. When you're ready, grab a small bucket of those allergic molecules and watch them disappear as they are surrounded by the

healthy, comforting molecules surrounding you . . . take your time . . . let the allergic molecules blend with yours while you stay healthy, calm, and comfortable.

14. Bask in your success of having blended the allergic molecules with your healthy, safe, and calming molecules . . . picture the blended healthy and happy you, no longer concerned at all about the allergy particles, completely safe and healthy . . . you're in a bubble of healthy, happy, and safe particles . . .

15. When you're ready, slowly lift up the plexiglass shield . . . keeping relaxed and comfortable, totally safe and healthy in your bubble . . .

16. Notice how the allergic molecules are slowly moving toward your safe and healthy bubble, but you don't mind because you feel safe and healthy, protected behind your bubble . . . and there you are, breathing easily and enjoying the fact that you no longer have any problems with the allergic particles . . . in fact, the two bubbles have met and blended and you continue to feel safe, comfortable, and healthy . . . realize that the allergic particles are now harmless and simply part of the things your body can handle easily and every day in a healthy and routine way . . . Take time to experience how good it feels to be free of things that used to bother you . . . to be totally in control of how good you feel . . . to be healthy, comfortable, and secure . . .

HYPNOSIS AND STORYTELLING

Hypnosis is an exaggerated form of body relaxation and focused attention that uses suggestion. It is easily learned and easily practiced once the method is learned. A hypnosis preschool family education program reduced physician visits for asthma, and parents reported increased confidence in self-management skills (Kohen & Wynne, 1997). Symptom severity was reduced as well. In this study, symptom severity was also reduced through storytelling, imagery, and relaxation. Many activities such as reading, driving, and watching TV can bring on a hypnotic state of relaxation and focused attention.

For a child diagnosed with asthma, try reading or telling calming stories, perhaps finding ideas in the preceding guided imagery script. For example, depending on the age of the child, tell a story about a fairy princess who can't breathe and who finds a wizard who provides her with a plexiglass shield from the dog (trees, flowers, or whatever) and she lives happily ever after. The idea is to tell the story in a monotone, using plenty of pauses and calming phrases. Talk to your local librarian to find stories that are relaxing and calming. Read them to children prior to bedtime or at times of stress to ward off asthma attacks. With adults, use age-appropriate stories.

EVALUATING TREATMENT ACTIONS

The client introduced at the beginning of this chapter provided the following specific examples of observed changes: "I make sure to give my cat and dog a bath every week and they now sleep in the laundry room." "I feel more in control since I've been saying a meditation." "I wrote a letter to my parents, but didn't mail it." "I listen to my relaxation tape at least twice a day; more when I'm under stress."

REFERENCES

Alm, J. S., Swartz, J., Lilja, G., Scheynius, A., & Pershagen, G. (1999). Atopy in children of families with an anthroposophic lifestyle. *Lancet, 353,* 1484–1488.

Baran, R. (2002). Nail cosmetics: Allergies and irritation. *American Journal of Clinical Dermatology, 3,* 547–555.

Barr, R. G., Wentowski, C. C., Geodstein, F., Somers, S. C., Stampfer, M. J., Schwartz, J., Speizer, F. E., & Camargo, C. A. (2004). Prospective study of postmenopausal hormone use and newly diagnosed asthma and chronic obstructive pulmonary disease. *Archives of Internal Medicine, 164,* 379–386.

Bee wise about allergy. (1998). *Clinical Advisor* (April), 47.

Bowler, R. P., & Crapo, J. D. (2002). Oxidative stress in allergic respiratory diseases. *Journal of Allergy and Clinical Immunology, 110,* 349–356.

Bt-treated crops may induce allergies. (1999). *Science News, 156,* 6.

Bush, R. K. (2002). Environmental controls in the management of allergic asthma. *Medical Clinics of North America, 86,* 973–989.

Carey, O. J., Cookson, J. B., Britton, J., & Tattersfield A. E. (1996). The effect of lifestyle on wheeze atrophy and bronchial hyperreactivity in Asian and white children. *American Journal of Respiratory and Critical Care Medicine, 154*(2, part 1), 537–540.

Carey, O. J., Locke, C., & Cookson, J. B. (1996). Effect of alterations of dietary sodium on the severity of asthma in men. *Thorax, 48,* 107–110.

Castes, M., Hagel, I., Palenque, M., Canelones, P., Corao, A., & Lynch, N. R. (1999). Immunological changes associated with clinical improvement of asthmatic children subjected to psychosocial intervention. *Brain and Behavioral Immunity, 13*(1), 1–13.

Challem, J. (2003). *The inflammation syndrome.* Hoboken, NJ: Wiley.

Chang, S. T. (1986). *The complete system of self-healing internal exercises.* San Francisco: Tao.

Chong, S. U., Worm, M., & Zuberbier, T. (2002). Role of adverse reactions to food in urticaria and exercise-induced anaphylaxis. *International Archives of Allergy and Immunology, 129*(1), 19–26.

Das, U. N. (2002). Essential fatty acids as possible enhancers of the beneficial actions of probiotics. *Nutrition, 18*(9), 786.

Davis, B. (1980). *Rapid healing foods.* West Nyack, NY: Parker.

Dayton, B. R. (1994). *An introduction to a gentle acupressure for caregivers.* Friday Harbor, WA: High Touch Network.

DePaepe, K., Hachem, J. P., Vanpee, E., Roseeuw, D., & Rogiers, V. (2002). Effect of rice starch as a bath additive on the barrier function of healthy but SLS-damaged skin and skin of atopic patients. *Acta Derm Venereology, 82,* 184–186.

Dorsch, W., Wagner, H., Bayer, T. S., Fessler, B., Hein, G., Ring, J., et al. (1988). Antiasthmatic effects of onions. *Biochemical Pharmacology, 37,* 4479–4486.

Ellwood, P., Asher, M. I., Bjorkstein, B., Burr, M., Pearce, N., & Robertson, C. F. (2001). Diet and asthma, allergic rhinoconjunctivitis and atopic eczema symptom prevalence: An ecological analysis of the International Study of Asthma and Allergies in Childhood (ISAAC) data. *European Respiratory Journal, 17,* 436–443.

Emelyanov, A., Fedoseev, G., Krasnoschekova, O., Abulimity, A., Trendeleva, T., & Barnes, P. J. (2002). Treatment of asthma with lipid extract of New Zealand green-lipped mussel: A randomised clinical trial. *European Respiratory Journal, 20,* 596–600.

Fogarty, A., Lewis, S., Weiss, S., & Britton, J. (2000). Dietary vitamin E, IgE concentrations and atopy. *Lancet, 356,* 1573–1574.

Gilliland, F. D., Berhane, K., Islam, T., McConnell, R., Ganderman, W. J., Gilliland, S. S., Avol, E., & Peters, J. M. (2003). Obesity and the risk of newly diagnosed asthma in school-age children. *American Journal of Epidemiology, 158,* 400–415.

Griffiths, G., Trueman, L., Crowther, T., Thomas, B., & Smith, B. (2002). Onions—a global benefit to health. *Phytotherapy Research, 16,* 603–615.

Griner, T., & Nunes, M. (1996). *What's really wrong with you? A revolutionary look at how muscles affect health.* Garden City Park, NY: Avery.

Gueck, T., Aschenbach, J. R., & Fuhrmann, H. (2002). Influence of vitamin E on mast cell mediator release. *Veterinary Dermatology, 13,* 301–305.

Halken, S., Host, A., Niklassen, U., Hansen, L. G., Nielsen, F., Pedersen, S., et al. (2003). Effect of mattress and pillow encasings on children with asthma and house dust mite allergy. *Journal of Allergy and Clinical Immunology, 111*(1), 169–176.

Halper, N. J. (1997). Guided imagery in the treatment of asthma. Http://altmed.od.nih.gov/oam/cgi-bin/research/search_simple.cgi. Accessed July 21, 1997.

Hasselmark, L., Malmgren, R., & Zetterstrom, O. (1993). Selenium supplementation in intrinsic asthma. *Allergy, 48,* 30–36.

Hodge, L., Salome, C. M., Peat, J. K., Haby, M. M., Xuan, W., & Woolcock, A. J. (1996). Consumption of oily fish and childhood asthma risk. *Medical Journal of Australia, 164,* 137–140.

Howland, J., Weinberg, J., Smith E., Laramie, A., & Kupka, M. (2002). Prevalence of allergy symptoms and associated medication use in a sample of college seniors. *Journal of the American College of Health, 51*(2), 67–70.

Kimata, H., Tai, H., Nakagawa, K., Yokoyama, Y., Nakajima, H., & Ikegama, Y. (2002). Improvement of skin symptoms and mineral imbalance by drinking deep sea water in patients with atopic eczema/dermatitis syndrome (AEDS). *Acta Medica, 45*(2), 83–84.

Kirjavainen, P. V., Salminen, S. J., & Isolauri, E. (2003). Probiotic bacteria in the management of atopic disease: Underscoring the importance of viability. *Journal of Pediatric Gastroenterology and Nutrition, 36,* 223–227.

Knekt, P., Kumpulainene, J., Jarvinen, R., Rissanen, H., Heliovaara, M., Reunanen, A., Hakulinen, T., & Aromaa, A. (2002). Flavonoid intake and risk of chronic diseases. *American Journal of Clinical Nutrition, 76,* 560–568.

Koh, K. J., Pearce, A. L., Marshman, G., Finlay-Jones, J. J., & Hart, P. H. (2002). Tea tree oil reduces histamine-induced skin inflammation. *British Journal of Dermatology, 147,* 1212–1217.

Kohen, D. P., & Wynne, E. (1997). Applying hypnosis in a program: Uses of storytelling, imagery and relaxation. *American Journal of Clinical Hypnosis, 39,* 169–181.

Kull, I., Wickman, M., Lilja, G., Nordvall, S. L., & Pershagen, F. (2002). Breast feeding and allergic diseases in infants—a prospective birth cohort study. *Archives of Disease in Childhood, 87,* 478–481.

Lecomte, J. (2002). Asthma and exercise. *Review of Medical Bruxism, 23,* A206–A210.

Leonard, R., & Sur, S. (2002). Asthma: Future directions. *Medical Clinics of North America, 86,* 1131–1156.

Liu, S., Manson, J. E., Buring, J. E., Stampfer, M. J., Willett, W. C., & Ridker, P. M. (2002). Relation between a diet with a high glycemic load and plasma concentrations of high-sensitivity C-reactive protein in middle-aged women. *American Journal of Clinical Nutrition, 75,* 492–498.

Manocha, R., Marks, G. B., Kenchington, P., Peters, D., & Salome, C. M. (2002). Sahaja yoga in the management of moderate to severe asthma: A randomised controlled trial. *Thorax, 57,* 110–115.

Martin, J., Donaldson, A. N., Villarroel, R., Parmar, M. K., Ernst, E., & Higginson, I. J. (2002). Efficacy of acupuncture in asthma: Systematic review and meta-analysis of published data from 11 randomised controlled trials. *European Respiratory Journal, 20,* 846–852.

Miraglia del Giudice, M., Jr., De Luca, M. G., & Capristo, C. (2002).

Probiotics and atopic dermatitis. A new strategy in atopic dermatitis. *Digestive and Liver Diseases, 34*(Suppl. 2), S68–S71.

Moneret-Vautrin, D. A. (2002). Optimal management of atopic dermatitis in infancy. *Allergy Immunology, 34,* 325–329.

Montalto, M., Arancio, F., Izzi, D., Cuoco, L., Curigliano, V., Manna, R., & Gasvarrini, G. (2002). Probiotics: History, definitions, requirements and possible therapeutic applications. *Ann Ital Med Int, 17,* 157–165.

Mundy, W. L. (1993). *Curing allergy with visual imagery.* Shawnee Mission, KS: Mundy and Associates.

Nathell, I., Jensen, I., & Larsson, K. (2002). High prevalence of obesity in asthmatic patients on sick leave. *Respiratory Medicine, 96,* 642–650.

National Asthma Education and Prevention Program Expert Panel. (1997). Guidelines for the diagnosis and management of asthma. Bethesda, MD: National Heart, Lung, and Blood Institute. Available at: www.nhlbi.nih.gov/guidelines/asthma/asthgdln.htm. Accessed August 13, 2002.

Nelsen, D. A., Jr. (2002). Gluten-sensitive enteropathy (celiac disease): More common than you think. *American Family Physician, 66*(12), 2259–2266.

Oosting, A. J., de Brun-Weller, M. S., Terreehorst, I., Tempels-Pavlica, Z., Aalberse, R. C., de Moncy, J. G., van Wijk, R. G., & Bruijnzeel-Koomen, C. A. (2002). Effect of mattress casings on atopic dermatitis outcome measures in a double-blind, placebo-controlled study: The Dutch mite avoidance study. *Journal of Allergy and Clinical Immunology, 110*(3), 500–506.

Parcell, S. (2002). Sulfur in human nutrition and applications in medicine. *Alternative Medicine Review, 7*(1), 22–44.

Pert, C. B., Dreher, H. E., & Ruff, M. R. (1998). The psychosomatic network: Foundations of mind–body medicine. *Alternative Therapy and Health Medicine, 4*(4), 30–41.

Reilly, D. T., Taylor, M. A., McSharry, C., & Aitchison, T. (1986). Is homeopathy a placebo response? Controlled trial of homeopathic potency, with pollen in hay fever as model. *Lancet, 344,* 1601–1606.

Ritz, T., & Steptoe, A. (2000). Emotion and pulmonary function in asthma: Reactivity in the field and relationship with laboratory induction of emotion. *Psychosomatic Medicine, 62*(6), 808–815.

Rockhill, B., Willett, W. C., Manson, J. E., Leitzmann, J. F., Stampfer, M. J., Hunter, D. J., & Colditz, G. A. (2001). Physical activity and mortality: A prospective study among women. *American Journal of Public Health, 91*(4), 578–583.

Romieu, I., Sienra-Monge, J. J., Ramirez-Aguilar, M., Tellez-Rojo, M. M., Moreno-Macias, H., Reyes-Riuz, N. I., del Rio-Navano, B. E., Riuz-Navarro, M. X., Hatch, G., slade, R., & Hernandez-Avila, M. (2002). Antioxidant supplementation and lung functions among children with asthma exposed to high levels of air pollutants. *American Journal of Respiratory and Critical Care Medicine, 166*(5), 703–709.

Ross, S. M. (2003). An integrative approach to eczema (atopic dermatitis). *Holistic Nurse Practitioner, 17*(1), 56–62.

Seeram, N. P., Momin, R. A., Nair, M. G., & Bourquin, L. D. (2001). Cyclooxygenase inhibitory and antioxidant cyanidin glycosides in cherries and berries. *Phytomedicine, 8,* 362–369.

Sellappan, S., Akoh, C. C., & Krewer, G. (2002). Phenolic compounds and antioxidant capacity of Georgia-grown blueberries and blackberries. *Journal of Agricultural and Food Chemicals, 50*(8), 2432–2438.

Shimizu, S. (1999). Pantothenic acid. *Nippon Rinsho, 57*(10), 2218–2222.

Smeeth, L., Boulis, M., Hubbard, R., & Fletcher, A. E. (2003). A population-based, case-control study of cataract and inhaled corticosteroids. *British Journal of Ophthalmology, 87,* 1247–1251.

Smith, C. M., Narrow, C. M., Kendrick, Z. V., & Steffen, C. (1987). The effect of pantothenate deficiency in mice on their metabolic response to fast and exercise. *Metabolism, 36*(2), 115–121.

Smith, J. M., Stone, A. A., Hurewitz, A., & Kaell, A. (1999). Effects of writing about stressful experiences on symptom reduction in patients with asthma or rheumatoid arthritis. *Journal of the American Medical Association, 281,* 304–309.

Souter, A., Seaton, A., & Brown, K. (1997). Bronchial reactivity and dietary antioxidants. *Thorax, 52,* 166–170.

Stögmann, W., & Kurz, H. (1996). Atopic dermatitis and food allergy in infancy and childhood. *Wiener Medizinische Wochenschrift, 146,* 411–414.

Tanner, J. O. (2001, October). Asthma vs. anti-inflammatory drugs. *Clinical Advisor,* p. 45.

Thomson, F., Masters, I. B., & Chang, A. B. (2002). Persistent cough in children and the overuse of medications. *Journal of Paediatric Child Health, 38,* 578–581.

Upritchard, J. E., Sutherland, W. H., & Mann, J. L. (2000). Effect of supplementation with tomato juice, vitamin E, and vitamin C on LDL oxidation and products of inflammatory activity in type 2 diabetes. *Diabetes Care, 23,* 733–738.

Wallengren, J. (2002). Cutaneous field stimulation of sensory nerve fibers reduces itch without affecting contact dermatitis. *Allergy, 57,* 1195–1199.

Yoon, S., Lee, J., & Lee, S. (2002). The therapeutic effect of evening primrose oil in atopic dermatitis patients with dry scaly skin lesions is associated with the normalization of serum gamma-interferon levels. *Skin Pharmacology and Applied Skin Physiology, 15*(1), 20–25.

CHAPTER 4

Alzheimer's Disease

Alzheimer's disease is one of the most common causes of dementia. To date, no effective medication has been found to treat the condition. However, many self-care measures have been shown to prevent and/or treat the symptoms of Alzheimer's.

HOLISTIC NURSING ASSESSMENT

Study the holistic nursing assessment for Mr. R., a 72-year-old resident in a nursing home, who has been diagnosed with Alzheimer's disease. Through talking with Mr. R. and listening to him talk, the nurse developed the following assessment.

Learning needs: "Where's my wife?"

Indicants of readiness to learn: Grabbed nurse's arm and looked in her eyes, making good eye contact.

Soul/spirituality symbol(s): Listens to church music.

Meaning of the condition: Not verbalized.

Relationships: "I've been waiting for you, Betty." (His dead wife was named Betty.)

Patterns/attitudes that may create dis-ease for this client: Refusal to deal with the world as it is may increase feelings of confusion.

Life purpose: Client indicates no life purpose except to reunite with dead wife.

Client strengths: Client is well-nourished and capable of showering and walking outside.

Ability to participate in care: Client has periods of confusion, but can participate during periods of lucidity.

Ethical dilemmas: Should the nurse enter the client's non–reality-based world in order to meet treatment goals (e.g., should the nurse pretend to be the client's wife so client will cooperate?).

Nurse–client process: The client believes the nurse is his dead wife. Continual reorientation to the nurse is necessary to build a relationship.

TIPS FOR CARETAKERS AND FAMILY MEMBERS

Cells in the adult brain appear capable of replacing lost or dysfunctional neurons and cells (Andrews & Andrews, 2003; Mattson et al., 2002), so by reducing stress, enhancing nutrition, and stimulating the brain, positive change is possible. Caregivers can follow each of these tips.

1. *Stay calm and listen.* It's easy to get upset when talking to someone who's agitated, but it's essential not to take that behavior personally. Let your loved one express frustrations. Even if the words don't make total sense, the speech and inflection may hold clues to what is meant.

2. *Use positive communication.* Speak slowly and clearly. Use words that are short, simple, and familiar and a gentle, relaxed tone of voice with positive, friendly facial expressions. Maintain eye contact, use touch and pointing to emphasize words, identify others by name, ask one question at a time, allowing for a response, avoid quizzing. Avoid interrupting, criticizing, correcting, and arguing. Walk away rather than get into an angry argument. Break instructions down into simple steps. Encourage the other person to continue to speak, even when he or she has difficulty. Avoid talking about the other person as if he or she isn't there. Offer assistance, but don't push.

3. *Encourage decision making.* Give your loved ones as much control over their daily lives as possible. Ask, "What do you want to wear today?" and hold up two outfits. Ask, "What do you want to eat for breakfast?" and hold up an egg and a box of cereal (or whatever choices there are). Do the same for lunch and dinner. It is

important to assume that some of what you say and do is getting through to your loved one. This gives the message that you care and respect the person.

4. *Structure the environment.* Provide signs, pictures, and familiar objects that can guide a family member who wanders. Offer toileting every two hours. Consider getting an ID bracelet or alarm device to ensure safer walking, designed to sound when your loved one rises from a bed or chair unassisted. Regular vision and hearing assessments to confirm that eyeglasses are clean and operational and hearing aids are working can decrease misinterpretation of the environment. Introduce yourself and your relationship regularly during the day and keep a clock nearby so you can say the time aloud, especially when you notice the memory of your loved one is failing. Photo albums with familiar pictures, favorite foods, personal memorabilia, and preferred music can provide comfort.

5. *Use a rocking chair.* An unpublished 1998 study by a geriatric nursing researcher at the University of Rochester found that rocking chairs calm dementia sufferers. The agitation caused by Alzheimer's is soothed by rocking. If you don't have a rocking chair you may want to consider getting one.

6. *Use a mirror for feedback.* Looking in a mirror can raise awareness and promote self-care in most individuals. In a study, for a small number of individuals, looking into the mirror initially aroused feelings of anger or despair, but they passed quickly and were followed by relief and calmness (Tabak, Bergman, & Alpert, 1996). Avoid using mirrors during a period of agitation.

7. *Serve the meal with the most calories at breakfast.* Because of alterations in circadian rhythms and behavioral difficulties, traditional large lunch or large supper meals do not work well and are apt to result in weight and memory loss and behavioral deterioration (Young, Binns, & Greenwood, 2001). Suggestions include green tea (noncaffeinated) and (1) peanut butter (preferably organic with no oil, salt, or sugar added), sunflower seeds and sliced banana on 4 slices of whole grain spelt, rice, or any nonwheat bread, and a large bowl of nonprocessed (preferably steel cut) oatmeal with bananas, 2 tablespoons of wheat germ, a handful of both sunflower and pumpkin seeds and soy or rice milk; (2) ½ block of tofu scrambled or stir fried in olive oil with at least 4 fresh vegetables (preferably broccoli, carrots, asparagus, peas, kale, cabbage, and/or parsley); or (3) 4–8 ounces of baked or canned fish (preferably sardines, mackerel, salmon, or bluefish) with at least 4 steamed vegetables, rice or baked potato, and a salad with homemade olive oil and cider

vinegar dressing. Consider eating the same food plan yourself. It will increase your energy and clear thinking, prevent Alzheimer's and other chronic diseases, and help you normalize your weight.

8. *Provide a vitamin and trace-mineral supplement at breakfast and make sure it includes vitamins E, C, and A, selenium, and zinc* to enhance memory, thinking, problem solving, and attention (Chandra, 2001), and protect against free radicals and neurodegeneration (Fang, Yang, & Wu, 2002).

9. *Omit animal proteins.* They contain saturated fats (meat, chicken, eggs, cheese, milk). At least one study linked high consumption of animal fats to Alzheimer's (Otsuka, Yamaguchi, & Ueki, 2002). Other items to avoid include sugary snacks and desserts, soft drinks and diet sodas, and all alcohol. They may be linked to Alzheimer's disease (Berrino, 2002) and when the stomach is filled with them, there is no room for the fresh fruit and vegetables, legumes, cereals, and fish that can enhance brain function (Kruman et al., 2002).

10. *Never use aluminum cooking pots or pans.* The element is toxic to the human brain (Perez-Granados & Vaquero, 2002).

11. *Always stir fry or bake food.* High intake of fats (fried foods, pastries, cakes, cookies, candy) may be associated with a higher risk of Alzheimer's disease and lack of clear thinking once it occurs (Goldman, Klatz, & Berger, 1999).

12. *Increase intake of dried beans and peas, peanuts/peanut butter, pumpkin seeds, sunflower seeds, soy products* (File et al., 2001), *and fresh vegetables, and decrease intake of sugar/sugary foods.* Degenerative disease in general, and Alzheimer's in particular, are linked to excessive dietary intake of sugar and refined carbohydrates and insufficient cereals, legumes, seeds, and vegetables (Berrino, 2002).

13. *Serve tea (preferably green and decaffeinated) and eliminate coffee.* Tea has polyphenols that protect against cell injury and neurodegeneration (Fang et al., 2002), and coffee can overstimulate.

14. *Try the following supplements,* which have been shown to protect against neurodegeneration: glutathione, arginine, citrulline, taurine, superoxide dismutase, catalase, glutathione reductase, and glutathione peroxidases (Fang et al., 2002).

15. *Turn off the TV, reduce noise levels, and make sure lighting is adequate* during mealtimes. One study showed enhanced light and reduced noise improved food intake levels (McDaniel, Hunt, Hackes, & Pope, 2001). Another study showed that quiet music can be soothing (Denney, 1997).

16. *Include mind stimulation in daily activities.* Puzzles, memory repetition games, music, developing other-handedness, reading aloud, and other fun brain twisters can enhance memory and thinking ability. Choose from the list below and find others or adapt them to the level of concentration of an Alzheimer-diagnosed family member. Do all activities together, so both caregiver and receiver participate. Use the other hand to brush teeth. Jot down notes or numbers. Buy a Rubik's cube and work on it . Do crossword puzzles in the newspaper or a puzzle book. Memorize a poem, starting with something short and familiar. Sketch a simple object together. Stand in front of a mirror and practice facial expressions. Read aloud from favorite books (Goldman et al., 1999).

17. *Get an aquarium* and place it in front of eating sites so the fish are clearly visible during meals. Weight increased significantly and less nutritional supplementation was needed when fish aquariums were introduced on specialized Alzheimer's units (Edwards & Beck, 2002).

18. *Take a walk together* outside in a pleasant and nurturing place before breakfast and after dinner to enhance appetite, improve mental function, calm the mind, firm the body, and prepare for calm sleep. If you can't go outside, walk the building, mall, stairs, or whatever is available wearing headsets playing calming music or a relaxation tape.

19. *Play a relaxation or self-hypnotic tape with positive affirmations* ("I am calm," "I am healthy," "I am strong," "I sleep well," etc., repeated with calming music) in the background all day long, even if the TV is on. The subconscious mind will hear and respond to the tape. Stress is one of the greatest robbers of brain function (Goldman et al., 1999).

WHAT TO DO IF NURSING HOME OR ASSISTED-LIVING CARE IS NEEDED

If Alzheimer's progresses to a point of great memory loss and combativeness, nursing home or assisted-living care may be necessary, although many of the measures listed below can also be instituted at home Family members can enhance a loved one's life by participating in care to enhance wellness. Tips include:

1. *Enlist the services of a gerontologic advanced practice nurse* (GAPN) who can treat urinary incontinence, pressure ulcers, depres-

sion, and aggressive behavior, as well as help families adjust to the transition to the nursing home. Nursing home residents who worked with a GAPN showed significantly less deterioration than residents who didn't work with a GAPN (Ryden et al., 2000). If this is not feasible or necessary, consult with a GAPN while working with a family or client.

2. *Make an audiotape.* Tape the music the client loves or ask the family to bring a loved music tape to the nursing home and play it in the dining room at mealtimes.

3. *Provide touch and ensure that additional touch is available for the client.* Show an aide or nursing technician how to massage the loved one's back, feet, or hands. Supervise the aide or technician at least the first time and randomly at other times to make sure the massage is performed in a competent and safe manner.

4. *Inquire about the exercise program at the nursing home.* If there is none, suggest one or make sure you provide some exercise opportunities when you visit.

5. *Incorporate all the tips suggested for at-home care.*

TREATMENT PLANNING: SETTING JOINTLY AGREED-UPON GOALS

Because clients may have periods of confusion and memory loss, use your ingenuity to learn client choices. In the case of the client discussed above, the following goals were agreed upon:

1. Provide foot massage
2. Enhance memory
3. Develop orienting resources

There are a number of things you can help clients and their families do to prevent and/or treat Alzheimer's. Provide the information presented earlier to family caregivers to improve both the client's and the caregiver's quality of life (Riviere et al., 2002). The more active clients are in self-care measures, the more likely they are to control their symptoms. Caregivers need to plan for time away from caretaking and for activities that reduce their stress. One study showed that a 12-month home-based exercise program improved physical activity levels and lowered stress for caregivers (Castro, Wilcox, O'Sullivan, Baumann, & King, 2002).

ADDITIONAL INFORMATION AND TREATMENTS TO SHARE WITH CLIENTS

NUTRITIONAL MEASURES

1. *Eat low-fat foods* (World Alzheimer Congress, 2000). Eliminate fried foods and those with saturated fats (meats, cheese, pastries, cakes, and pies). Eat primarily low-fat foods including fruits, vegetables, and whole grains, but have at least 2 tablespoons of olive oil a day on salad or via peanut or other nut butters to maintain mind–body functions.

2. *Eat foods high in vitamin B12.* A deficiency in vitamin B12 and an overabundance of homocysteine (a type of amino acid, a building block of protein that can injure blood vessel linings) can cause dementia and severe nerve damage (Kruman et al., 2002). With age, the digestive tract becomes less efficient in absorbing vitamin B12. It may be important to eat more foods containing B12 in order to overcome the lack of efficiency of the digestive tract (Russell, 2000). Foods high in this vitamin include sardines, mackerel, trout, herring, eggs, nutritional yeast, crabs, crayfish, clams, oysters, sea vegetables (kombu, dulse, kelp, wakame), and fermented soyfoods (tempeh, natto, and miso). There's another reason to eat soy foods— they enhance memory (File et al., 2001).

3. *Eat at least five fruits and vegetables every day.* Oxidative stress probably plays a key role in the dementia that occurs in Alzheimer's disease. Plant foods contain flavonoids, powerful antioxidant substances (Commenges et al., 2000).

4. *Eat foods rich in folate.* A lack of this important substance may be involved in the development of Alzheimer's (Wang et al., 2001). It makes sense to eat foods rich in folate including asparagus, desiccated or fresh liver, fresh dark green uncooked vegetables, wheat bran, turnips, potatoes, orange juice, black-eyed peas, lima beans, watermelon, oysters, and cantaloupe.

5. *Drink more green tea.* It exerts a protective effect against brain injury (Hong et al., 2000).

6. *Reduce intake of aluminum.* Drink filtered or distilled water. Aluminum in drinking water is correlated with Alzheimer's disease (Rondeau, Commenges, Jacquin-Gadda, & Dartigues, 2000). Fluoridated drinking water may be especially bad because aluminum-fluoride, which is used to fluoridate drinking water, alters nerves and blood vessels in the brain (Van der Voet, Schiijns, & de Wolff, 1999; Varner, Jensen, Horvath, & Isaacson, 1998). Minerals compete with each other in the body. By increasing consumption of magne-

sium and/or magnesium-rich foods, there will be less chance of aluminum absorption. Magnesium-rich foods include whole grain breads and cereals, fresh peas, brown rice, soy flour, wheat germ, nuts, Swiss chard, figs, green leafy vegetables, and citrus fruit.

7. *Drink grape juice.* This beverage is a rich source of flavonoids, which have greater antioxidant efficacy than does vitamin E, and is a potent protector against oxidative stress, reducing the risk of free radical damage and chronic disease (O'Byrne, Devaraj, Grundy, & Jialal, 2002).

8. *Use supplements that have been shown to be effective.* Pycnogenol is a supplement that may prevent and/or treat neurodegenerative conditions such as Alzheimer's disease (Liu, Lau, Peng, & Shah, 2000). *Acetyl-L-carnitine* is another supplement to consider. It contains both acetyl and carnitine, both of which have neurobiological properties that have been shown to have beneficial effects in Alzheimer's disease (Pettegrew, Levine, & McClure, 2000). Antioxidants can function as powerful protectants.

The progression of Alzheimer's of moderate to severe impairment is slowed equally well with *vitamin E* or selegiline, a monoamine oxidase inhibitor (Sano et al., 1997). Vitamin E (alpha-tocopherol) in both its natural and synthetic form has been shown to protect neurons against the oxidative cell death caused by Alzheimer's disease (Behl, 2000). *Vitamin C* is another antioxidant that can help. Supplementation with *vitamin C and E together* significantly decreases oxidation, a factor in Alzheimer's disease (Kontush et al., 2001). Older men, aged 71 to 93, who took both vitamin C and E supplements at least once a week were 88% less likely to have vascular dementia (speech, language, and visual disturbances; paralysis and mental impairment) and a 20% greater chance of having better cognitive function than those who didn't, even 4 years later (Helmer et al., 1999). Participants in the study who took the supplements over a 6-year period showed a 75% greater chance of better mental performance. Alzheimer's is associated with deficiency of a brain chemical, acetylcholine. *Lecithin* (made from soy) and *choline* (a supplement) are precursors to this chemical, so taking them daily could help.

ENVIRONMENTAL ACTIONS

Delete any sources of aluminum in the living environment. Switch to iron, stainless steel, glass, or porcelain-coated cookware. Aluminum is toxic to the brain (Perez-Granados & Vaquero, 2002). Discontinue the use of spray-on antiperspirants, hair sprays, cleaning solutions, hobby sprays, paint, and glues. Inhaled aluminum may be completely absorbed because the olfactory nerves in the nasal cavity lead directly to the brain. Reduce consumption of drugs that contain aluminum, including antacids and buffered aspirin.

HERBS

Try gingko biloba, an herb that has been shown to be useful and safe in the treatment of Alzheimer's. Used for thousands of years in traditional Chinese medicine, this herb now has been shown to treat failing memory, age-related dementias, and poor blood flow to the head and brain (McKenna, Jones, & Hughes, 2001). Healthy participants who took gingko biloba showed significant improvements in speed of working memory and processing information (Stough, Clarke, Lloyd, & Nathan, 2001). The herb has a significant effect on the central nervous system and may treat insufficient blood flow to the brain (Itil & Martorano, 1995). Gingko is equally effective as cholinesterase inhibitors, including donepezil, rivastigmine, and metrifonate (Wettstone, 2000). It also benefits Alzheimer's patients by improving thinking and social function (LeBars et al., 1997). Note: The use of any herbs needs to be carefully coordinated with other medications. Be sure to consult with a health care practitioner who is an expert in herbs, as ginkgo can interact with aspirin and anti-platelet drugs and can increase clotting time. If gingko can be taken, follow the dosage directions on the bottle.

WEIGHT LOSS

Eat low-fat foods and increase exercise. Although most age-related dementia is due to Alzheimer's, the second most frequent cause is high blood pressure. *Eat breakfast.* Skipping breakfast can mean eating more in the evening and binge-eating episodes. Eating more in the evening after dinner, especially when one is less active, can turn the extra calories to fat. Also, counsel clients to take a stress reduction class to learn how to control stress and anger, and consider massage, which can lower the body's level of cortisol, an indicator of stress.

EXERCISE

1. *Exercise the mind.* Adults with hobbies that exercise their minds such as reading, doing jigsaw puzzles, or playing chess or

bingo are protected more than twice as much from Alzheimer's disease as those whose leisure is limited to TV watching (Wilson et al., 2002). Unused brain power is lost brain power. Every day be sure to read, do a puzzle, play a musical instrument or a board game, knit, or do woodwork.

2. *Exercise the body.* Physical activities such as baseball, football, bike riding, swimming, walking, or skating also stimulate the brain and may help ward off Alzheimer's (Francese, Sorrell, & Butler, 1997). At home, dancing, walking, and mild stretching can be employed. It is best to complete the activity regularly, at the same time of day and in the same vicinity, to minimize confusion.

3. *Seated range of motion exercise programs can be beneficial for frail elders.* This type of exercise can help improve energy, circulation, stamina, and mood (Arkin, 1999). Memory loss, mobility, balance, flexibility, and knee and hip strength improved in a three-times-a-week program (Lazowski, 1999; Sobel, 2001).

SMOKING CESSATION

Smoking raises homocysteine and depletes antioxidant vitamins that may protect the brain. Stopping smoking could help to prevent the development of Alzheimer's.

MUSIC

Listening to preferred music can work better than medication for agitated movement (Clark, Lipe, & Bilbrey, 1997; Gerdner, 1997, 2000). Find out what kind of music is preferred and play it in the background at all times and/or at the first sign of agitation.

TOUCH

1. *Approach an agitated person in a gentle, unhurried manner.*

2. *If feasible, hold the client's hands and talk softly to reduce agitation.*

3. *Gently stroke from ear lobe to chin* in an unhurried manner to bring calm, stimulate memory, and reduce pacing, wandering, and resisting in individuals with Alzheimer's (Gerdner & Buckwalter, 1994).

4. *Use massage to enhance relaxation and reduce blood pressure.* Gentle hand massage using lotion with a scent familiar to the client can reduce anxiety and agitation and lower the body's level of cortisol, an indicator of stress (Kilstoff, 1998). Ask family to bring lotion

that is familiar to the client to the nursing home and ask the staff to use it with the client. Teach family members and caregivers to use a lotion familiar to the person with Alzheimer's; hold some in their hands to warm it, and then gently massage the back. Massage with lotion can increase alertness and contentment, reduce stress levels and agitation, and improve sleep. Family caregivers providing massage reported that their loved one's sleeping patterns improved too, and that they themselves felt more calm and less stressed. Foot massage with acupressure reduced patient wandering and increased periods of calm (Sutherland, 1999). If a family member is a resident in a nursing home, suggest that clients ask to receive foot massage. If there are no nurses or massage therapists available to give a foot massage, clients can investigate having one come into the nursing home on a consultant basis after coordinating this with the physician. Teach family members how to give foot massages. Therapeutic touch may also be useful. It can reduce agitated behavior (as measured by pacing) in persons with Alzheimer's by decreasing cortisol, a measure of hyperresponsiveness to stress (Woods & Dimond, 2002).

ACUPRESSURE

Hold index, middle, and fourth fingers of the right hand on the top of the shoulder just below the side of the neck; find the same spot with the left hand or teach the client to perform the procedure. Hold until pulsation is felt in all three fingers, then move straight up to a spot on the bony ridge that runs along the back of the head, then to a spot above the eyes in the middle of the forehead, then back to the bony ridge across the back of the head, ending with spots directly below at the points just before the neck ends (Dayton, 1994).

AFFIRMATIONS

For clients who are unable to read or respond to affirmations, it may be helpful for the nurse to say them aloud to the client in a calm and positive voice. Use the statements that appear to soothe clients and avoid those that agitate. As each client is unique, this may be a trial and error process. The idea is to provide positive thoughts to balance (or overcome) the negative ones in the client's perception.

Some affirmations that might be helpful to say or write at least 20 times a day are: "I forgive and release the past." "I accept a life of complete joy." "I move forward into a new and better way of experiencing life." These sayings should be written on 3 x 5 cards and put in prominent places.

EVALUATING TREATMENT GOALS

The client's daughter provided the following evaluation comments: "I've been giving him a foot or hand massage every day; he tells me which one he wants. I read to him from his favorite books and that seems to calm him. I put up signs around the house so he can find the bathroom and bedroom and that seems to make him less agitated."

REFERENCES

Andrews, J. C., & Andrews, N. C. (2003). Counseling Alzheimer's patients and their families. *Clinician Reviews, 13*(4), 56–62.

Arkin, S. M. (1999). Elder rehab: A student-supervised exercise program for Alzheimer's patients. *Gerontology, 39,* 729–735.

Behl, C. (2000). Vitamin E protects neurons against oxidative cell death in vitro more effectively than 17-beta estradiol and induces the activity of the transcription factor NF-kappaB. *Journal of Neural Transmission, 107,* 393–407.

Berrino, F. (2002). Western diet and Alzheimer's disease. *Epidemiology and Prevention, 26,* 107–115.

Castro, C. M., Wilcox, S., O'Sullivan, P., Baumann, K., & King, A. C. (2002). An exercise program for women who are caring for relatives with dementia. *Psychosomatic Medicine, 64,* 458–468.

Chandra, R. K. (2001). Effect of vitamin and trace-element supplementation on cognitive function in elderly subjects. *Nutrition, 17,* 709–712.

Clark, M. E., Lipe, A. W., & Bilbrey, M. (1997). Use of music to decrease aggressive behaviors in people with dementia. *Journal of Gerontological Nursing, 24*(7), 10–17.

Commenges, D., Scotet, V., Renaud, S., Jacquin-Gadda, H., Barberger-Gateau, P., & Dartigues, J. F. (2000). Intake of flavonoids and risk of dementia. *European Journal of Epidemiology, 15,* 357–363.

Dayton, B. R. (1994). *An introduction to a gentle acupressure for caregivers.* Friday Harbor, WA: High Touch Network.

Denney, A. (1997). Quiet music: An intervention for mealtime agitation. *Journal of Gerontologic Nursing, 23*(7), 16–23.

Edwards, N. E., & Beck, A. M. (2002). Animal-assisted therapy and nutrition in Alzheimer's disease. *Western Journal of Nursing Research, 24,* 697–712.

Fang, Y. Z., Yang, S., & Wu, G. (2002). Free radicals, antioxidants, and nutrition. *Nutrition, 18,* 872–879.

File, S. E., Jarrett, N., Fluck, E., Duffy, R., Casey, K., & Wiseman, H. (2001). Eating soya improves human memory. *Psychopharmacology, 157,* 430–436.

Francese, T., Sorrell, J., & Butler, F. R. (1997). Effects of regular exercise on muscle strength and functional ability of late stage Alzheimer's residents. *American Journal of Alzheimer's Disease, 12,* 122–127.

Gerdner, L. (1997). An individualized music intervention for agitation. *Journal of the American Psychiatric Nurses Association, 3,* 177–184.

Gerdner, L. (2000). Effects of individualized versus classical "relaxation" music on the frequency of agitation in elderly persons with Alzheimer's disease and related disorders. *International Journal of Psychogeriatrics, 12*(1), 49–65.

Gerdner, L. A., & Buckwalter, K. C. (1994). Assessment and management of agitation in Alzheimer's disease and related disorders. *Journal of Gerontological Nursing, 20*(4), 11–19.

Goldman, R., Klatz, R., & Berger, L. (1999). *Brain fitness.* New York: Doubleday.

Helmer, C., Damon, D., Letenneur, L., Fabrijoale, C., Barberger-Gateau, P., Lafont, S., Fuhrer, R., Antonucci, T., Commenges, D., Orgogozo, J. M., & Dartigues, J. F. (1999). Marital status and risk of Alzheimer's disease: A French population-based cohort study. *Neurology, 53,* 1953–1958.

Hong, J. T., Ryu, S. R., Kim, H. J., Lee, J. K., Lee, S. H., Kim, D. B., et al. (2000). Neuroprotective effect of green tea extract in experimental ischemia-reperfusion brain injury. *Brain Research Bulletin, 53,* 743–749.

Itil, T., & Martorano, D. (1995). Natural substances in psychiatry (Ginkgo biloba in dementia). *Psychopharmacology Bulletin, 31*(1), 147–158.

Kilstoff, K. (1998). New approaches to health and well-being for dementia day-care clients, family caregivers, and day-care staff. *International Journal of Nursing Practice, 4*(2), 70–83.

Kontush, A., Mann, U., Arlt, S., Ujeyl, A., Luhrs, C., Muller-Thomsen, T., & Beisiegel, U. (2001). Influence of vitamin E and C supplementation on lipoprotein oxidation in patients with Alzheimer's disease. *Free Radicals in Biological Medicine, 31,* 345–354.

Kruman, I. I., Kumaravel, T. S., Lohani, A., Pedersen, W. A., Cutler, R. G., Kruman, Y., et al. (2002). Folic acid deficiency and homocysteine impair DNA repair in hippocampal neurons and sensitize them to amyloid toxicity in experimental models of Alzheimer's disease. *Journal of Neuroscience, 22,* 1752–1762.

Lazowski, D. A. (1999). A randomized outcome evaluation of group exercise programs in long term care institutions. *Journal of Gerontology, 54,* M621–M628.

LeBars, P. L., Katz, M. M., Berman, N., Itil, T. M., Freedman, A. M., & Schatzberg, A. F. (1997). A placebo-controlled, double-blind randomized trial of an extract of gingko biloba for dementia. *Journal of the American Medical Association, 278,* 1327–1332.

Liu, F., Lau, B. H., Peng, Q., & Shah, V. (2000). Pcynogenol protects vascular endothelial cells from beta-amyloid-induced injury. *Biology Pharmacy Bulletin, 23*, 735–737.

Luchsinger, J. A., Tang, M. X., Shea, S., & Mayeux, R. (2002). Caloric intake and the risk of Alzheimer's disease. *Archives of Neurology, 59*, 1258–1263.

Masaki, K. H., Losonczy, K. G., Izmirlian, G., Foley, D. J., Ross, G. W., Petrovich, H., Havlik, R., & White, L. R. (2000). Association of vitamin E and C supplement use with cognitive function and dementia in elderly men. *Neurology, 54*, 1265–1272.

Mattson, M. P., Duan, W., Chan, S. L., Cheng, A., Haughey, N., Gary D. S., et al. (2002). Neuroprotective and neurorestorative signal transduction mechanisms in brain aging: Modification by genes, diet and behavior. *Neurobiological Aging, 23*, 695–705.

McDaniel, J. H., Hunt, A., Hackes, B., & Pope, J. F. (2001). Impact of dining room environment on nutritional intake of Alzheimer's residents: A case study. *American Journal of Alzheimers Disease and Other Dementias, 16*, 297–302.

McKenna, D. J., Jones, K., & Hughes, K. (2001). Efficacy, safety, and use of ginkgo biloba in clinical and preclinical applications. *Alternative Therapies in Health and Medicine, 7*(5), 70–86; 88–90.

O'Byrne, D. J., Devaraj, S., Grundy, S. M., & Jialal, I. (2002). Comparisons of the antioxidant effects of Concord grape juice flavonoids alpha-tocopherol n markers of oxidative stress in healthy adults. *American Journal of Clinical Nutrition, 76*, 1367–1374.

Otsuka, M., Yamaguchi, K., & Ueki, A. (2002). Similarities and differences between Alzheimer's disease and vascular dementia from the viewpoint of nutrition. *Annals of the New York Academy of Science, 977*, 155–161.

Perez-Granados, A. M., & Vaquero, M. P. (2002). Silicon, aluminum, arsenic, and lithium: Essentiality and human health implications. *Journal of Nutrition and Aging, 6*, 154–162.

Pettegrew, J. W., Levine, J., & McClure, R. J. (2000). Acetyl-L-carnitine physical-chemical, metabolic and therapeutic properties: Relevance for its mode of action in Alzheimer's disease and geriatric depression. *Molecular Psychiatry, 5*, 616–632.

Riviere, S., Gillette-Guyonnet, S., Andrieu, S., Nourhashemi, F., Lauque, S., Cantet, C., Salva, A., et al. (2002). Cognitive function and caregiver burden: Predictive factors for eating behaviour disorders in Alzheimer's disease. *International Journal of Geriatric Psychiatry, 17*, 950–955.

Rondeau, V., Commenges, D., Jacquin-Gadda, H., & Dartigues, J. F. (2000). Relation between aluminum concentrations in drinking water and Alzheimer's Disease: An 8-year follow-up study. *American Journal of Epidemiology, 152*(1), 59–66.

Russell, R. M. (2000). The aging process as a modifier of metabolism. *American Journal of Clinical Nutrition, 72*, 529S–532S.

Ryden, M. B., Snyder, M., Gross, C. R., Savik, K., Pearson, V., Kirchbaum, K.,

& Mueller, C. (2000). Value-added outcomes: The use of advanced practice nurses in long-term care facilities. *Gerontologist, 40,* 654–662.

Sano, M., Ernesto, C., Thomas, R. G., Klauber, M. R., Schafter, K., Grundman, M., et al. (1997). A controlled trial of Selegiline, Alpha-Tocopherol, or both as treatment for Alzheimer's disease. *The New England Journal of Medicine, 336,* 1216–1222.

Sobel, B. P. (2001). Bingo vs. physical intervention in stimulating short-term cognition in Alzheimer's disease patients. *American Journal of Alzheimers Disease and Other Dementias, 16,* 115–120.

Stough, C., Clarke, J., Lloyd, J., & Nathan, P. J. (2001). Neuropsychological changes after 30-day Gingko biloba administration in healthy participants. *International Journal of Neuropsycho-Pharmacology, 4,* 131–134.

Sutherland, J. (1999). Foot acupressure and massage for patients with Alzheimer's disease and related dementias. *Image: Journal of Nursing Scholarship, 31,* 347–348.

Tabak, N., Bergman, R., & Alpert, R. (1996). The mirror as a therapeutic tool for patients with dementia. *International Journal of Nursing Practice, 2,* 155–159.

Van der Voet, G. B., Schiijns, E., & de Wolff, F. A. (1999). Fluoride enhances the effect of aluminum chloride on interconnections between aggregates of hippocampal neurons. *Archives of Physiology and Biochemistry, 107*(1), 15–21.

Varner, J. A., Jensen, K. F., Horvath, W., & Isaacson, R. L. (1998). Chronic administration of aluminum-fluoride or sodium-fluoride to rats in drinking water: Alterations in neuronal and cerebrovascular integrity. *Brain Research, 784*(1–2), 284–298.

Wang, H. X., Wahlin, A., Basun, H., Fastbom, J., Winblad, B., & Fratiglioni, L. (2001). Vitamin B12 and folate in relation to the development of Alzheimer's disease. *Neurology, 56,* 1188–1194.

Wettstone, A. (2000). Cholinesterase inhibitors and gingko extracts—are they comparable in the treatment of dementia? Comparison of published placebo-controlled efficacy studies of at least six months' duration. *Phytomedicine, 6,* 393–401.

Wilson, B. S., Bennett, D. A., Bienias, J. L., Aggarwal, N. T., Mendes De Leon, C. F., Morris, M. C., et al. (2002). Cognitive activity and incident AD in a population-based sample of older persons. *Neurology, 59,* 1910–1914.

Woods, D. L, & Dimond, M. (2002). The effect of therapeutic touch on agitated behavior and cortisol in persons with Alzheimer's disease. *Biological Research in Nursing, 4,* 104–114.

World Alzheimer Congress. (2000). AD risk increases with high-fat diet. *Clinician Reviews, 10*(11), 132.

Young, K. W., Binns, M. A., & Greenwood, C. E. (2001). Meal delivery practices do not meet needs of Alzheimer patients with increased cognitive and behavioral difficulties in a long-term care facility. *Journal of Gerontology and Biological Science in Medical Sciences, 56,* M656–M561.

CHAPTER 5

Arthritis

Arthritis is an inflammation of the joints. The most common forms are rheumatoid arthritis and osteoarthritis. A treatment program includes medication, physical and/or occupational therapy, and weight control. The physician will often prescribe NSAIDS (non-steroidal anti-inflammatory drugs), acetaminophen (Tylenol), Aleve, or prednisone. All have dangerous side effects, including hip fracture, intestinal bleeding, death, decreased collagen deposition, and tuberculosis (Lapane, Spooner, & Mucha, 2001; Lystbaek, Svendsen, & Hesler, 1995; Manicourt & Druetz-Van Egeren, 1994; Muscara, McKnifhet, & Asfaha, 2000).

HOLISTIC NURSING ASSESSMENT

The nurse wrote up the following holistic nursing assessment after interviewing Mrs. B., a 45-year-old woman, diagnosed with rheumatoid arthritis. The client is overweight and smokes a pack or more of cigarettes a day. Let the results provide you with ideas for assessing other clients with arthritis.

Client learning needs: "I'm in pain all the time."

Indicants of readiness to learn: "Can you help me?"

Soul/spirituality symbol(s): "I go to church on Sunday, isn't that enough?"

Meaning of the condition to client: "I can't get around much anymore. This disease has set me back. Sometimes I don't even feel like getting up in the morning."

Relationship needs/effects as perceived by client: "My husband never wants to make love anymore. I guess he thinks I'm too sick."

Patterns/attitudes that may create dis-ease for this client: Client uses negative affirmations including, "I'll always be in pain," and "I'm never going to get any sleep."

Life purpose: States no life purpose. Facial expression and body language indicate frustration.

Client strengths: Can ask for help and is able to get around with the help of a cane.

Ability to participate in care: Complains of pain continually, but asks for help with pain.

Ethical dilemmas: Trying to get the client to stop smoking even though she wants to work on being pain free.

Nurse–client process: Client is critical of nurse's actions. May be feeling unloved and self-critical.

TREATMENT PLANNING: SETTING JOINTLY AGREED-UPON GOALS

Goals that were jointly agreed-upon for the client discussed above include:

1. Learn pain reduction measures.
2. Lose weight.
3. Stop eating foods that aggravate arthritis.
4. Stop smoking.

Acceptance of condition/attitude change: The client chose the following affirmation to use to replace the resentment she feels for having been sexually abused by her uncle: "I now choose to love and approve of myself." Client agreed to say the affirmation at least 20 times a day.

Facilitating the healing process/healing intention formulation: From a list of meditative statements, client chose the following one to assist in the healing process: "I see others with love." Client will repeat the meditative statement while in a relaxed state before arising and before retiring. Nurse will use centering and caring nonverbal communication to enhance client healing.

Creating a sacred space: Client plans to use softer lights in her office and play calming music in the background all day while she works.

Integrative practices planned: Client gave away the meat, eggs, and oils that a food diary she kept for a week showed increased her pain. She has bought more fresh fruits, vegetables, and grains.

Role model strategies: Nurse brought in recipes using fresh vegetables and grain dishes she prepares to share with the client.

Protection plan: Taught client how to use guided imagery to picture a protective green light around herself prior to meeting other people.

Family strategies: Client plans to confront her uncle about his abusive behavior either in person or through a ritual.

Life issues/life purpose work: Client wants to volunteer to work in a women's shelter, teaching little girls to be safe and what to do if someone molests them.

Treatment possibilities/considerations: For clients with arthritis, work in collaboration with them to choose holistic approaches that will work for them.

ADDITIONAL INFORMATION AND TREATMENTS TO SHARE WITH CLIENTS

NUTRITIONAL APPROACHES

Children suffering from juvenile arthritis have reduced serum levels of beta-carotene, retinol, and zinc compared with healthy children (Helgeland, Svendsen, Forre, & Haugen, 2000). Low serum selenium and vitamin E may be risk factors for rheumatoid arthritis (Knekt et al., 2000) and so can eating meat (Grant, 2000), because the iron and nitrites contribute to inflammation (Darlington & Stone, 2001).

Arthritis is rare in poorer countries where fresh fruits, vegetables, whole grains, and legumes are staples. Research supports the connection between diet and arthritis, which for years was considered quackery. The Arthritis Foundation now considers a healthy diet an important factor. Being overweight (stressing the workload joints must bear), injury, smoking, and repeated overuse of certain joints are associated with osteoarthritis.

Clients suffering from rheumatoid arthritis often eat too much total fat and too little fish and fiber. Their diets are also deficient in pyridoxine, zinc, and magnesium. This suggests that regular supplementation with multivitamins and trace elements may be needed or foods rich in these nutrients be eaten (Kremer & Bigaouette, 1996). Other nutritional approaches include the following:

1. *Use a food symptom diary* to find out and eliminate the foods that create or increase symptoms. Wheat, corn, milk/dairy products, and beef are common irritants. In a column next to the foods, write down mood/feelings thirty minutes after eating each item. Mood has been correlated with symptoms (Schanberg et al., 2000; Zautra et al., 1997, 2001).

2. *Focus meals around healthy foods.* Change eating patterns to focus on whole grains, fresh vegetables, and fruits, and on reducing (and preferably eliminating) sugar, refined carbohydrates (doughnuts, muffins, cakes, pies, candy, potato chips, jellies, jello, custard, pudding, white bread, anything prepared from a mix, prepared or semi-prepared cereals), and saturated fats (meat, hard cheese, ice cream, and other dairy products, unless they are nonfat). The antioxidants in a vegan diet can be especially protective. A "living foods" (LF) regimen of berries, fruits, vegetables and roots, nuts, germinated seeds, and sprouts provides a rich source of carotenoids and vitamins C and E and can reduce the immunoreactivity to food antigens that set off arthritic inflammation (Hafstrom et al., 2001). In two separate studies, rheumatoid arthritis clients eating the LF diet reported a decrease in joint stiffness and pain, and an improvement in their self-experienced health; these findings were supported by objective measures (Hanninen et al., 2000) and weight loss (McDougall, Bruce, Spiller, Westerdahl, & McDougall, 2002).

3. *Eat soy foods and drinks and take avocado to reduce pain.* These foods help reduce pain as they rebuild cartilage (Muller-Fassbender, Bach, Haase, Rovati, & Setnikar, 1994).

4. *Try a vegetable/fruit juice fast.* A fast for 3 or 4 days, using no nightshade foods (tomatoes, potatoes, eggplant, and peppers), followed by a vegetarian diet, has shown a significant long-term effect (Kjeldsen-Kragh, 1999; Muller, de Toledo, & Resch, 2001). Cut the tops and bottoms off carrots and beets before juicing them. Grape juice is a richer source of flavonoids than vitamin E and can protect cells against oxidative stress and reduce the risk of free radical damage (O'Byrne, Devaraj, Grundy, & Jialal, 2002).

5. *Drink several glasses of one or more of the following fresh juices daily to help heal arthritic joints.* Space the juices through the day, leaving at least an hour, preferably 2 hours, between each combination. Because all fiber is removed from the vegetables and fruits, they are easy to digest. Dilute the juices with filtered water and sip them slowly, enjoying their fresh taste: (a) celery juice, (b) 10 ounces of carrot and 2 ounces of celery combined, (c) 5 or 6 large carrots or enough to make 10 ounces of juice intermixed with juiced

pieces of ½ fresh beet and 1 medium-sized cucumber (take the skin off the cucumber if it's been waxed). Drink 2 glasses of fresh grapefruit juice daily in the morning. Use these last two juices by themselves for a day: (a) every 30 minutes, add the juice of half a lemon to a glass of water and drink, (b) drink the juice of one orange every 2 hours followed by a glass of filtered water.

6. *Eat more fish, especially sardines, herring, Atlantic mackerel, salmon, lake trout, sturgeon, anchovies, and bluefin tuna.* Adding fish oils to the diet can reduce pain and stiffness (Hansen et al., 1996; Rennie, Hughes, Lang, & Jebb, 2003; Shapiro et al., 1996) by protecting against degradative and inflammatory aspects of joint tissue metabolism (Curtis et al., 2002). Reduce or eliminate meat. Meat eaters have more joint symptoms (Grant, 2000).

7. *If sensitive, avoid foods from the nightshade family* (see #4, as well as paprika, strawberries, mushrooms, cayenne and tobacco) for 1 month. Reintroduce each one slowly to see if it affects symptoms. Keep a food/symptom diary, writing down reactions ½ hour after eating one of the nightshade family foods.

8. *Add vitamin B6 foods.* Pain, swelling, and stiffness are associated with low levels of vitamin B6 (Frisco, Jacques, Wilson, Rosenberg, & Selhub, 2001). For more of this nutrient, eat sunflower seeds, toasted wheat germ, brown rice, soybeans, white beans, liver, chicken, mackerel, salmon, tuna, bananas, walnuts, peanuts, sweet potatoes, and cooked cabbage.

9. *Eat foods containing copper.* A deficiency of this mineral can exacerbate arthritic symptoms. Foods rich in copper are almonds, avocados, barley, beans, dandelion greens, and lentils.

10. *Eat foods rich in pantothenic acid.* This B-vitamin can reduce arthritis symptoms. Foods that contain pantothenic acid include soy flour, sunflower seeds, dark buckwheat, sesame seeds, brewer's yeast, peanuts, lobster, wheat bran, broccoli, mushrooms, eggs, oysters, sweet potatoes, and cauliflower.

11. *Avoid the artificial sweetener Aspartame.* It is found in many bottled or canned drinks and foods. It may make arthritis symptoms worse.

12. *Eat half a fresh pineapple daily for 1 to 3 weeks.* At least one study (Walker, Bundy, Hicks, & Middleton, 2002) showed that the bromelain in the fruit can reduce pain and swelling. Use fresh pineapple, which contains the necessary enzyme.

13. *Eat foods containing sulfur* (garlic, onions, Brussels sprouts, and cabbage) to help regenerate and rebuild cartilage cells, reduce inflammation, and relieve pain (Parcell, 2002).

14. *Eat fresh cherries* (Davis, 1980).

15. *Drink at least 8 glasses of water every day.* Other fluids are good, too, but drink plain water to get properly hydrated. When human tissue gets dry, tough, shrunken, and brittle, it needs to be softened, filled, and gently flexed to rebuild. Pain is often due to dehydration, so when you have pain, drink two glasses of water to reduce symptoms.

16. *Use fish oil, olive oil, and evening primrose oil.* These oils can protect against inflammatory reactions of arthritis (Darlington & Stone, 2001).

17. *Drink green tea.* It is rich in antioxidants that offset arthritis symptoms (Anthony et al.,1999).

18. *Avoid foods with high glycemic load* (rapidly digested and absorbed carbohydrates such as cake, pie, candy, doughnuts) as they are associated with an increased risk of ischemic heart disease (Liu et al., 2002) and other complications in diabetes (Nagaraj et al., 1996).

SUPPLEMENTS

1. *Take a copper supplement if foods high in the mineral are not ingested.* A deficiency of copper may exacerbate arthritic symptoms (Kremer & Bigaouette, 1996). If a chosen vitamin/mineral supplement has no copper in it, and foods high in this mineral are not eaten (almonds, avocados, barley, beans, dandelion greens, lentils), it is important to take a copper supplement of 2 mg daily with food.

2. *Evening primrose and borage seed oils may help.* Tender and swollen joints were reduced in study participants who took gamma-linolenic acid as opposed to a group taking a placebo (sugar pill). Black currant seed oil may also may reduce inflammation and joint tissue injury (Leventhal, Boyce, & Zurier, 1994).

3. *Take vitamins and other supplements to relieve pain and protect cells from injury due to oxidation.* Taking vitamins E and C in combination with indomethacin, sulfasalazine alone, and/or indomethacin alone controlled symptoms more effectively than drugs alone (Helmy, Shohayeb, Helmy, & el-Bassiouni, 2001). Consider leaving pain medication behind entirely. Taking vitamin C, beta-carotene, selenium, and poly-unsaturated fatty acids can ameliorate the symptoms of rheumatoid arthritis and related conditions (Darlington & Stone, 2001). A vitamin supplement of 6400 micrograms of folate and 20 micrograms of cobalamin worked as well as NSAID, had fewer side effects (none), and cost less (Flynn, Irvin, & Krause, 1994). Take antioxidants that protect cells from injury and prevent rheumatoid arthritis, including glutathione, arginine, citrulline, taurine, creatine,

zinc, vitamin A, and antioxidant enzymes such as superoxide dismutase, catalase, glutathione reductase, and glutathione peroxidases (Fang, Yang, & Wu, 2002).

4. *Increase intake of vitamin D.* Low intake of vitamin D is associated with an increased risk for progression of osteoarthritis of the knee (Leventhal et al., 1994). To enhance intake of this vitamin, spend at least 20 minutes in the sunshine every day, eat fish, take cod liver oil, or eat vitamin D-enriched foods. *SAMe* is a supplement to look into for pain, healing, and depression.

5. *Take SAMe or glucosamine.* The main components of cartilage are chondroitin sulfate, collagen, and proteoglycans. SAMe (S-adenosylmethionine) is synthesized from the amino acid methionine and is found throughout the body. SAMe protects chondrocytes, the cells that manufacture the main components of cartilage, against wear and tear on the joints. By taking SAMe, production of proteoglycans improves, and cartilage can be better maintained and repaired (McAlindon et al., 1996; Parcell, 2002). In several trials, SAMe worked just as well as naproxen, ibuprofen, and indomethacin, but had fewer side effects (Domijan, 1989; Konig, 1987). SAMe worked faster and with more significant improvements than antidepressants and with fewer reported adverse effects (Bell, Plon, Bunney, & Potkin, 1988; Vahora & Malek-Ahmadi, 1988). No studies have shown any reason not to use SAMe, as long as the normal daily dose recommended by Murray (1,200 to 1,600 mg divided in several doses for 21 days, then reduced to 400 mg a day) is followed (Murray, 1996). Another option is *glucosamine sulfate.* It has also been shown to reduce pain as well as NSAIDs, and with fewer and less damaging side effects (Muller-Fassbender, 1987) and to delay progression of knee osteoarthritis (Pavelka, Gatterova, & Olejarova, 2002).

HERBS

Australian aborigines have used indigenous herbs to treat arthritis for many years. Because there is no financial incentive, no clinical trials have been completed, but four herbs might be worth investigating: lemon myrtle, aniseed myrtle, mountain pepper, and wild rosella (Williams, 1998).

MASSAGE

Massage the suboccipital muscles at the base of the skull. When the rectus capitus becomes spastic, it irritates the sphenoid sinus and histamine may be released, producing inflammation, irritation, and pain in the joints (Griner & Nunes, 1996). See p. 43 for the appropriate massage technique.

Because skin is a living, absorbing organ, gently massaging aching joints with castor oil, garlic oil, or olive oil will provide soothing. For an even more soothing oil, add 10 drops of rosemary essential oil, 10 drops of eucalyptus oil, 5 drops of ginger oil, and 5 drops of peppermint to an ounce of sweet almond, jojoba, or olive oil. (All can be obtained at a health food store.) Put some of the oil mixture in the palm of the hand and gently and soothingly rub the sorest spot, moving to other sore areas when ready. Pay special attention to a spot that may be especially sore and can even result in spasms in the rest of the body, and the muscles on and below the bony shelf at the back of the head (suboccipital muscles).

Rub grated onion, garlic, or uncooked potato on inflamed joints. These substances can draw out heat and reduce swelling. Experiment and find which ones work.

ACUPUNCTURE

A randomized trial compared the effectiveness of acupuncture with advice and exercises on the symptomatic treatment of osteoarthritis of the hip. A significantly greater treatment effect (relieved pain and enhanced functionality) was found after 6 weeks of treatment with acupuncture than for the same period of time providing only advice and exercises (Haslam, 2001).

AFFIRMATIONS

Affirmations written on 3 x 5 cards can be put in prominent places around the home and workplace, including mirrors, desk drawers, or wherever they might be seen and read many times a day. Some suggestions are: "I let others be themselves and I am free." "I am full of love and forgiveness. "I see others through loving eyes." "I feel love toward myself and others." "My joints are healing, my body is well." "I picture all negative thoughts and feelings flowing out of me."

EXERCISE

1. *Yoga* may help. In one study, a yoga group of clients met for 8 weeks with an instructor while another group with osteoarthritis of

the hands received no yoga. The yoga group improved significantly more than the control group in pain, tenderness, and finger range of motion (Garfinkle, Schumacher, Husain, Levy, & Reshetar, 1994).

2. *Dance* has been shown to reduce pain, depression, anxiety, fatigue, and tension (Noreau, Martineau, Roy, & Belzile, 1995; Perlman et al., 1990). Ask clients to keep exercise moderate. Running more than 20 miles a week can create, not prevent, osteoarthritis (Cheng et al., 2000).

3. *Strength training* in adults 55 years or older works well for osteoarthritis, according to a randomized controlled trial. High intensity, home-based training can produce substantial improvements in pain, strength, physical function, and quality of life (Baker et al., 2001).

4. *Other exercises* that can be helpful include rotating each toe, ankle, knee, hips, waist, shoulders, elbows, wrists, and each finger, first clockwise and then counterclockwise Ask clients to squeeze the fingers together and hold, then open them as wide as possible. Repeat several times before doing the same with the toes.

The American Chiropractic Association (n.d.) suggests exercises for fingers:

- With your palm flat on a table, raise and lower your fingers one by one.
- Make an "O" by touching your thumb to each of the other fingertips, one at a time.
- Crumple a sheet of newspaper into a small ball with one hand.
- Squeeze a small rubber ball or sponge.
- Pick up coins or buttons of assorted sizes.
- Keep time to music with each finger by drumming with extended fingers.
- Rest the hand on a table and spread the fingers wide and then bring them together.
- Flip balls of paper with the fingers or flip a lightweight book or folded newspaper off extended fingers.

If the client is unable to complete the exercises, a friend or family member can bend and straighten the affected fingers gently, never forcing movement. Whether doing these exercises alone or with an assistant, stop if any movement causes severe pain or if soreness persists for more than twenty minutes. Other exercises to use to stretch and enhance comfort include the following:

A. To strengthen the muscles that help support the back and legs, sit in a chair and press the buttocks together. Hold for five seconds, relax, and repeat. Work up gradually to 20 repetitions a day.

B. Lie in bed and bend each knee to the chest, then pull both knees to the chest and hold for six seconds. Repeat, gradually increasing to 10 repetitions.

C. Lie on the back. While counting to five, move the feet and legs in the air as if riding a bicycle. Relax and repeat, gradually increasing to 10 repetitions a day.

D. To stretch the hips, lie on the stomach in bed or on a padded floor. Raise one leg and foot off the bed or floor, keeping the knee straight. Hold for five seconds. Repeat, working up to 10 repetitions. Repeat with the other leg.

For more exercises, see Sobel and Klein, 1995.

5. *Hula or Tai Chi* can increase flexibility, increase circulation, and reduce pain. Dancing is also helpful (Perlman et al., 1990; Van Deusen & Harlowe, 1987).

6. *Strength-building exercises* may help.

A. Sit, stand, or lie down. With the right hand close to the right armpit and palm facing front, slowly move the hand away from the chest and extend it straight out, leading with the heel of the hand. Breathe normally, keeping the fingers relaxed, and push as if pushing the air away from the body. Repeat 7 times. Repeat 7 times with the left hand.

B. Lie on the stomach, holding the body up by bending the elbows and keeping a steady but light pressure on the arms. Stay focused and hold this position for several seconds while relaxing the mind. Slowly turn the head to look at the heel of the right foot. While inhaling, picture the air coming in through that foot, traveling up the leg and through the body to the right arm and down the fingers. While exhaling, picture the air flowing back out the arm, down the right leg and out the right toes. Turn the head the other way and repeat, using the left foot, leg, and arm. Repeat both sides for a total of 7 times each. Keep the mind focused on the flow of energy through the body, feeling the circulation increasing and gently flowing (Chang, 1986).

SUPPORT GROUP

Encourage clients to spend time with individuals who make them feel appreciated and loved and stop spending time with people who don't.

COUNSELING

Clients who have been sexually abused as children have a two- to three-fold increased disease risk if they've had multiple abuse episodes (Stein & Barrett-Connor, 2000). Refer clients to a psychiatric/mental health nurse practitioner or psychologist you trust and encourage them to start weekly sessions to help them resolve their feelings. It could be an important factor in preventing arthritis and/or reducing its effects. Other signs for which a referral may be useful are depression or inability to lose weight or stop smoking.

WARM PACKS/SOAKS

1. *Soak a piece of unbleached and undyed flannel cloth in warmed castor oil* and place it on affected joints. Keep it on for 15–20 minutes while lying down and relaxing.

2. *Soak feet in hot epsom-salt water.*

3. *Submerge the affected part in hot water.* Move the joint(s) back and forth. Take two to three baths a day and rest in bed for a short time afterwards (Davis, 1980).

RELAXATION

1. *Self-regulatory techniques, such as progressive muscle relaxation, guided imagery, and meditative breathing can lead to substantial reduction of pain intensity* for patients with juvenile rheumatoid arthritis (Walco, Varni, & Ilowite, 1992), and in adults with rheumatoid arthritis (O'Leary, Shoor, Lorig, & Holman, 1990).

2. *Guided imagery can be used to picture the joints being soothed one by one, from the neck to the toes, by a cool, healing salve or liquid.* Picturing painful joints healthy and relaxed can also work. For an example of a combination of relaxation, guided imagery, and self-hypnosis that can be recorded, see pp. 97–98.

3. *Soak in a warm tub.*

4. *Brush the skin all over with a body brush before taking alternate cold and warm showers.*

5. *Take an afternoon nap* to relax the body

6. *Try acupuncture or acupressure* to relax the body and help it use its own internal healing mechanisms.

7. *Therapeutic touch is also useful.* It has been shown to reduce pain and improve function in osteoarthritis of the knee (Gordon, Merenstein, D'Amico, & Hudgens, 1998).

8. *Provide a relaxation tape* with guided imagery or ask clients to make or purchase one and listen to it morning and evening each day.

GENTLE ACUPRESSURE

Hold the 2nd, 3rd, and 4th fingers of each hand on the inside of the affected knee until pulsation is felt in all three fingers; then move to the bony prominence at the back of the hips, then to the middle of the instep, then to the bottom of the big toe, then to the top of the shoulder where the outside of the neck ends, finishing with the inside edge of the bottom ribs (Dayton, 1994).

WRITING

Writing about stressful experiences can relieve arthritic symptoms (Smith, Stone, Hurewitz, & Kaell, 1999). For best results, ask clients to spend at least 20 minutes on three consecutive days writing about the most stressful events.

HERBS

Some herbs that may help include *feverfew, lemon myrtle, aniseed myrtle, mountain pepper, and wild rosella. White willow bark* is available in capsules and works as well as aspirin, and does not have the digestive and bleeding side effects. Consult an herbologist or health care practitioner with special knowledge of the use of herbs prior to trying these or any herbs. Also, always inform your doctor or health care professional of any herbs or supplements you are taking or thinking about taking.

WALKING AIDS

Investigate the use of crutches, special soles and shoes, splints, and braces (Ravaud, 2002).

EVALUATING TREATMENT GOALS

The effect of holistic nursing treatments were evaluated a month after treatment began by asking the client described above to provide specific examples of observed changes. The client reported the following changes: "Thanks to your help, I haven't had a cigarette in a month, I'm on a vegetarian food plan, and I've lost 10 pounds. Listening to the relaxation tape you made me has helped me sleep better and feel better about myself."

REFERENCES

American Chiropractic Association (n.d.). *Corrective finger exercises.* ACA FORM No. E-4.

Anthony, D. D., Gupta, S., Ahmad, N., Lee, M., Kumar, G. K., & Hasan, M. (1999). Prevention of collagen-induced arthritis in mice by a polyphenolic fraction from green tea. *Proceedings of the National Academy of Sciences, 96,* 4524–4529.

Baker, R. R., Nelson, M. E., Felson, D. T., Layne, J. E., Sarno, R., & Roubenoff, R. (2001). The efficacy of home based progressive strength training in older adults with knee osteoarthritis: A randomized controlled trial. *Journal of Rheumatology, 28,* 1655–1665.

Bell, K. M., Plon, L., Bunney, W. E. Jr., & Potkin, S. G. (1988). S-adenosyl-methionine treatment of depression: A controlled clinical trial. *American Journal of Psychiatry, 145,* 1110–1114.

Chang, S. T. (1986). *The complete system of self-healing internal exercises.* San Francisco: Tao.

Cheng, Y., Macera, C. A., Davis, D. R., Ainsworth, B. E., Troped, P. J., & Blair, S. N. (2000). Physical activity and self-reported, physician-diagnosed osteoarthritis: Is physical activity a risk factor? *Journal of Clinical Epidemiology, 53,* 315–322.

Curtis, C. L., Rees, S. G., Cramp, J., Flannery, C. R., Hughes C. E., Little, C. B., et al. (2002). Effects of n-3 fatty acids on cartilage metabolism. *Proceedings of the Nutrition Society, 61,* 281–289.

Darlington, L. G., & Stone, T. W. (2001). Antioxidants and fatty acids in the amelioration of rheumatoid arthritis and related disorders. *British Journal of Nutrition, 85,* 251–269.

Davis, B. (1980). *Rapid healing foods.* West Nyack, NY: Parker.

Dayton, B. R. (1994). *An introduction to a gentle acupressure for caregivers.* Friday Harbor, WA: High Touch Network.

Domijan, Z., Vrhovac, B., & Dumgi, T. (1989). A double-blind trial of adernetionine vs. Naproxen in activated gonarthritis. *International Journal of Clinical Pharmacology and Toxicology, 27,* 329–333.

Fang, Y. Z., Yang, S., & Wu, G. (2002). Free radicals, antioxidants, and nutrition. *Nutrition, 18,* 872–879.

Flynn, M. A., Irvin, W., & Krause, G. (1994). The effect of folate and cobalamin on osteoarthritic hands. *Journal of the American College of Nutrition, 13,* 351–356.

Frisco, S., Jacques, P. F., Wilson, P. W., Rosenberg, I. H., & Selhub, J. (2001). Low circulating vitamin B(6) is associated with elevation of the inflammation marker C-reactive protein independently of plasma homocysteine levels. *Circulation, 103*(23), 2788–2791.

Garfinkle, M. S., Schumacher, H. R., Husain, A., Levy, M., & Reshetar, R. A. (1994). Evaluation of a Yoga based regimen for treatment of osteoarthritis of the hands. *Journal of Rheumatology, 21,* 2341–2343.

Gordon, A., Merenstein, J. H., D'Amico, F., & Hudgens, D. (1998). The effects of therapeutic touch on patients with osteoarthritis of the knee. *Journal of Family Practice, 47(4),* 271–277.

Grant, W. B. (2000). The role of meat in the expression of rheumatoid arthritis. *British Journal of Nutrition, 84,* 589–595.

Griner, T., & Nunes, M. (1996). *What's really wrong with you? A revolutionary look at how muscles affect health.* Garden City Park, NY: Avery.

Hafstrom, I., Ringertz, B., Spangberg, A., von Zweigbergk, L., Brannemark, S., Nylander, I., et al. (2001). A vegan diet free of gluten improves the signs and symptoms of rheumatoid arthritis: The effects of arthritis correlate with a reduction in antibodies to food antigens. *Rheumatology, 40,* 1175–1179.

Hanninen, K. K., Rauma, A. L., Nenonen, M., Torronen, R., Hakkinen, A. S., Adlercreutz, H., et al. (2000). Antioxidants in vegan diet and rheumatic disorders. *Toxicology, 155*(1–3), 45–53.

Hansen, G. V., Nielsen, L., Kluger, E., Thysen, M., Emmertsen, H., Stengaard-Pedersen, K., et al. (1996). Nutritional status of Danish rheumatoid arthritis patients and effects of a diet adjusted in energy intake, fishmeal, and antioxidants. *Scandinavian Journal of Rheumatology, 25,* 325–330.

Haslam, R. (2001). A comparison of acupuncture with advice and exercises on the symptomatic treatment of osteoarthritis of the hip—a randomised controlled trial. *Acupuncture Medicine, 19*(1), 19–26.

Helgeland, M., Svendsen, E., Forre, O., & Haugen, M. (2000). Dietary intake and serum concentrations of antioxidants in children with juvenile arthritis. *Clinical Experiments in Rheumatology, 18,* 637–641.

Helmy, M., Shohayeb, M., Helmy, M. H., & el-Bassiouni, E. A. (2001). Antioxidants as adjuvant therapy in rheumatoid disease. *Arzneimittelforschung, 5*(4), 293–298.

Kjeldsen-Kragh, J. (1999). Rheumatoid arthritis treated with vegetarian diets. *American Journal of Clinical Nutrition, 70*(3 Suppl.), 594S–600S.

Knekt, P., Heliovaara, M., Aho, K., Alfthan, G., Marniemi, J., & Aromaa, A. (2000). Serum selenium, serum alpha-tocopherol, and the risk of rheumatoid arthritis. *Epidemiology, 11,* 402–405.

Konig, B. (1987). A long-term (two years) clinical trial with S-adenosylmethionine for the treatment of osteoarthritis. *American Journal of Medicine, 83*(SA), 89–94.

Kremer, J. M., & Bigaouette, J. (1996). Nutrient intake of patients with rheumatoid arthritis is deficient in pyridoxine, zinc, copper and magnesium. *Journal of Rheumatology, 23,* 990–994.

Lapane, K. L., Spooner, J. J., & Mucha, L. (2001). Effect of steroidal anti-inflammatory drug use on the rate of gastrointestinal hospitalizations among people living in long-term care. *Journal of the American Geriatric Society, 49,* 577–584.

Leventhal, L. J., Boyce, E. G., & Zurier, R. B. (1994). Treatment of rheumatoid arthritis with gammalinolenic acid. *Annals of Internal Medicine, 119,* 867–873.

Liu, S., Manson, J. E., Buring, J. E., Stampfer, M. J., Willett, W. C., & Ridker, P. M. (2002). Relation between a diet with a high glycemic load and plasma concentrations of high-sensitivity C-reactive protein in middle-aged women. *American Journal of Clinical Nutrition, 75,* 492–498.

Lystbaek, B. B., Svendsen, L. B., & Hesler, L. (1995). Paracetamol poisoning. *Nordic Medicine, 110,* 156–159.

Manicourt, D., & Druetz-Van Egeren, A. (1994). Effects of tenoxicam and aspirin on the metabolism of proteoglycans and hyaluronan in normal and osteoarthritic human and articular cartilage. *British Journal of Pharmacology, 113,* 1113–1120.

McAlindon, T. E., Felson, D. T., Zhang, Y., Hanna, M. T., Aliabadi, P., Weissman, B., Rush, D., Wilson, P. W., & Jacques, P. (1996). Relation of dietary intake and serum levels of vitamin D to progression of osteoarthritis of the knee among participants in the Framingham Study. *Annals of Internal Medicine, 125*(1), 353–359.

McDougall, J., Bruce, B., Spiller, G., Westerdahl, J., & McDougall, M. (2002). Effects of a low fat, vegan diet in subjects with rheumatoid arthritis. *Journal of Alternative and Complementary Medicine, 8*(1), 71–75.

Muller, H., de Toledo, F. W., & Resch, K. L. (2001). Fasting followed by vegetarian diet in patients with rheumatoid arthritis: A systematic review. *Scandinavian Journal of Rheumatology, 30*(1), 1–10.

Muller-Fassbender, H. (1987). Double-blind clinical trial of S-adenosylmethionine versus ibuprofen in the treatment of osteoarthritis. *American Journal of Medicine, 83*(5A), 81–83.

Muller-Fassbender, H., Bach, G. L., Haase, W., Rovati, L. C., & Setnikar, I. (1994). Glucosamine sulfate compared to ibuprofen in osteoarthritis of the knee. *Osteoarthritis Cartilage, 2*(1), 61–69.

Murray, M. T. (1996). *Encyclopedia of nutritional supplements.* Roseville, CA: Primar.

Muscara, M., McKnifhet, W., & Asfaha, S. (2000). Wound collagen deposition in rats: Effects of an NO-NSAID and a selective COX-2 inhibitor. *British Journal of Pharmacology, 129*(4), 81–83.

Nagaraj, R. H., Kern, T. S., Sell, D. R., Fogarty, J., Engerman, R. L., & Monnier, V. N. (1996). Evidence of a glycemic threshold for the formation of pentosidine in diabetic dog lens but not in collagen. *Diabetes, 45,* 587–594.

Noreau, L., Martineau, H., Roy, L., & Belzile, M. (1995). Effects of a modified dance-based exercise on cardiorespiratory fitness, psychological state and health status of persons with rheumatoid arthritis. *American Journal of Physical Medicine and Rehabilitation, 74*(1), 19–27.

O'Bryne, D. J., Devaraj, S., Grundy, S. M., & Jialal, I. (2002). Comparison of the antioxidant effects of Concord grape juice flavonoids alpha-tocopherol n markers of oxidative stress in healthy adults. *American Journal of Clinical Nutrition, 76,* 1367–1374.

O'Leary, A., Shoor, S., Lorig, K., & Holman, H. R. (1990). A cognitive-behavioral treatment for rheumatoid arthritis. *Health Psychology, 7,* 527–544.

Parcell, S. (2002). Sulfur in human nutrition and applications in medicine. *Alternative Medicine Review, 7*(1), 22–44.

Pavelka, K., Gatterova, J., & Olejarova, M. (2002). Glucosamine sulfate use and delay of progression of knee osteoarthritis: A 3-year, randomized, placebo-controlled, double-blind study. *Archives of Internal Medicine, 162,* 2113–2123.

Perlman, S. G., Connell, K. J., Clark, A., Robinson, M. S., Conlon, P., Gecht, M., Caldron, P., & Sinacore, J. M. (1990). Dance-based aerobic exercise for rheumatoid arthritis. *Arthritis Care Research, 3*(1), 29–35.

Ravaud, P. (2002). Non-drug treatments for osteoarthritis. *Presse Med, 31*(39, Pt. 2), 4S10–4S12.

Rennie, K. L., Hughes, J., Lang, R., & Jebb, S. A. (2003). Nutritional management of rheumatoid arthritis: A review of the evidence. *Journal of Human Nutrition and Diet, 16,* 97–109.

Schanberg, L. E., Sandstrom, M. J., Starr, K., Gil, K. M., Lefebvre, C., Keefe, F. J., et al. (2000). The relationship of daily mood and stressful events to symptoms in juvenile rheumatic disease. *Arthritis Care Research, 13*(1), 33–41.

Shapiro, J. A., Koepsell, T. D., Voigt, L. F., Dugowson, C. E., Kestin, M., & Nelson, J. (1996). Diet and rheumatoid arthritis in women: A possible protective effect of fish consumption. *Epidemiology, 7,* 256–263.

Smith, J. M., Stone, A. A., Hurewitz, A., & Kaell, A. (1999). Effects of writing about stressful experiences on symptom reduction in patients with asthma or rheumatoid arthritis. *Journal of the American Medical Association, 281,* 1328–1330.

Sobel, D., & Klein, A. C. (1995). *Arthritis: What exercises work.* New York: St. Martin's Press.

Stein, M. B., & Barrett-Connor, E. (2000). Sexual assault and physical health: Findings from a population-based study of older adults. *Psychosomatic Medicine, 62,* 838–843.

Vahora, S. A., & Malek-Ahmadi, P. (1988). S-adenosylmethionine in the treatment of depression. *Neuroscience and Biobehavioral Review, 12,* 139–141.

Van Deusen, J., & Harlowe, D. (1987). The efficacy of the ROM Dance Program for adults with rheumatoid arthritis. *American Journal of Occupational Therapy, 41*(2), 90–95.

Walco, G. A., Varni, J. W., & Ilowite, N. T. (1992). Cognitive-behavioral pain management in children with juvenile rheumatoid arthritis. *Pediatrics, 89*(6, pt. 1), 1075–1079.

Walker, A. F., Bundy, R., Hicks, S. M., & Middleton, R. W. (2002). Bromelain reduces mild acute knee pain and improves well-being in a dose-dependent fashion in an open study of otherwise healthy adults. *Phytomedicine, 9,* 681–686.

Williams, D. G. (1998). An international breakthrough in the treatment of arthritis. *Alternatives, 7*(17), 129–133.

Zautra, A. J., Hoffman, J., Potter, P., Matt, K. S., Yocum, D., & Castro, L. (1997). Examination of changes in interpersonal stress as a factor in disease exacerbations among women with rheumatoid arthritis. *Annals of Behavioral Medicine, 19,* 279–286.

CHAPTER 6

Cancer

There are numerous types of cancer, all of which have multiple causes. Basic medical treatments for cancer include radiation, chemotherapy, and surgery. All have their risks and uses.

HOLISTIC NURSING ASSESSMENT

the holistic nursing assessment below was completed by a nurse after she interviewed Mrs. T., a 35-year-old woman, who was dying from lung cancer. Use the following format when working with clients diagnosed with cancer to help you decide what treatments may be most beneficial for each unique client with whom you work.

Client learning needs: "I don't have any control over this."

Indicants of readiness to learn: "I'm going to die, aren't I?"

Soul/spirituality symbol(s): "I brought my collection of angels with me to the hospital. They will protect me."

Meaning of the condition to client: "Death would be a relief after all this pain."

Relationship needs/effects as perceived by client: "How will my husband get along without me?"

Patterns/attitudes that may create dis-ease for this client: Client uses negative affirmations, including, "I'll always be in pain," and "I'm afraid of dying." Client is overweight and was left at an orphanage at birth by her mother, a young teenager.

Life purpose: Client states, "I just want this suffering to be over. I'm so stressed out." Facial expression and body language indicate hopelessness.

Client strengths: Client trusts nurse enough to confide.

Ability to participate in care: Client complains of pain continually, but is able to choose whether she wants therapeutic touch or relaxation therapy.

Ethical dilemmas: Deciding whether to discuss self-fulfilling prophecies with the physician, who keeps telling the client she only has a month to live.

Nurse–client process: Client is clingy and dependent, constantly asking for reassurance.

TREATMENT PLANNING: SETTING JOINTLY AGREED-UPON GOALS

Goals that were jointly agreed upon for the client discussed above include:

1. Use affirmations to change negative expectations.
2. Ask for pain measures as needed.
3. Write a letter to her birth mother sharing feelings.

Acceptance of condition/attitude change: From the following affirmations, the client chose one to use to replace the resentment she feels for having been abandoned by her birth mother: "I lovingly release the past. It has no hold over me. I choose to fill my world with joy and peace." Client agreed to say the affirmation at least 20 times a day.

Facilitating the healing process/healing intention formulation: From a list of meditative statements, client chose the following one to assist in the healing process. "I deserve loving attention." Client will repeat the meditative statement while in a relaxed state before arising and before retiring. Nurse will use centering and caring nonverbal communication to enhance client healing.

Creating a sacred space: Client asked her husband to bring in her favorite CDs and a silk robe to wear that makes her feel pampered and special. Directed the nurse on how to display her angel collection near her bed and back light it so she could see them at all hours of the day and night.

Integrative practices planned: Client has asked her adoptive parents and brothers and sisters to gather at her bedside for a reenactment of their lives together.

Role model strategies: Facilitated family gathering and helped each person voice his or her statements of caring for the client.

Protection plan: Suggested client picture angels at her door and inside her room to assist in peaceful sleep and recuperation.

Family strategies: Each day client dictates portions of the letter she would like to send to her birth mother.

Life issues/life purpose work: Client is beginning to discuss the many acts of kindness she has offered to others in her journey through life.

Treatment possibilities/considerations: For clients dealing with cancer, work in collaboration with them to cho0se holistic approaches that will work for them.

ADDITIONAL INFORMATION AND TREATMENTS TO SHARE WITH CLIENTS

ACTIONS CLIENTS CAN TAKE PRIOR TO SURGERY

1. *Take milk thistle between meals for a week before and two weeks after surgery.* Many drugs can damage the liver. This herb will support healthy liver function (Ladas & Kelly, 2003).

2. *Eat plenty of foods that are high in fiber to enhance good bowel function, including plenty of whole grains, fresh fruits, and vegetables* (Li et al., 2003).

3. *Take vitamin A,* 15,000 IU (not beta-carotene) for several weeks before surgery and 50,000 IU the two days before surgery, unless pregnant, in which case don't take more than 15,000 IU a day (McKay & Miller, 2003).

4. *Take vitamin E* 400 IU, and an extra 1,000 to 2,000 mg of vitamin C, but stop at the point of diarrhea (McKay & Miller, 2003),

5. *Take 200 mcg of selenium* (Berger et al., 1996).

6. *Take 15 mg extra of zinc* (Berger et al., 1996).

7. *Drink lots of green tea.* Green tea helps speed wound healing.

8. *Take glutamine* (500 mg twice a day) between meals for a week before surgery and two weeks after surgery. It can speed up healing, help detoxify the liver and kidneys, and keep the digestive system healthy (Mindell & Hopkins, 1998).

FOR WOMEN

1. *Encourage breast feeding* in mothers to lower their risk for breast cancer (Newcomb et al., 1999).

2. *Avoid wearing push-up bras and never wear a bra for more than 12 hours a day.* Not wearing a bra gives the lymph system every chance to filter out toxins. Clients who complain of red marks or indentations near the bra line should be encouraged to get a larger bra that does not constrict breast tissues or feel tight and to omit wearing a bra when at home or whenever possible (Singer & Grismaijer, 1995).

3. *Use breast massage.* See p. 97—the Deer—for directions (For Women and Men: Exercise).

4. *Avoid taking estrogen after menopause;* it increases risk of breast cancer, and the longer estrogen is taken, the greater the risk (Ross, Paganini-Hill, Wan, & Pike, 2000).

5. *Avoid taking oral contraceptives.* They increase the risk of early-onset breast cancer before the age of 45.

6. *Avoid red and/or processed meats, sweets, french fries, and refined grains.* Women who had the highest intake of these items had a 1.46 relative risk for developing colon cancer, compared to women who followed a prudent eating plan of more fruits, vegetables, legumes, fish, poultry, and whole grains, and who had an inverse relationship to colon cancer (Fung et al., 2003).

7. *Eat lots of vegetables and fruits and take a stress vitamin* (vitamins B and C). Taking high levels of vitamin C and beta carotene decreased the risk of death in women due to breast cancer, especially those who ate a high fat diet (Bagga, Capone, & Wang, 1997; Freudenheim, Marshall, & Vena, 1996).

8. *Eat foods high in folate and vitamin B6.* Circulating levels of folate and vitamin B6 may reduce the risk of developing breast cancer (Zhang et al., 2003). Food sources of these B vitamins include sunflower seeds, toasted wheat germ, brown rice, soybeans, chicken, salmon, tuna, bananas, walnuts, peanuts, sweet and white potatoes, cooked cabbage, asparagus, orange juice, black-eyed peas, lima beans, watermelon, oysters, and cantaloupe.

9. *Use only olive oil on salads and for cooking.* A high consumption of olive oil was significantly related to a lower risk of breast cancer, whereas eating saturated fats (meat and dairy products, fried foods, and products with cottonseed oil in them) prior to developing cancer is highly correlated with dying from the disease (Bagga et al., 1997; Trichopoulou et al., 1995).

10. *Avoid polyunsaturated fats (fried foods, salad oils that aren't olive oil), and white wine.* Both are associated with breast density, a significant risk factor for breast cancer (Hayes et al., 1999).

11. *Eat plenty of omega-3 fatty acids, found in fish and fish oil.* They can protect against breast cancer (Rose, 1997).

12. *Eat more soy products and fiber.* Both are associated with a reduction in risk for endometrial cancer (Goodman et al., 1997).

13. *Obtain sufficient vitamin D* (through food, supplements, or sunshine). This vitamin's metabolites may reduce breast cancer risk (Garland, Garland, & Gorham, 1999).

14. *Reduce exposure to magnetic fields.* Avoid living or working close to power lines, or near radio, TV, and microwave transmitters (e.g., cellular phone towers), or radar units; restrict close exposure to computer screens (unless laptops), television sets, and microwave ovens; and avoid using electric blankets. In a study of 1.1 million women, those who were exposed to a potential magnetic field had an increased risk of breast cancer (Milham, 1996), as did female flight attendants (Rafnsson, Tulinius, Jonasson, & Hrafnkelsson, 2001).

15. *Take coenzyme Q10.* In one study, women with breast cancer had lower levels of this enzyme. The researchers theorized that malignant cells may consume more coenzyme Q10, so taking this supplement may protect breast tissue (Portakal et al., 2000).

16. *Avoid gaining weight, especially after menopause.* Losing unneeded weight can contribute to the prevention of breast cancer (Chiu et al., 1996; Lee et al., 1997.)

17. *Remain physically active.* It helps in losing weight and is also linked with a 30% risk reduction in breast cancer in postmenopausal women (Friedenreich, Bryant, & Courneya, 2001), and a 30–50% reduction in younger women (Bernstein, Henderson, Hanisch, Sullivan-Halley, & Ross, 1994).

18. *Use reverse osmosis-filtered drinking water.* Chlorination by-products are linked with cancer incidence among postmenopausal women (Doyle et al., 1997).

19. *Avoid powdering the genital area.* Women who do use powder have an increased risk for ovarian cancer (Cramer et al., 1999). Using corn starch may be okay (Whysner & Mohan, 2000).

20. *Seek psychotherapy if sexually abused.* One study found that past sexual assault was associated with an increased risk for breast cancer (Stein & Barrett-Connor, 2000). Find a mental health nurse practitioner or psychologist with experience in these matters.

21. *Avoid exposure to pesticides.* They increase the risk of breast cancer (Mathur, Bhatnagar, Sharma, Acharya, & Sexana, 2002;

Moysich et al., 1998). Instead, use boric acid, diatomaceous earth, sprays made of citrus oils, garlic, alcohol, or soapy water, and use natural pest control such as praying mantises.

22. *If you must color your hair, use only one method.* Women with exclusive use of just one method of hair coloring application (rinses, dyes, bleaching, or frosting) are less likely to develop breast cancer than are women who use more than one method (Cook, Malone, Daling, Voigt, & Weiss, 1999).

23. *Avoid drinking wine.* The risk of breast cancer was highest (by 2.5 times increased risk) among women who reported drinking wine on a weekly or daily basis, especially beginning on or before the age of 40 (Lenz, Goldberg, Labreche, Parent, & Valois, 2002).

FOR MEN

1. *Eat fish and/or take fish oil capsules.* Numerous epidemiological studies and at least one prospective study (Aronson et al., 2001) show omega-3 fatty acids in fish oil prevent the development and progression of prostate cancer.

2. *Investigate herbs that can enhance prostate health:* saw palmetto, pygeum, stinging nettle, zinc alanine, glycine, and glutamic acid. Before taking saw palmetto, have a PSA test, which examines the antibodies that accompany prostate cancer, but be aware that this test overdiagnoses prostate cancer. In one study (Etzioni et al., 2002) between 29% and 44% of men were overdiagnosed and may have received surgery or radiation treatment for prostate cancer that would never have progressed to threaten their health. Explore the use of Silymarin (milk thistle). It acts as an antiproliferative agent and has potential in prostate cancer treatment (Zi et al., 2000).

3. *Eat more tomatoes.* The lycopene in tomatoes has a potentially protective effect (Norrish et al., 2000; Willis & Wians, 2003).

4. *Eat more citrus fruit.* Citrus and citrus oils may protect against prostate cancer (Pienta, Naik, & Alchtar, 1995).

5. *Drink more water.* Dehydration is one of the greatest stresses on the prostate.

6. *Eat foods that contain zinc or take zinc picolinate daily.* Zinc regulates testosterone levels in the prostate and may prevent cancer of the prostate, whereas surgery or radiation may not. Environmental exposure to lead may be a risk factor for prostate cancer because it reduces the level of zinc, which acts as a cellular growth protector (Siddiqui, Srivastava, & Mehrotra, 2002). To decrease this risk, stay away from lead in gasoline (or pumping it), paints, joints in food

cans, drinking water that comes through lead pipes, eating canned tomatoes in quantity, foods containing phytate that interfere with zinc absorption (dried beans, whole grains, and peanut butter), fried potatoes, fast foods, imitation meats, rich desserts, and alcohol. Foods high in zinc include oysters, herring, liver, eggs, nuts, wheat germ, and red meats.

7. *Eat more soy and soy products.* Soy contains an antioxidant isoflavone called genistein that may help fight prostate cancer (Nagata, 2000).

8. *Eat more legumes* (peanuts, chickpeas, black beans, kidney beans, lentils, mung beans, navy beans, peas, pinto beans, soybeans, split peas), yellow-orange vegetables, and cruciferous vegetables (broccoli, kale, cauliflower, Brussels sprouts). They can help nourish and protect you.

9. *Eat less fat.* High fat intake increases risk of prostate cancer (Veierod, Laake, & Thelle, 1997).

10. *Eat fewer dairy products.* Consuming large amounts of calcium in dairy products may put men at higher risk for prostate cancer. Skim milk was the dairy food found to be most strongly related to risk (Chan et al., 2001).

11. *Eat fruits and nuts.* Men who consumed the most boron, an element found in nuts and fruits, had a 64% lower risk of prostate cancer. One serving of peanuts or almonds and 3.5 servings of fruits put men in the low risk group (Cui, Winton, Zhang, Rainey, et al., 2004). Grapes are also protective, as is grape seed extract (Tyagi, Agarwal, & Agarwal, 2003).

12. *Avoid consuming alcoholic beverages, especially beer.* Consumption of alcoholic beverages increases the risk of colorectal cancer and the evidence most strongly implicates beer (Sharpe, Siemiatycki, & Rachet, 2002).

13. *Take a selenium supplement.* Selenium has a positive effect in reducing the incidence or preventing the occurrence of prostate cancer (Willis & Wians, 2003). Because American soils have been depleted of this nutrient, the only way to obtain it is to take a supplement. **Caution:** be sure not to exceed the recommended dosage on the bottle.

14. *Take a vitamin E supplement and eat foods high in the substance.* Vitamin E has been shown to reduce the incidence of prostate cancer (Willis & Wians, 2003). Food sources include wheat germ, peanuts, outer leaf of cabbage, leafy portions of broccoli and cauliflower, raw spinach, asparagus, whole grain rice or oats, cold pressed wheat germ or safflower oil, cornmeal, eggs and sweet potatoes (Clark, 1996).

NUTRITIONAL APPROACHES FOR MEN AND WOMEN

1. *Lose weight if overweight and limit consumption of refined carbo-hydrates* (breads, pastas, sugary foods, and candies). Eat less fat, especially saturated fat (animal food products, especially pork, red meat, and processed meats). Low-fat diets reduce estrogen production for women and testosterone production for men: these are the sex hormones that can stimulate tumor production. Toxic chemicals also collect in the fatty tissues in the body, so even if a tumor is not sex hormone-related or stimulated, losing weight and eating low fat is a good plan.

2. *Fight free radicals, enhance the immune system, and even prevent disease* (Kris-Etherton et al., 2002) by eating more fresh or frozen fruits, vegetables, seeds (sunflower, pumpkin), fish, poultry, potatoes, green tea, olive oil, peanuts and other legumes (baked or boiled beans), berries (Roy et al., 2002), grapes (Katsuzaki et al., 2003), seeds (especially flaxseed), papaya (Rimbach et al., 2000), bell and black peppers (El Hamss, Idaomar, Alonso-Moraga, & Munoz, 2003), and onions (Irion, 1999).

A. *Eat soy foods daily,* such as four ounces of tofu or an eight-ounce glass of soy milk. Soy contains genistein, which prevents malignant angiogenesis, the development of blood vessels that promote cancer growth. Genistein may also encourages normal cell growth in some types of cancer cells. Soy and increased fiber consumption can also reduce the risk of endometrial cancer (Goodman et al., 1997) and ovarian and breast cancer (Lu, Anderson, Grady, & Nagamani, 2001). Soybeans and peanuts have also decreased prostate, colon, breast, oral, pharyngeal, pancreatic, and stomach cancers.

B. *Choose fish (it contains omega-3 fatty acids that suppress the growth of tumor cells) over meat every time.* Red meat, particulary processed meat or beef, is associated with prostate cancer, as well as breast cancer (Kushi & Giovannucci, 2002). Meat is also linked with colorectal cancer, adenocarcinoma, and ovarian and endometrial cancer. Even when eating fish, eat a moderate amount, about the size of the palm of the hand, per meal. Too much protein stresses kidneys and liver.

C. *Avoid sugar.* Adding sugar to coffee or tea and drinking nondiet carbonated soft drinks was associated with intestinal cancers (Wu, Yu, & Mack, 1997). Sugar is also associated with biliary tract cancer and colon cancer risk (Slattery, Edwards, Boucher, Anderson, & Caan, 1999). Eating highly processed foods, especially those containing a lot of sugar, is associated with breast cancer.

D. *Eat more garlic and onions.* Garlic produces various seleno amino acids that are potentially bioactive, organic, selenium-containing phytochemicals (Irion, 1999). Garlic may protect against bladder and prostate cancer (Riggs, DeHaven, & Lamm, 1997), stomach cancer, and aflatoxin-induced toxicity (Abdel-Wahhab & Aly, 2003). If garlic is offensive or upsets the stomach, take Kyolic non-odor capsules available at health food stores. Both garlic and onions contain organo-sulfur compounds that have anticarcinogenic actions (Kris-Etherton et al., 2002).

E. *Eat foods containing lycopene.* They can reduce the incidence of cancer of the breast, cervix, colon, esophagus, mouth, pancreas, and rectum (Barnes, Sfakianos, Coward, & Kirk, 1996). These foods include tomatoes, watermelon, guava, apricots, and pink grapefruit. Even ketchup and tomato paste will help. Lutein, a carotenoid found in dark, leafy greens and broccoli, also protects against colon cancer.

F. *Use only olive oil.* Switch from corn and safflower oil (they help mammary tumors grow) and take a fish oil supplement or eat a lot of fish to protect against breast cancer. Another oil that protects is sesame oil. A study demonstrated that it decreased risk of stomach cancer (Yo, 1997).

G. *Get a juicer.* Vegetable juices are more easily digested than whole vegetables and can help cleanse the body of the toxicities of chemotherapy or radiation. Vegetables can also protect against proliferation of cancer cells. In a study, spinach showed the highest inhibitory effect, followed by cabbage, red pepper, onion, and broccoli (Chu, Sun, Wu, & Liu, 2002). Use carrot juice as a base. Be sure to wash the vegetables and cut the tops and ends off the carrots first. Carrot juice contains vitamins A, B, C, D, E, G, and K. It helps promote appetite and is an aid to digestion and healing. Add 1–2 ounces of raw spinach to the carrot juice to cleanse and regenerate body tissues. Drink 4–6 glasses of water-diluted carrot or carrot and spinach juice a day. Carrot, beet, and cucumber juice is a combination especially helpful for reducing fever and helping detoxify the body. Alternate the carrot juice drinks with nutritional fruit drinks. For example, make a smoothie in a blender. Combine plain yogurt with active acidophilus cultures, banana, pineapple juice, and cherries (frozen or fresh, preferably organically grown). Try a green drink several times a week: fill half a blender with fresh spinach, kale, and/or endive; add a cup of fresh parsley; fill the blender to the top with pineapple juice and add 1–2 teaspoons of cider vinegar; blend and chew each mouthful carefully.

H. *Avoid fried foods.* Use low-fat cooking methods such as steaming, broiling, or baking.

I. *Eat fresh pineapple or get bromelain tablets* at the health food store. Bromelain can decrease metastasis of cancer cells, enhance the absorption of drugs, reduce inflammation, and reduce healing time, including that necessary for surgical wounds (Batkin, Taussig, & Szekerezes, 1998; "Bromelain," 1998; Taussig & Batkin, 1998).

J. *Eat more citrus fruits and cherries.* These foods have monoterpenes that have anticarcinogenic actions (Kris-Etherton et al., 2002).

3. *Eat yogurt with active cultures or take acidophilus;* both exhibit anti-tumor qualities by stimulating the immune system (Montalto et al., 2002).

4. *Drink tea.* A growing body of evidence suggests that moderate consumption of tea may protect against several forms of cancer. Green tea is good. Kombucha tea may also increase life span and has potent anti-oxidant and immunopotentiating activities (Sai et al., 2000) and is available at health food stores.

5. *Sprinkle a little turmeric on food.* This spice has strong anticarcinogenic effects for the skin, stomach, colon, small intestine, breast, and tongue (Ren & Lien, 1997).

6. *Take a daily multivitamin to get enough folic acid every day.* According to Harvard's long-running Nurses Health Study, folic acid reduces the risk of colon cancer and birth defects. Most cases of colon cancer can be prevented by taking 1800 mg of calcium and 800 IU of vitamin D regularly (Garland et al., 1999).

7. *Eat foods high in vitamin A.* Retinoids and carotenoids have been shown to prevent tumors in the head, neck, and lung (Hinds, West, & Knight, 1997; Lotan, 1997). Foods high in vitamin A include carrots (cooked or as juice), broccoli, kale, turnip greens, watercress, beets, dandelion greens, spinach, eggs, papayas, parsley, red peppers, fish liver oils, sweet potatoes, pumpkin, yellow squash, apricots, and cantaloupes (Clark, 1996).

8. *Eat seaweed.* The seaweeds wakame, hiziki, and kombu have been shown to prevent the absorption and reabsorption of toxic agents (Morita & Nakano, 2002).

9. *Eat rice bran products.* Phytonutrients from rice bran have shown promising disease-preventing and health-related benefits (Jariwalla, 2001).

10. *Take vitamin C supplements.* After exposure to many toxic chemicals, including chemotherapy and radiation, natural killer (NK) immune protective function can be decreased significantly. Vitamin C in high oral dose (granulated buffered vitamin C in water at a dosage of 60 mg/Kg body weight) was capable of enhancing NK activity up to tenfold in 78% of patients tested (Heuser & Vojdani, 1997).

11. *Take an L-arginine supplement.* This semi-essential amino acid is involved in ammonia detoxification, hormone secretion, and immune modulation (Appleton, 2002) and has been shown to increase protein synthesis and growth cells (Brittenden et al., 1994). The supplement can also potentiate chemotherapy (Heys et al., 1998).

HERBS

Investigate the use of natural agents that have been shown to defend against tumor cells including marshmallow (the herb, not the candy!), licorice (again, not the candy!), panax ginseng, psyllium seed, aloe vera gel, dang gui, astragalus, dan shen, pishen fang, shen xue tang, milk thistle, Echinacea purpurea (Boik, 1997), witch hazel bark, rosemary, jasmine tea, sage, slippery elm, black walnut leaf, Queen Anne's lace, and linden flower (Choi, Choi, Han, Bae, & Chung, 2002; Nagasawa, Watanabe, Yoshida, & Inatomi, 2001).

ESSENTIAL OIL

Chamomile essential oil has been shown to be an effective antimutagen (Hernandez-Ceruelos, Madrigal-Bujaidar, & de la Cruz, 2002).

ALOE

Freeze-dried aloe whole leaf powder was shown in an animal study to prevent pancreatic neoplasms (Furukawa et al., 2002).

ENVIRONMENTAL ACTIONS

1. *Limit radiation exposure* as much as possible and find alternative measures to all X-rays, mammograms, frequent air travel, electromagnetic exposure (home appliances, television screens,

office equipment, and outside electric power lines, including using cellular phones or being within one meter of a cellular phone in the on position). Radiation is associated with an increased risk for cancer.

2. *Limit exposure to environmental carcinogens: estrogens from plastics (containers, plastic wrap, etc.), herbicides, and pesticides.* Use wax paper or glass containers, and natural insect repellents such as soapy water/garlic and vegetable oil (on plants to ward off insects), boric acid (either mixed with honey into a syrup and placed in ant hills, or as a powder to eliminate roaches), citronella or catnip oil (to ward off mosquitoes). Pesticides increase risk for genetic and fetal damage, soft tissue sarcomas, non-Hodgkin's lymphoma, breast cancer, and Hodgkin's disease (A. S. Hoar et al., 1990; S. K. Hoar et al., 1986; Mathur et al., 2002; Morrison et al., 1992).

3. *Stop using permanent or semi-permanent hair dyes.* Use of permanent hair dyes is also correlated with bladder cancer (Gago-Dominguez, Castelao, Yuan, Yu, & Ross, 2001) and Hodgkins lymphoma (Holly, Lele, & Bracci, 1998). Use henna, or natural coloring such as chamomile (for blonde hair). Use highlighting mousses (available at health food stores), and natural coloring agents such as black tea. Check out other natural products to color the hair or keep natural coloring.

4. *Avoid drinking alcohol.* Alcohol from liquor and white wine is correlated with an increase in basal cell carcinoma of the skin for both women and men. Alcohol increases the risk of death from cancer of the liver and breast (Singer, 2002).

5. *Drink only water that has been filtered by reverse osmosis or has been distilled.* Exposure to chlorination by-products in drinking water is associated with increased risk of colon cancer (Doyle et al., 1997) and bladder cancer (Vena, 1993).

6. *Avoid smoking and smoky places.* Both are correlated with lung cancer and some other cancers. And think twice before using nicotine patches, sprays, or gum to quit smoking. Stanford University researchers have found that nicotine impairs the growth of new blood vessels and dramatically increases the number of times cells divide. The researchers found that when mice with certain types of human cancers were given nicotine, the tumors grew (Natori, Sate, Washida, Hirata, et al., 2003). Instead of using nicotine as a quit-smoking aid, use behavioral methods such as hypnosis or affirmations.

EXERCISE

1. *Exercise daily* to exert a protective effect on the immune system and enhance body functioning and mood. It may even reduce the risk of endometrial, colon, and breast cancer (Batty & Thune, 2000; Friedenreich et al., 2001; Frisch et al., 1985; Lee et al., 1997; Martinez et al., 1997). Exercise also increases circulation (bringing nutrition to cells and moving waste products out), and reduces stress, fatigue, anxiety, anger, fear, and depression.

2. *Set a regular time of day to exercise and stick to it.* Start each session with stretching exercises to ready the body by using an exercise book or videotape at an appropriate level of proficiency, start walking a short distance, then build up gradually until walking 20 or 30 minutes a day, and slow down when unable to talk with comfort while walking. Stop and consult an exercise specialist at the first sign of pain and be sure to report symptoms to primary health care providers. Always wear walking sneakers and use good posture. Jogging and running put stress on the joints and may not be the right forms of exercise. If necessary, consult a fitness coach to find the right exercise.

3. *Practice internal exercises.* These simple movements can both treat dis-ease and prevent it by energizing the internal organs and the immune system and aiding in hormonal balance (Chang, 1986). Complete the exercises on arising and prior to retiring each day.

A. *The Crane:* Lie on a mat on the floor or on a bed. Place the hands, palms down, on the lower abdomen. Keep the mouth closed and inhale easily through the nostrils, exhaling slowly while pressing the hands down lightly on the abdomen. Slowly inhale and extend the abdomen outward like a balloon, keeping the chest still. Work up to 12 rounds of inhaling and exhaling.

B. *The Turtle:* Sit or stand and bring the chin down onto the chest while stretching the top of the head upward and slowly inhaling. Let the shoulders relax downward. Slowly exhale while slowly bringing the back of the skull down as if to touch the back of the neck. Let the chin be pulled upward and the throat stretch slightly while the shoulders are pulled up toward the ears. Repeat up to 12 times, moving in a relaxed and thoughtful way, keeping the mind focused on the movements and keeping the fingers clasped around the thumbs and the eyes gently closed.

C. *The Deer for Women:* While sitting, rub the hands together vigorously and place them on the breasts, focusing on the sensation of heat. Rub the breasts slowly in outward circular motions, so the right hand makes a counter-clockwise circle and the left hand makes a clockwise circle 36 times.

D. *The Deer for Men:* Sit or stand and alternately squeeze, hold, and then relax the anus as if trying to stop the stream of urine through anal muscle contraction. (Chang, 1986).

REDUCE STRESS

Stress encourages free radicals to form. This leads to a weakened immune system and increases the risk for at least one form of cancer (Fackelmann & Raloff, 1993).

1. *Write about feelings.* Get in touch with submerged anger and feelings of joy. Pennebaker (1989; Pennebaker, Kiecolt-Glaser, & Glaser, 1988) demonstrated the healing power of expressing emotions by writing about them and how this expression can enhance the immune system. Purchase a blank journal and write about traumatic events or upsetting issues. Put in all the details of what happened, and all thoughts and feelings.

2. *Discuss thoughts and feelings about cancer* with nurse or someone else client trusts.

3. *Use touch therapies.* Touch therapy (TT) has been shown to decrease anxiety and stress (Gagne & Toye, 1994) and TT and massage therapy have been shown to significantly enhance comfort scores for clients receiving bone marrow transplant (Smith, Reeder, Daniel, Baramee, & Hagman, 2003).

4. *Use a relaxation tape.* Use the relaxation script that follows or adapt it. A combination of progressive muscle relaxation training and guided imagery training can significantly reduce depression and enhance quality of life (Sloman, 2002).

SAMPLE RELAXATION SCRIPT

Directions: Speak slowly in a calm, monotone voice to enhance the positive effects. I am letting my body sink into the comfort and safety of this bed (chair, floor, etc.), feeling the sensations of the bed (chair, floor, etc.) against my body, breathing in comfort and relaxation, beginning to let go, to relax, to let my breathing move slowly and without effort to my center, my abdominal area, where I feel calm and serene . . . I breathe in relaxation and comfort as a sooth-ing color and breathe out whatever it's time to let go of as another color (pause up to 2 minutes) . . . Each time I inhale, I am 100 times more relaxed and comfortable than I was. It is so easy and effortless to be relaxed and comfortable . . . calm . . . serene . . . peaceful . . . (pause 1–2 minutes) . . . I am breathing in relaxation and comfort and breathing out whatever it is time to let go of . . . (pause 1–2 minutes) . . . I am scanning my body now, looking for any areas that need more relaxation and comfort, and the next time I take a breath, I will send a wave of relaxation to that area . . . (pause for 3 minutes) . . . I will continue to breathe in relaxation and comfort as a color and breathe out whatever it is time to let go of as a color until I am com-pletely relaxed . . . knowing I am safe and relaxed, drifting or sinking, whatever feels right for me . . . When I am ready, I will picture myself very small, small enough to go inside my ear or nose or some other way, taking a fantastic journey through the tissues of my body, maybe turning on a tiny flashlight so I can see very clearly what is going on in my tissues . . . picturing all the tissues healthy, pink, and functioning perfectly . . . continuing to breathe in relaxation and healing as a color . . . Sending relaxation, healing and health to my entire body . . . (pause up to 4 minutes) . . . I am ready to come back through time and space now and return to the here and now, bring-ing with me everything I learned and all the healing and health-gen-erating knowledge I've accumulated . . . knowing that I can return to this state of comfort, relaxation, and healing anytime I want to, sim-ply by breathing in relaxation and comfort as a color and breathing out whatever it is time to let go of as another color . . . In just a minute, this tape will end and I will either open my eyes and feel energized and healthy, ready to go about my day's activities, or I will continue to rest and fall into a peaceful sleep, whichever is right for me at this moment . . . I will listen to this tape many times a day until I have put into action all the healing capabilities of my mind and body and have advanced to a higher level of being.

ACUPRESSURE

To enhance the life force, gently touch the inside of the right knee with the right hand and the inside of the left knee with the left hand, paying attention to the pulsations in the fingers. When pulse is felt in the 2nd, 3rd, and 4th fingers, hold the middle of the instep on each foot (Dayton, 1994). To prevent tension build-up, knead shoul-der muscle to open blocked meridians, massage the arms, and prac-tice the turtle and crane. (See p. 96 for directions.)

AFFIRMATIONS

Write one or more affirmations on 3 x 5 cards and carry or post in important places in home or office. "I am healing with each breath I take." "It's getting easier and easier to be healthy and free." "Nothing can harm me." "I am safe and secure." "It is okay to feel anger; I can use my anger in a constructive way."

TREATMENT EVALUATION

1. Client reported using only positive affirmations for the past week.
2. Client asked for therapeutic touch, listened to her relaxation tape, and hasn't had any pain medication for three days.
3. Client has started a letter to her birth mother, sharing feelings.

REFERENCES

Abdel-Wahhab, M. A., & Aly, S. E. (2003). Antioxidants and radical scavenging properties of vegetable extracts in rats fed aflatoxin-contaminated diet. *Journal of Agriculture and Food Chemistry, 51,* 2409–2414.

Appleton, J. (2002). Arginine: Clinical potential of a semi-essential amino. *Alternative Medicine Review, 7,* 512–522.

Aronson, W. J., Glaspy, J. A., Reddy, S. T., Reese, D., Heber, D., & Bagga, D. (2001). Modulation of omega-3/omega-6 polyunsaturated ratios with dietary fish oils in men with prostate cancer. *Urology, 58,* 283–288.

Bagga, D., Capone, S. & Wang, H. (1997). Dietary modulation of Omega-3/Omega-6 poly-unsaturated fatty acid ratios in patients with breast cancer. *Journal of the National Cancer Institute, 89,* 1123–1131.

Barnes, S., Sfakianos, J., Coward, L., & Kirk, M. (1996). Soy isoflavonoids and cancer prevention: Underlying biochemical and pharmacological issues. *Advanced Experimental and Medical Biology, 401,* 87–100.

Batkin, S., Taussig, S. J., & Szekerezes, J. (1998). Antimetastatic effect of bromelain with or without its proteolytic and anticoagulant activity. *Journal of Cancer Research and Clinical Oncology, 114,* 507–508.

Batty, D., & Thune, I. (2000). Does physical activity prevent cancer? Evidence suggest protection against colon cancer and probably breast cancer. *British Medical Journal, 321,* 1424.

Berger, M. M., Cavadini, C., Chiolero, R., & Dirren, H. (1996). Copper, selenium and zinc status and balances after major trauma. *Journal of Trauma, 40,* 103–109.

Bernstein, L., Henderson, B. E., Hanisch, R., Sullivan-Halley, J., & Ross, R. K. (1994). Physical exercise and reduced risk of breast cancer in young women. *Journal of the National Cancer Institute, 86,* 1403–1408.

Boik, J. (1997). *Cancer & natural medicine: A textbook of basic science and clinical research.* Princeton, MN: Oregon Medical Press.

Brittenden, J., Heys, S. D., Miller, I., Sarkar, T. K., Hutcheon, A. W., Needham, G., et al. 1994). Dietary supplementation with L-arginine in patients with breast cancer receiving multimodality treatment: Report of a feasibility study. *British Journal of Cancer, 69,* 918–921.

Bromelain. (1998) *Alternative Medicine Review, 3,* 302–305.

Chan, J. M., & Giovannucci, E. L. (2001). Dairy products, calcium, and vitamin D and risk of prostate cancer. *Epidemiology Review, 23*(1), 87–92.

Chang, S. T. (1986). *The complete system of self-healing.* San Francisco: Tao.

Chiu, B. C.-H., Cerhan, J. R., & Folson, A. R. (1996). Diet and risk of non-Hodgkin's lymphoma in older women. *Journal of the American Medical Association, 275,* 1315–1321.

Choi, H. R., Choi, J. S., Han, Y. N., Bae, S. J., & Chung, H. Y. (2002). Peroxynitrite scavenging activity of herb extracts. *Phytotherapy Research, 16,* 364–367.

Chu, Y. F., Sun, J., Wu, X., & Liu, R. H. (2002). Antioxidant and antiproliferative activities of common vegetables. *Journal of Agriculture and Food Chemistry, 50,* 6910–6916.

Clark, C. C. (1996). *Wellness practitioner: Concepts, research, and strategies.* New York: Springer Publishing Co.

Cook, L. S., Malone, K. E., Daling, J. R., Voigt, L. F., & Weiss, N. S. (1999). Hair product use and the risk of breast cancer in young women. *Cancer Causes and Control, 10,* 551–559.

Cramer, D. W, Liberman, R., Titus-Ernstoff, L., Welch, W. R., Greenberg, E. R., Baron, J. A., & Harlow, B. L. (1999). Genital talc exposure and risk of ovarian cancer. *International Journal of Cancer, 81,* 351–356.

Cui, Y., Winton, M. I., Zhang, Z. F., Rainey, C., Marshall, J., De Kernion, J. B., et al. (2004). Dietary boron intake and prostate cancer risk. *Oncology Reports, 11,* 887–892.

Dayton, B. R. (1994). *An introduction to a gentle acupressure for caregivers.* Friday Harbor, WA: High Touch Network.

Doyle, T. J., Zheng, W., Cerhan, J. R., Hong, C. P., Sellers, T. A., Kushi, L. H., & Folsom, A. R. (1997). The association of drinking water source and chlorination by-products with cancer incidence among postmenopausal women in Iowa: A prospective cohort study. *American Journal of Public Health, 87,* 1168–1176.

El Hamss, R., Idaomar, M., Alonso-Moraga, A., & Munoz, S. A. (2003). Antimutagenic properties of bell and black peppers. *Food Chemistry and Toxicology, 41*(1), 41–47.

Etzioni, R., Penson, D. F., Legler, J. M., diTommaso, D., Boer, R., Gann, P. H., et al. (2002). Overdiagnosis due to prostate-specific antigen screening: Lessons from U.S. prostate cancer incidence trends. *Journal of the National Cancer Institute, 94,* 981–990.

Fackelmann, K. A., & Raloff, J. (1993). Psychological stress linked to cancer. *ScienceNews, 144,* 23–29.

Freudenheim, J. L., Marshall, J. R., & Vena, J. E. (1996). Premenopausal breast cancer risk and intake of vegetables, fruits and related nutrients. *Journal of the National Cancer Institute, 88,* 340–348.

Friedenreich, C. M., Bryant, H. E., & Courneya, K. S. (2001). Case-control study of lifetime physical activity and breast cancer risk. *American Journal of Epidemiology, 154,* 336–347.

Frisch, R. E., Wyshak, G., Albright, N. L., Albright, T. E., Schiff, I., Jones, K. P., et al. (1985). Lower prevalence of breast cancer and cancers of the reproductive system among former college athletes compared to non-athletes. *British Journal of Cancer, 52,* 885–891.

Fung, T., Hu, F. B., Fuchs, C., Giovannucci, E., Hunter, D. J., Stampfer, M. J., & Colditz, G. H. (2003). Major dietary patterns and the risk of colorectal cancer in women. *Archives of Internal Medicine, 163,* 309–314.

Furukawa, F., Nishikawa, A., Chihara, T., Shimpo, K., Beppu, H., Kuzuya, H., et al. (2002). Chemopreventive effects of Aloe arborescens on N-nitrosobis (2-oxopropyl) amine-induced pancreatic carcinogenesis in hamsters. *Cancer Letter, 178,* 117–122.

Gagne, D., & Toye, R. C. (1994). The effects of therapeutic touch and relaxation therapy in reducing anxiety. *Archives of Psychiatric Nursing, 8,* 184–189.

Gago-Dominguez, M., Castelao, J. E., Yuan, J. M., Yu, M. C., & Ross, R. K. (2001). Use of permanent hair dyes and bladder cancer risk. *International Journal of Cancer, 91,* 575–579.

Garland, C. F., Garland, F. C., & Gorham, E. D. (1999). Calcium and vitamin D: Their potential roles in colon and breast cancer prevention. *Annals of the New York Academy of Science, 889,* 107–119.

Goodman, M. T., Wilkens, L. R., Hankin, J. H., Lyu, L. C., Wu, A. H., & Kolonel, L. N. (1997). Association of soy and fiber consumption with the risk of endometrial cancer. *American Journal of Epidemiology, 146*(4), 294–306.

Hayes, R. B., Ziegler, R. G., & Gridley, G. (1999). Dietary factors and risks for prostate cancer among blacks and whites in the United States. *Cancer Epidemiology Biomarkers for Prevention, 8*(1), 25–34.

Hernandez-Ceruelos, A., Madrigal-Bujaidar, E., & de la Cruz, C. (2002). Inhibitory effect of chamomile essential oil on the sister chromatid exchange induced by daunorubicin and methyl methanesulfonate in mouse bone marrow. *Toxicology Letter, 135*(1–2), 103–110.

Heuser, G., & Vojdani, A. (1997). Enhancement of natural killer cell activity and T and B cell function by buffered vitamin C in patients exposed to toxic chemicals: The role of protein kinase-C. *Immunopharmacology and Immunotoxicology, 19,* 291–312.

Heys, S. D., Ogston, K., Miller, I., Hutcheon, A. W., Walker, L. G., Sarker, T. K., et al. (1998). Potentiation of the response to chemotherapy in patients with breast cancer by dietary supplementation with L-arginine: Results of a randomised controlled trial. *International Journal of Oncology, 12*(1), 221–225.

Hinds, T. S., West, W. L., & Knight, E. M. (1997). Carotenoids and retinoids: A review of research, clinical, and public health applications. *Journal of Clinical Pharmacology, 37,* 551–558.

Hoar, A. S., Weisenburger, D. D., Babbitt, P. A., Saal, R. C., Vaught, J. B., Cantor, K. P., & Blair A. (1990). A case-control study of non-Hodgkin's lymphoma and the herbicide 2,4-dichloro phenoxyacetic acid (2,4-D) in East Nebraska. *Epidemiology, 1,* 349–356.

Hoar, S. K., Blair A., Holmes, F. F., Boysen, C. D., Robel, R. J., Hoover, R., & Fraumeni, J. F. (1986). Agricultural herbicide use and risk of lymphoma and soft-tissue sarcoma. *Journal of the American Medical Association, 256,* 1141–1147.

Holly, E. A., Lele, C., & Bracci, P. M. (1998). Hair-color products and risk for non-Hodgkin's lymphoma: Population-based study in the San Francisco Bay area. *American Journal of Public Health, 88,* 1767–1773.

Irion, C. W. (1999). Growing alliums and brassicase in selenium-enriched soils increases their anticarcinogenic potentials. *Medical Hypotheses, 53,* 232–235.

Jariwalla, R. J. (2001). Rice-bran products: Phytonutrients with potential applications in preventive and clinical medicine. *Drugs in Experimental and Clinical Research, 27*(1), 17–26.

Katsuzaki, H., Hibasami, H., Ohwaki, S., Ishikawa, K., Imai, K., Date, K., et al. (2003). Cyanidin 3-0-beta-D-glucoside isolated from skin of black Gycine max and other anthocyanins isolated from skin of red grape induce apoptosis in human lymphoid leukemia Molt 4B cells. *Oncology Reports, 10,* 297–300.

Kris-Etherton, P. M., Hecker, K. D., Bonanome, A., Coval, S. M., Binkoski, A. E., Hilpert, K. F., et al. (2002). Bioactive compounds in foods: Their role in the prevention of cardiovascular disease and cancer. *American Journal of Medicine, 113*(Suppl. 9B), 71S–88S.

Kushi, L., & Giovannucci, E. (2002). Dietary fat and cancer. *American Journal of Medicine, 113*(Suppl. 9B), 63S–70S.

Ladas, E. J., & Kelly, K. M. (2003). Milk thistle: Is there a role for its use as an adjunct therapy in patients with cancer? *Journal of Alternative & Complementary Medicine, 9,* 411–416.

Lenz, S. K., Goldberg, M. S., Labreche, F., Parent, M. E., & Valois, M. F. (2002). Association between alcohol consumption and postmenopausal breast cancer: Results of a case-control study in Montreal, Quebec, Canada. *Cancer Causes and Control, 13,* 701–710.

Li, J., Kaneko, T., Qin, L. Q., Wang, J., & Wang, Y. (2003). Effects of barley intake on glucose tolerance, lipid metabolism, and bowel function in women. *Nutrition, 19,* 926–929.

Lotan, R. (1997). Roles of retinoids and their nuclear receptors in the development and prevention of upper aerodigestive tract cancers. *Environmental Health Perspectives, 105*(Suppl. 4), 985–988.

Lu, L. J., Anderson, K. E., Grady, J. J., & Nagamani, M. (2001). Effects of an isoflavone-free soy diet on ovarian hormones in premenopausal women. *Journal of Clinical Endocrinology and Metabolism, 86,* 3045–3052.

MacKay, D., & Miller, A. L. (2003). Nutritional support for wound healing. *Alternative Medicine Review, 8,* 359–377.

Martinez, M. E., Giovannucci, E., Spiegelman, D., Hunter, D. J., Willett, W. C., & Colditz, G. A. (1997). Leisure-time physical activity, body size, and colon cancer in women: Nurses' Health Study Research Group. *Journal of the National Cancer Institute, 89,* 948–955.

Mathur, V., Bhatnagar, P., Sharma, R. G., Acharya, V., & Sexana, R. (2002). Breast cancer incidence and exposure to pesticides among women orginating from Jaipur. *Environment International, 28,* 331–336.

Milham, S. Jr. (1996). Increased incidence of cancer in a cohort of office workers exposed to strong magnetic fields. *American Journal of Industrial Medicine, 30,* 702–704.

Mindell, E., & Hopkins, V. (1998). *Prescription alternatives.* New Canaan, CT: Keats.

Montalto, M., Arancio, F., Izzi, D., Cuoco, L., Curigliano, V., Manna, R., & Gasbarrini, G. (2002). Probiotics: History, definition, requirements and possible therapeutic applications. *Annals of Italian Internal Medicine, 17,* 157–165.

Morita, K., & Nakano, T. (2002). Seaweed accelerates the excretion of dioxin stored in rats. *Fukuoka Institute of Health and Environmental Sciences, 50,* 910–917.

Morrison, H. I., Wilkins, K., Semenciw, R., Mao, Y., & Wigle, D. (1992). Herbicides and cancer. *Journal of the National Cancer Institute, 84,* 1866–1871.

Moysich, K. B., Ambrosone, C. B., Vena, J. E., Shields, P. G., Mendola, P., Kostyniak, P., et al. (1998). Environmental organochlorine exposure and postmenopausal breast cancer risk. *Cancer Epidemiological Biomarkers and Prevention, 7,* 181–188.

Nagasawa, H., Watanabe, K., Yoshida, M., & Inatomi, H. (2001). Effects of gold banded lily (Lilium auratum Lindl) or Chinese milk etch (Astragalus sinicus L) on spontaneous mammary tumourigenesis in SHN mice. *Anticancer Research, 21,* 2328–2338.

Nagata, C. (2000). Ecological study of the association between soy product intake and mortality from cancer and heart disease in Japan. *International Journal of Epidemiology, 29,* 832–836.

Narrish, A. E., Jackson, R. T., Sharpe, S. J., & Skeaff, C. M. (2000). Men who consume vegetable oils rich in monounsaturated fat: Their dietary patterns and risk of prostate cancer. *Cancer Causes and Control, 11,* 609–615.

Natori, T., Sata, M., Washida, M., Hinata, Y., Nagai, R., & Makunchi, M. (2003). Nicotine enhances neovascularization and promotes tumor growth. *Molecules and Cells, 16,* 143–146.

Newcomb, P. A., Egan, K. M., Titus-Ernstoff, L., Trentham-Dietz, A.,

Greenberg, E. R., Baron, J. A., et al. (1999). Lactation in relation to post-menopausal breast cancer. *American Journal of Epidemiology, 150,* 174–182.

Pennebaker, J. W. (1989). Confession, inhibition, and disease. In L. Berkowitz (Ed.), *Advances in experimental social psychology, Volume 22* (pp. 211–133). New York: Academic Press.

Pennebaker, J. W., Kiecolt-Glaser, J. K., & Glaser R. (1988). Disclosure of traumas and immune function: Health implications for psychotherapy. *Journal of Clinical and Consulting Psychology, 63,* 787–792.

Pienta, K. J., Naik, H., & Alchtar, A. (1995). Inhibition of spontaneous metastasis in rat prostate cancer model by oral administration of modified citrus pectin. *Journal of the National Cancer Institute, 87,* 348–353.

Portakal, O., Ozkaya, O., Erden, I. M., Bozan, B., Kosan, M., & Sayek, L. (2000). Coenzyme Q10 concentrations and antioxidant status in tissues of breast cancer patients. *Clinical Biochemistry, 33,* 279–284.

Rafnsson, V., Tulinius, H., Jonasson, J. G., & Hrafnkelsson, J. (2001). Risk of breast cancer in female flight attendants: A population-based study. *Cancer Causes and Control, 12,* 95–101.

Ren, S., & Lien, E. J. (1997). Natural products and derivatives as cancer chemopreventive agents. In E. Jucker (Ed.), *Progress in drug research, Volume 48* (pp. 147–170). Basel, Switzerland: Birkhauser Verlag.

Riggs, D. R., DeHaven, I., & Lamm, D. L. (1997). Allium Sativum (garlic) treatment for murine traditional cell carcinomas. *Cancer, 79,* 1987–1994.

Rimbach, G., Park, Y. C., Guo, W., Moini, H., Qureshi, N., Saliou C., et al. (2000). Nitric oxide synthesis and TNF-alpha secretion in RAW 264,7 Macrophages: Mode of action of a fermented papaya preparation. *Life Sciences, 67,* 679–694.

Rose, D. P. (1997). Dietary fat, fatty acids and breast cancer. *Breast Cancer, 4*(1), 7–16.

Ross, R. K., Paganini-Hill, A., Wan, P. C, & Pike, M. C. (2000). Effect of hormone replacement therapy on breast cancer risk: Estrogen versus estrogen plus progestin. *Journal of the National Cancer Institute, 92,* 328–332.

Roy, S., Khanna, S., Alessio, H. M., Vider, J., Bagchi, D., Bagchi, M., & Sen, C. K. (2002). Anti-angiogenic property of edible berries. *Free Radical Research, 36,* 1023–1031.

Sai, R. M., Anju, B., Pauline, T., Dipti, P., Kain, A. K., Mongia, S. S., et al. (2000). Effect of kombucha tea on chromate (VI)-induced oxidative stress in albino rats. *Journal of Ethnopharmacology, 71*(1–2), 235–240.

Sharpe, C. R., Siemiatycki, J., & Rachet, B. (2002). Effects of alcohol consumption on the risk of colorectal cancer among men by anatomical subsite (Canada). *Cancer Causes and Control, 13*(5), 483–491.

Siddiqui, M. K., Srivastava, S., & Mehrotra, P. K. (2002). Environmental exposure to lead as a risk for prostate cancer. *Biomedical and Environmental Sciences, 15,* 298–305.

Singer, M. V. (2002). Effect of ethanol and alcoholic beverages on the gastrointestinal tract in humans. *Romanian Journal of Gastroenterology, 11,* 197-204.

Singer, S. R., & Grismaijer, S. (1995). *Dressed to kill: The link between breast cancer and bras.* Garden City Park, NY: Avery.

Slattery, M. L., Edwards, S. L., Boucher, K. M., Anderson, K., & Caan, B. J. (1999). Lifestyle and colon cancer: An assessment of factors associated with risk. *American Journal of Epidemiology, 150,* 869–877.

Sloman, R. (2002). Relaxation and imagery for anxiety and depression control in community patients with advanced cancer. *Cancer Nursing, 25,* 432–435.

Smith, M. C., Reeder, F., Daniel, L., Baramee, J., & Hagman, J. (2003). Outcomes of touch therapies during bone marrow transplant. *Alternative Therapies in Health and Medicine, 9*(1), 40–49.

Stein, M. B., & Barett-Connor, E. (2000). Sexual assault and physical health: Findings from a population-based study of older adults. *Psychosomatic Medicine, 62,* 838–843.

Taussig, S. J., & Batkin, S. (1998). Bromelain, the enzyme complex of pineapple (Ananas comosus) and its clinical application: An update. *Journal of Ethnopharmacology, 22,* 191–203.

Trichopoulou, A., Katsouyanni, K., Stuver, S., Tzala, L., Gnardellis, C., Rimm, E., et al. (1995). Consumption of olive oil and specific food groups in relation to breast cancer risk in Greece. *Journal of the National Cancer Institute, 87,* 110–116.

Tyagi, A., Agarwal, R., & Agarwal, C. (2003). Grape seed extract inhibits EGF-induced and constitutively active mitogenic signaling but activates JNK in human prostate carcinoma DU145 cells: Possible role in antiproliferation and apoptosis. *Oncogene, 22,* 1302–1316.

Veierod, M. B., Laake, P., & Thelle, D. S. (1997). Dietary fat intake and risk of prostate cancer: A prospective study of 25,708 Norwegian men. *International Journal of Cancer, 73,* 634–638.

Vena, J. E. (1993). Bladder cancer and chlorinated tap water. *Archives of Environmental Health, 48,* 191.

Whysner, J., & Mohan, M. (2000). Perineal application of talc and cornstarch powders: Evaluation of ovarian cancer risk. *American Journal of Obstetrics and Gynecology, 182,* 720–724.

Willis, M. S., & Wians, F. H. (2003). The role of nutrition in preventing prostate cancer: A review of the proposed mechanism of action of various dietary substances. *Clinica Chimica Acta, 330*(1–2), 57–83.

Wu, A. H., Yu, M. C., & Mack, T. M. (1997). Smoking, alcohol use, dietary factors, and risk of small intestinal adenocarcinoma. *International Journal of Cancer, 70,* 512–517.

Yo, A. (1997). Diet and stomach cancer in Korea. *International Journal of Cancer, 10*(Suppl. 10), 7–9.

Zhang, S. M., Wilett, W. C., Selhub, J., Hunter, D. J., Giovannucci, E. L.,

Holmes, M. D., et al. (2003). Plasma folate, vitamin B6, vitamin B12, homocysteine, and risk of breast cancer. *Journal of the National Cancer Institute, 95,* 373–380.

Zheng, T., Holford, T. R., Mayne, S. T., Owens, P. H., Ward, B., Carter, D., Dubrow, R., et al. (1999). Beta-benzene hexachloride in breast adipose tissue and risk of breast carcinoma. *Cancer, 85,* 2212–2218.

Zheng, T., Holford, T. R., Mayne, S. T., Tessari, J., Ward, B., Carter, D., et al. (2000). Risk of female breast cancer associated with serum polychlorinated biphenyls and 1,1-dichloro-2,2'-bis(p-chlorophenyl)ethylene. *Cancer Epidemiological Markers and Prevention, 2,* 167–174.

Zheng, W., Kushi, L. H., Potter, J. D., Sellers, T. A., Doyle, T. J., Bostick, R. M., et al. (1995). Dietary intake of energy and animal foods and endometrial cancer incidence: The Iowa women's health study. *American Journal of Epidemiology, 142,* 388–394.

Zi, S., Zhang, J., Agarwal, R., & Pollak, M. (2000). Silibinin up-regulates insulin-like growth factor-binding protein 3 expression and inhibits proliferation and androgen-independent prostate cancer cells. *Cancer Research, 60,* 5617–5620.

CHAPTER 7

Carpal Tunnel Syndrome

Carpal tunnel syndrome (CTS) is the leading occupational hazard of the computer age. The condition results when repetitive action compresses or damages the median nerve in the wrist. The medical treatment for CTS is to discontinue any tasks that require forceful flexing of the wrist. A cock-up split is used to help relieve night pain and take pressure off the nerve. Local corticosteroid injections may give temporary relief. The doctor will recommend surgery if symptoms continue. The operation includes decompressing the median nerve at the wrist.

HOLISTIC NURSING ASSESSMENT

Study the holistic nursing assessment for Mrs. T., a 56-year-old client diagnosed with carpal tunnel syndrome, that follows. Working in collaboration with your clients with CTS, adapt it as necessary.

Client learning needs: "I've only been working at a computer for a few months, but I suppose I should have expected something like this."

Indicants of readiness to learn: "There must be something you can do to help the pain."

Soul/spirituality symbol(s): "I pray to the Virgin Mary. She helps me."

Meaning of the condition to client: "I don't know why I got this. Stella has been on the computer for years and she doesn't have it."

Relationship needs/effects as perceived by the client: "My husband left me for his secretary. Do you believe it? I worked for years to put him through medical school and now he leaves me."

Patterns/attitudes that may create dis-ease for this client: Client uses negative affirmations (e.g., "This is so frustrating," and "My wrists keep burning and burning").

Life purpose: Client indicates no life purpose except to get better and see her ex-husband "burn in hell for what he's done."

Client strengths: Able to verbalize feelings and is willing to discuss a plan of care.

Ability to participate in care: Client has periods of pain, but expresses interest in learning and changing mental and work patterns.

Ethical dilemmas: None yet identified.

Nurse–client process: The client talks in an angry tone to the nurse, but apologizes, "It's not your fault."

TREATMENT PLANNING: SETTING JOINTLY AGREED-UPON GOALS

In the case of the client discussed above, the following goals were agreed upon:

1. Reduce pain level.
2. Reduce angry feelings toward ex-husband.
3. Plan for a healthier work environment.
4. Enhance healing.

TREATMENT

Acceptance of condition/attitude change: The client chose the following affirmation to use to replace the frustration she feels: "I now choose to be joyous and free." Client agreed to write or say the affirmation at least 20 times each day.

Facilitating the healing process/healing intention formulation: From a list of meditative statements, client chose the following one to assist in the healing process: "I am flexible and at ease." Nurse asked client to meditate on the words while in a relaxed state. Nurse will use caring nonverbal communication, centering, and a meditative state to enhance client healing, will verbalize observed patterns that may be holding the client back and offer alternate approaches.

Creating a sacred space: Client requested that her arms and hands be rubbed with warm scented massage oil. Agreed to use sage to cleanse the energy of the working space.

Encouraging re-storying: Client states she doesn't know how to tell stories, but agreed to write in a journal about her relationship with her husband and how she feels about what he did.

Integrative practices planned: Client stated she wanted to learn specific exercises that might help with the pain in her wrists. She is developing a script to be used to develop a guided imagery and relaxation tape.

Role model strategies: Nurse showed client several exercises to use to reduce pain.

Protection plan: Client agreed to picture the Virgin Mary beside her, protecting her.

Family strategies: Client started writing a letter to her ex-husband. Plans to have a burning ritual of their marriage license.

Life issues/life purpose Work: Client has purchased a journal and has started to write about forgiveness.

Treatment possibilities/considerations: Client is considering surgery for her wrists, but is afraid it might not help. Other suggested treatments appear below. Most are evidence-based.

ADDITIONAL INFORMATION AND TREATMENTS FOR CLIENTS

NUTRITION

1. *Increase intake of B-vitamins.* Several studies have shown an association between vitamin B6 deficiency and carpal tunnel syndrome (Feuerstein et al., 1999; Frisco, Jacques, Wilson, Rosenberg, & Selhub, 2001; Shizukuishi, Nishii, & Folkers, 1981). Foods rich in B-vitamins are sunflower seeds, whole wheat flour, rolled oats, green peas, soybeans, lima beans, crab meat, brown rice, asparagus, raisins, wheat germ, chicken, hazelnuts, peanuts, hickory nuts, spinach, kale, peas, salmon, prunes, lentils, tuna, turkey, rabbit, white beans, mackerel, bananas, walnuts, sweet potatoes, cooked cabbage,

sardines, trout, herring, sea vegetables (kombu, dulse, kelp, wakame) fermented soy products (tempeh, natto, miso), turnips, cantaloupe, buckwheat, lobster, broccoli, and cauliflower.

2. *Eat more foods high in vitamin C.* This vitamin is important in healing (Goode, Burns, & Walker, 1992). Foods to concentrate on are green peppers, honeydew melon, Brussels sprouts, strawberries, papaya, watercress, raspberries, parsley, raw cabbage, blackberries, onions, sprouts, and tomatoes.

3. *Magnesium for healing.* This mineral works with calcium to ensure good muscle movement (Clark, 1996). For more of this essential substance, eat figs, green leafy vegetables, citrus fruits, whole grain breads and cereal, brown rice, wheat germ, and soy flour.

4. *Try essential fatty acids.* These essential structural components of every cell's membrane regulate the function of membrane-bound enzymes, and control the electrolyte, energy, and water balance of the cell. They also mediate eicosanoids; an increased formation of these compounds correlates with inflammation (Adam, 1995). Increase intake of fish (mackerel, salmon, herring, whitefish, and tuna), walnuts, Brazil nuts, sunflower and pumpkin seeds, oil (canola, olive and flaxseed), and green leafy vegetables.

5. *Vitamin A is important to healing.* It is a potent antioxidant that has been shown to protect against and prevent many chronic illnesses (Fang, Yang, & Wu, 2002). Foods high in vitamin A include carrots, broccoli, kale, turnip greens, watercress, beets, dandelion greens, spinach, eggs, papaya, parsley, red peppers, pumpkin, yellow squash, apricots, and cantaloupes (Clark, 1996).

6. *Zinc enhances healing.* Zinc deficiency has been associated with delayed wound healing (Andrews & Gallagher-Allred, 1999) and may play a role in neurogenic inflammation (Scholzen, Stander, Riemann, Brzoska, & Luger, 2003). Some foods rich in zinc are pumpkin seeds, whole grains, oysters, herring, liver, eggs, nuts, and wheat germ.

7. *Avoid foods high in oxalic acid because they can promote joint problems.* Eat only raw asparagus, beets, beet greens, rhubarb, spinach, Swiss chard, and cabbage. Cooked, they contain oxalate acid.

8. *Avoid salt and salty foods.* They promote water retention and can aggravate the condition.

9. *Avoid caffeine and smoking.* They both constrict blood vessels.

10. *Eat half a fresh pineapple daily* for one to three weeks. The bromelain in the fresh (not canned) fruit can reduce pain and swelling (Hale, Greer, & Sempowski, 2002). If fresh pineapple is not available, take 250 to 500 milligrams of a bromelain supplement three times a day before meals.

11. *Eat foods that assist nerve function. Lecithin* supplies choline and inositol, both of which are important for nerve function, emulsifying fats, and mood (Westerlund, Ostlund-Lindqvist, Sainsbury, Shertzer, & Sjoquist, 1996). Take lecithin in granular form (1 tablespoon 3 times a day before meals; follow directions on the bottle) or capsules (1,200 mg 3 times a day before meals). It is derived from soybeans. *Grape seed extract* is a powerful anti-inflammatory and antioxidant (Castillo et al., 2000). Follow the directions on the label. *Primrose oil* contains essential fatty acids necessary for nerve function (Yoon, Lee, & Lee, 2002). Follow the directions on the bottle.

ACUPUNCTURE

Laser acupuncture has been shown to reduce carpal tunnel pain, even for failed surgical release cases. Inflammation also decreased (Branco & Naeser, 1999).

HAND BRACE

A hand brace was shown to significantly improve carpal tunnel syndrome symptoms after four weeks (O'Connor, Marshall, & Massy-Westropp, 2003).

YOGA

A randomized, single-blind controlled trial examined the effects of yoga on carpal tunnel syndrome in a geriatric center and at an industrial site. Participants in the yoga groups had significant improvement in grip strength and pain reduction (Garfinkle et al., 1999).

RANGE OF MOTION EXERCISES

Range of motion exercises appeared to be associated with less pain and fewer days to return to work in comparison to splinting (Feuerstein et al., 1999). Some range of motion exercises follow. Choose one or two in collaboration with the client. Directions to share with clients include: Start small and gently. Work up to more repetitions and more exercises. Do these exercises the first thing in the morning, and then hourly during the work day when engaged in repetitive wrist movements. When wearing a wrist splint, remove it to do the exercises, then replace it.

1. Rub palms together gently. Let palms face each other, an inch apart. Feel the energy between them.

2. Stretch arms out in front and gently shake the wrists.

3. Stand with arms outstretched in front and gently flex wrists up and down in each direction for 2 minutes.

4. Rotate wrists in circles for 3 minutes, moving first clockwise and then counterclockwise.

5. Bend elbows, resting hands on shoulders while breathing in. Then, exhaling, stretch arms out in front. Repeat 5 times.

6. Bend elbows out to the sides, resting hands gently on the top of shoulders while breathing in. Exhale and stretch the arms out to the side.

7. Hold both arms up toward the ceiling, letting the fingers stretch upward. Picture ligaments and tissues relaxing and healing.

8. Keeping elbows bent and hands on shoulders, inhale and draw elbows up in front of face and above the head. Exhale, lowering elbows back down in a circular movement.

9. Hold palms together with fingers touching but spread apart slightly. Exhale and press palms and fingers against each other. Inhale and breathe in, relaxing the hands, but keeping them touching. Repeat up to 5 times.

10. Hold the palm of right hand in front of chest in a *stop* motion. Exhale and use left fingers to gently pull right fingers back. Inhale and release fingers. Repeat several times. Repeat with other hand.

11. Massage each finger, starting with the little finger and working across to the thumb. Start at the base of each finger and use thumb and index finger and then pull out the end of each finger.

12. Rest little fingers lightly on a table or desk or on the thighs. Gently lower hands to stretch the fingers. Repeat with each finger.

13. Rub hands together and then gently shake wrists out.

INVESTIGATE HERBS

There are many herbs that could help. Consult with an herb book and/or an expert in the use of herbs before use.

1. *Use turmeric as a spice on all food.* It is very mild, yet packs a wallop because its anti-inflammatory activity is comparable to using steroids. If taking aspirin or nonsteroidal anti-inflammatory drugs (Tylenol, Advil and so on), don't mix them with turmeric.

2. *Aloe vera, devil's claw, yarrow, and yucca* can all restore flexibility and reduce inflammation.

3. *Butcher's broom* can relieve inflammation.

4. *Capsicum* (cayenne pepper) relieves pain and is a catalyst for other herbs.

5. *Parsley is a natural diuretic.* Put fresh parsley in salads, soups, stews, and entrees. Chew it well at the end of a meal and it will provide many vitamins and minerals as well as freshen the breath (Worwood, 1991).

6. *Use gingko biloba,* either as a tea or capsule. It can improve circulation and aid in nerve function.

7. *Marshmallow root* soothes and softens tissues and promotes healing.

8. *Skullcap may relieve muscle spasms and pain.*

PROTECT THE BODY WHILE WORD PROCESSING

1. Use an adjustable chair and place feet flat on the floor.

2. Avoid bending the wrists; angle the arms 90 degrees before extending them on the keyboard.

3. Take a break from typing every thirty minutes; set a timer if necessary. Take a walk and let the eyes relax and move up and down and from side to side, using peripheral vision, and letting the eyes linger on pleasant shapes.

4. Position the screen 18 to 28 inches away from the eyes at a 15 degree angle.

5. Avoid using laptops; they're not designed for prolonged use.

6. Use correct ambient or full-spectrum natural lighting.

7. Blink regularly.

8. Perform eye exercises throughout the day by visually tracing a horizontal figure eight or tracing diagonals from left to right and right to left with the eyes several times from top to bottom.

9. Use a computer shield that reduces glare and EMF emissions (Steinman, 1997).

AFFIRMATIONS

In collaboration with the client, choose one of the affirmations below to help change negative attitudes. Ask client to say or write the phrase 20 times a day and write it on 3 x 5 cards and put them in places where they'll be read often:

- I choose to create a life that is happy and peaceful
- I forgive everyone who has harmed me in any way
- I am calm

ACUPRESSURE

1. Press the point in the middle of inner wrist, $2\frac{1}{2}$ finger-widths above the wrist crease. Apply steady penetrating finger pressure for 2–3 minutes every hour or every other hour.

2. Let thumb slide around the wrist and let it come to rest on the acupoint on the upper side of the wrist in the depression between the tendons. Make several rotations into this point, pressing in the direction of the elbow (Castleman, 2000).

3. Hold the 2nd, 3rd, and 4th fingers of the right hand in the middle of the backside of the hip bone until pulsation is felt in all fingers; do the same with the left hand and left hip bone, then move to holding the bony prominence that runs across the back of the head, ending with the inside edge of the bottom rib (Dayton, 1994).

MASSAGE

In carpal tunnel syndrome, the flexor pollicus longus presses against the median nerve, producing pain in the wrist and hand (Griner & Nunes, 1996). Use the massage technique on p. 43 to release the spasm in the flexor pollicus longus in the wrist and ask the client to do a return demonstration and use the treatment daily.

AROMATHERAPY/MASSAGE

Fill styrofoam or heavy paper cups with water and freeze. Cut the cup down so that the ice is protruding. Massage over sore areas in circular movements. Massage arms and hands for relief. Start at the top of the arms and work down to fingers, being gentle with wrist, hands, and fingers. Work down again, this time with a gentle movement, barely touching the skin. Work down and out the fingertips, going a few inches beyond the end of fingers.

To enhance the effect, mix 10 drops of rosemary, 10 drops of lavender, and 10 drops of peppermint essential oil in 2 tablespoons of vegetable oil and massage the hands and wrists with the mixture.

SMOKING CESSATION

Stop smoking. It constricts your blood vessels and that, in turn, impedes blood flow to your wrists and hands.

WEAR A SPLINT OR GLOVES

Wear a splint during the day or at night. Find them in drugstores and medical supply stores. Make sure the wrist is almost straight and in about the same position as when writing with a pen. Make sure the splint fits properly. Be aware that doing range of motion exercises (see above) can reduce pain more effectively than a splint. If hands are cold, wear cotton gloves to warm them and improve circulation. If gloves get in the way of typing, cut off the fingers.

INCREASE CIRCULATION

To increase circulation, immerse hands and wrists in hot water for 3 minutes, then in cold water for 30 seconds. Repeat 3–5 times once or twice a day.

EVALUATING TREATMENT

The client rated herself at the beginning and end of sessions on a scale of 1 (no pain) to 10 (intense pain). After working on her affirmation and meditation and receiving therapeutic touch, she consistently rated herself a 3 at the end of our sessions. Client has finished writing her letter to her ex-husband, but decided instead of sending it to burn it in a ritual in her back yard. Client has arranged her work environment to reduce repetitive injury to her wrists.

REFERENCES

Adam, O. (1995). Review: Anti-inflammatory diet in rheumatic diseases. *European Journal of Clinical Nutrition, 49,* 703–717.

Andrews, M., & Gallagher-Allred, C. (1999). The role of zinc in wound healing. *Advances in Wound Care, 12,* 137–138.

Branco, K., & Naeser, M. A. (1999). Carpal tunnel syndrome: Clinical outcome after low-level laser acupuncture, microamps transcutaneous electrical nerve stimulation, and other alternative therapies—an open protocol study. *Journal of Alternative and Complementary Medicine, 5*(1), 5–26.

Castillo, J., Benavente-Garcia, O., Lorente, J., Alcarez, M., Redondo, A., Ortuno, A., et al. (2000). Antioxidant and radioprotective effects against chromosomal damage induced in vivo x-rays of flovan-3-ols (Procyanidins) from grape seeds. *Journal of Agricultural and Food Chemistry, 48,* 1738–1745.

Castleman, M. (2000). Carpal tunnel syndrome. *Blended medicine* (pp. 179–183). Emmaus, PA: Rodale, distributed by St. Martin's Press.

Clark, C. C. (1996). *Wellness practitioner.* New York: Springer Publishing Co.

Dayton, B. R. (1994). *An introduction to a gentle acupressure for caregivers.* Friday Harbor, WA: High Touch Network.

Fang, Y. Z., Yang, S., & Wu, G. (2002). Free radicals, antioxidants and nutrition. *Nutrition, 18,* 872–879.

Feuerstein, M., Burrell, L. M., Miller, V. I., Lincoln, A., Huang, G. D., & Berger, R. (1999). Clinical management of carpal tunnel syndrome: A 12-year review of outcomes. *American Journal of Industrial Medicine, 35,* 232–245.

Frisco, S., Jacques, P. F., Wilson, P. W., Rosenberg, I. H., & Selhub, J. (2001). Low circulating vitamin B(6) is associated with elevation of the inflammation marker C-reactive protein independently of plasma homocysteine levels. *Circulation, 103,* 2788–2791.

Garfinkle, M. S., Singhai, A., Katz, W. A., Allan, D. A., Reshetar, R., & Schumacher, H. R., Jr. (1998). Yoga-based intervention for carpal tunnel syndrome: A randomized trial. *Journal of the American Medical Association, 280,* 1601–1603.

Goode, H. F., Burns, E., & Walker, H. E. (1992). Vitamin C depletion and pressure sores in elderly patients with femoral neck fracture. *British Medical Journal, 305,* 925–927.

Griner, T., & Nunes, M. (1996). *What's really wrong with you? A revolutionary look at how muscles affect health.* Garden City Park, NY: Avery.

Hale, I. P., Greer, P. K., & Seinpowski, G. D. (2002). Bromelain treatment alters leukocyte expression of cell surface molecules involved in cellular adhesion and activation. *Clinical Immunology, 104,* 183–190.

O'Connor, D., Marshall, S., & Massy-Westropp, N. (2003). Non-surgical treatment (other than steroid injection) for carpal tunnel syndrome. *Cochrane Database System Review, 1,* CD003219.

Scholzen, T. E., Stander, S., Riemann, H., Brzoska, T., & Luger, T. A. (2003). Modulation of cutaneous inflammation by Angiotensin-converting enzyme. *Journal of Immunology, 170,* 3866–3873.

Shizukuishi, S., Nishii, S., & Folkers, K. (1981). Distribution of vitamin B6 deficiency in university students. *Journal of Nutrition Science Vitaminology, 27,* 193–197.

Steinman, D. (1997, March). Healthy computing. *Let's Live,* pp. 51–53.

Westerlund, C., Ostlund-Lindqvist, A. M., Sainsbury, M., Shertzer, H. G., & Sjoquist, P. O. (1996). *Biochemical Pharmacology, 51,* 1397–1402.

Yoon, S., Lee, J., & Lee, S. (2002). The therapeutic effect of evening primrose oil in atopic dermatitis patients with dry scaly skin lesions is associated with the normalization of serum gamma-interferon levels. *Skin Pharmacology and Applied Skin Physiology, 15*(1), 20–25.

Worwood, V. A. (1991). *The complete book of essential oils & aromatherapy.* San Rafael, CA: New World Library.

CHAPTER 8

Chronic Fatigue Syndrome

One explanation for chronic fatigue syndrome (CFS) is that it is an intensified form of hypoglycemia or abnormally low blood sugar. Because the sphenoid sinus controls metabolism, the suboccipital muscles must be relaxed to allow healthy metabolism to occur (Griner & Nunes, 1996). A psychoanalytic explanation for chronic fatigue syndrome includes viewing the body as a battleground for the fight to separate from the mother (Simpson, 1997). Symptoms of CFS resemble the flu and other viral infections, so it is often mistaken for one of them. Because there are so many symptoms, sufferers often complain of being misunderstood by their physicians (Ax, Gregg, & Jones, 1997). Immunoglobulin and hydrocortisone have shown limited positive effects, but the evidence was inconclusive (Whiting, Banall, & Sowden, 2001).

HOLISTIC NURSING ASSESSMENT

Study the holistic nursing assessment for one client diagnosed with chronic fatigue syndrome, Ms. Z., a 30-year-old single woman. Working in collaboration with clients who suffer from CFS, adapt it as necessary.

Client learning needs: "I'm just so tired all the time. I'd like to be able to exercise."

Indicants of readiness to learn: "I don't have the energy and I don't know what to do about it."

Soul/spirituality symbol(s): "I read the Bible."

Meaning of the condition to client: "I used to have a lot of energy. This is a real challenge for me."

Relationship needs/effects as perceived by the client: "I live with my mother and she's always telling me what to do."

Patterns/attitudes that may create dis-ease for this client: Client uses negative affirmations (e.g., "I just can't do things anymore," and "I'm tired all the time").

Life purpose: "I want to get back to teaching again. That's what I think I do well."

Client strengths: Wants to find more energy and is willing to discuss a plan of care.

Ability to participate in care: Client has periods of high fatigue, but expresses interest in learning and changing mental and work patterns.

Ethical dilemmas: "I want to get my own apartment, but my mother needs me."

Nurse–client process: Client states she wants to change, but shows signs of resistance about what she must do to change.

TREATMENT PLANNING: SETTING JOINTLY AGREED-UPON GOALS

In the case of the client discussed above, the following goals were agreed upon:

1. Change eating patterns to enhance energy.
2. Discuss pros and cons of getting own apartment.
3. Begin a workable exercise program.

TREATMENT

Acceptance of condition/attitude change: To counter negative thoughts and feelings, ask the client to say or write the following affirmation daily: "I am filled with energy and enthusiasm." "I love what I do." "Everything interests me." Client agreed to write the affirmations on 3 x 5 cards and say the words at least 20 times each day.

Facilitating the healing process/healing intention formulation: From a list of meditative statements, client chose the following one to assist in the healing process: "I am filling up with energy and enthusiasm, and agree to meditate on the words while in a relaxed state." Nurse will use caring nonverbal and verbal communication, centering, will use a meditative state to enhance client healing, and to verbalize observed patterns that may be holding the client back and offer alternate approaches.

Creating a sacred space: Client built a healing fountain and uses prayer to create a sacred space.

Encouraging re-storying: Client is writing in a journal about her relationship with her mother and telling stories about teaching kindergartners.

Integrative practices planned: Client stated she wanted to learn specific lifestyle changes that can help her, including nutrition, exercise, and stress management.

Role model strategies: Showed client how to develop a relaxation/guided imagery tape to enhance energy.

Protection plan: Client pictures "the Lord protecting me."

Family strategies: Client is writing a script of what to say to her mother about her life choices.

Life issues/life purpose work: Client has purchased a journal and has started to write about fatigue and resistance to change.

Treatment possibilities/considerations: Other suggested treatments appear below. Most are evidence-based.

OTHER HOLISTIC NURSING INTERVENTIONS

NUTRITION

1. *Increase intake of B-vitamins.* Deficiency in these nutrients is correlated with CFS (Werbach, 2000). Foods rich in B-vitamins include sunflower seeds, whole wheat flour, rolled oats, green peas, soybeans, lima beans, crab meat, brown rice, asparagus, raisins, wheat germ, chicken, hazelnuts, peanuts, hickory nuts, spinach, kale, peas, salmon, prunes, lentils, tuna, turkey, rabbit, white beans, mackerel, bananas, walnuts, sweet potatoes, cooked cabbage, sardines, trout, herring, sea vegetables (kombu, dulse, kelp, wakame) fermented soy products (tempeh, natto, miso), turnips, cantaloupe, buckwheat, lobster, broccoli, and cauliflower.

2. *Eat more foods high in vitamin C.* This vitamin is often deficient in CFS (Werbach, 2000). Foods to concentrate on are green peppers, honeydew melon, Brussels sprouts, strawberries, papaya, watercress, raspberries, parsley, raw cabbage, blackberries, onions, sprouts, and tomatoes.

3. *Take in magnesium-rich foods.* Deficiencies in magnesium are correlated with CFS (Werbach, 2000). For more of this essential substance, eat figs, green leafy vegetables, citrus fruits, whole grain breads and cereal, brown rice, wheat germ, and soy flour.

4. *Essential fatty acids may also help.* They are essential structural components of every cell's membrane; regulate the function of membrane-bound enzymes; and control the electrolyte, energy, and water balance of the cell. They also are often deficient in CFS clients (Werbach, 2000). Increase intake of fish (mackerel, salmon, herring, whitefish, and tuna), walnuts, Brazil nuts, sunflower and pumpkin seeds, oils (canola, olive, and flaxseed), and green leafy vegetables.

5. *Eat high-zinc foods.* Zinc deficiency has been associated with CFS (Werbach, 2000). Some foods rich in zinc are pumpkin seeds, whole grains, oysters, herring, liver, eggs, nuts, and wheat germ.

6. *Obtain tryptophan, carnitine, and coenzyme Q10 in capsule form.* These three nutrients are often deficient in CFS clients (Werbach, 2000).

7. *Increase intake of iron-rich foods* (Werbach, 2000). Foods rich in iron include kidney beans, molasses, whole grain breads and cereals, beets, cherries, red cabbage, spinach, cucumbers, tomato juice, fish, coconuts, blackberry juice, and green leafy vegetables.

8. *Replace good bacteria.* Insufficient "good bacteria" in the gut can lead to yeast infections. Replace them. This is especially important during and after taking antibiotics. Take *L. Acidophilus, lactobacillus, bifidobacteria* or other capsules or powders of live good bacteria. Some plain yogurts contain active cultures that can overpower candida and replace its colonies. Read package information carefully to make sure the cultures are active and the product does not contain sugar, which promotes candida growth.

9. *Starve yeast by eating well.* Foods that support the immune system include soy and fish protein, lots of fresh vegetables, olive oil, nuts (without oil), seeds (sunflower, pumpkin, sesame), legumes (dried beans and peanuts), whole grains (if tolerated), and small amounts of fruit (if tolerated). Avoid all saturated fats (meat, cheese, eggs) sweets, refined flours and cereals, caffeine (coffee, tea, chocolate), alcohol, dairy products (unless you eat them prior to sleep; they contain tryptophan, an amino acid known for its sedative effects),

salt (unless you have low blood pressure), any mold-containing foods if you are sensitive (e.g., MSG, food dyes, food colors, preservatives, mushrooms, and aged cheeses and wines), and allergic foods (those that bloat, give you gas, make you feel tired, give you a headache or other negative symptoms after you eat them).

10. *Start a food/reaction diary* . List everything eaten or drunk for a week. In a column alongside the food, write feelings and bodily reactions for an hour after eating. Notice patterns. Eliminate foods that evoke a negative reaction.

11. *At the first sign of pain, drink one or two glasses of water.* Dehydration is a common source of pain. Taking 1,000 mg of vitamin C either in capsule or powder form (in juice or water) can also relieve pain. For pain that moves around, try 1,000 mg vitamin C and 50 mg L-lysine. Both are available in your local health food store.

12. *Replace minerals lost through perspiration.* Precious minerals and vitamins can be lost in sweat, leading to weakness, fatigue, nausea, and bone and muscle pain. First try a mineral juice, such as V-8. Consider taking a multimineral and a multivitamin that contains at least 50 mg of the major B-vitamins, selenium, and less than 15 mg of iron. Take both because no multivitamin will be large enough to contain sufficient amounts of the minerals needed.

EXERCISE

Challenge erroneous beliefs about avoiding exercise and activity and *use graded aerobic exercise to reduce CFS symptoms.* Graded aerobic exercise proved useful for CFS when compared to participation in flexibility exercises and relaxation therapy (Fulcher & White, 1997).

MASSAGE

1. *Start by working with the hands.* Gently massage them, working deep in the webbing between each finger. Use the thumb to work up the inside of your palm and work out each finger with thumb and index finger. Use the index fingernail to poke the end of each finger. End by pulling down and out the hand with other hand and then shaking the hand just worked on as if flicking water off it. Repeat with the other hand.

2. *Work the feet.* Repeat the same massage with each foot, only work in the depression underneath the ball of the foot a third of the way along the sole. This is a general tonic point that can revive the spirit and enhance energy. If the client is unable to accomplish

the moves, the nurse can complete the massage or a partner, friend, massage therapist, or reflexologist can be employed.

3. *For neck and head pain,* work along, above, and below the bony ridge along the back of the head where it meets the neck. When membranes around the sphenoid sinus openings swell shut and pressure builds, chronic fatigue, among other conditions, can result (Griner & Nunes, 1996). Massage above and below the band of bone at the back of the head, working gently but more intensely wherever pain is experienced. Search for sore spots and give them loving massage. Work fingers up and through the scalp, locating any sore spots and working with them gently until they release and pain leaves. If pain increases, stop and consult with a massage therapist.

4. *Work across shoulders,* down the arms, across the chest and abdomen, and down the legs and feet.

GENTLE ACUPRESSURE

Place the 2nd, 3rd, and 4th fingers of the right hand on the inside of the right knee and the 2nd, 3rd, and 4th fingers of the left hand on the inside of the left knee. Hold until pulsation is evident in all six fingers, then hold a spot above the shoulder blades, the middle of the instep, the bottom of the big toe, behind the knee, and the spot on either side of the spinal column just below where the neck attaches to the shoulder (Dayton, 1994).

HERBS AND SUPPLEMENTS

1. *Try Echinacea purpurea and Panax ginseng.* They have been shown to enhance the immune system in individuals with CFS (see, Broumand, Sahl, & Tilles, 1997).

2. *Investigate* kombucha tea (to offer renewed energy), and ginger, licorice root, and Siberian ginseng to decrease fatigue and weakness.

3. *To kill yeast infections* try 3–5 teaspoons of grapefruit seed extract (GSE) in a quart of liquid (Landis, 1997), or echinacea root, garlic, Pau d'arco bark, oak bark, or astragalus.

4. *Try black cohosh for sleeping problems, night sweats, and irritability,* which are characteristic of perimenopause. Check a reliable herb text prior to beginning any herb.

5. *Consider taking malic acid and magnesium hydroxide.* At least one study found that this combination reduced muscle pain while increasing endurance (Abraham & Flechas, 1992).

Cognitive Therapy

Use cognitive-behavioral methods to challenge erroneous client beliefs (Prins et al., 2001). Cognitive-behavioral therapy was shown to be more effective in reducing fatigue than a guided support group and was more effective in changing beliefs than was relaxation therapy (Deale, Chalder, & Wessely, 1998). Based on these findings it may be wise to refer the client to a nurse psychotherapist or psychologist skilled in the method.

Aromatherapy

Use essential oils to stimulate or relax. A few drops of essential lavender oil in a warm bath can prepare for refreshing sleep. Oil of lemon can help clients unwind and prevent night sweats and fevers. Lemon and lavender combine to produce a refreshing sleep. Mix these two essential oils in an aromatic infuser. A few sniffs of oil of rosemary can take away early morning sluggishness. A sniff of oil of orange or oil of sweet orange can refresh and uplift. Although the oils are safe, a few may irritate the skin and should be used in a carrier oil such as sweet almond oil. Avoid oils if pregnant or breast feeding. If you plan to use essential oils, purchase a textbook (e.g., Landis, 1997) and follow it, or find a health care practitioner knowledgeable in their use.

Stress Reduction

Depending on the client's response, use relaxation therapy, guided imagery, self-hypnosis, or touch to assist in stress reduction. Avoid multiple vaccinations performed over a short period of time. They are associated with a diffuse myalgia and chronic fatigue (Gherardi, 2003).

EVALUATING TREATMENT

Client used a scale of 1 (no/none) to 10 (extreme amount) every week to evaluate change in eating patterns, exercise, fatigue, stress, relationship with mother, and decision to move into an apartment. Over time, by the end of 6 months, the client gradually noted positive changes in all behaviors.

REFERENCES

Abraham, G. E., & Flechas, J. D. (1992). Malic acid reduces muscle pain while increasing endurance in CFS and FM. *Journal of Nutritional Medicine, 3,* 49–59.

Ax, S., Gregg, V. N., & Jones, D. (1997). Chronic fatigue syndrome: Sufferers' evaluation of medical support. *Journal of Social Medicine, 90,* 250–254.

Dayton, B. R. (1994). *An introduction to a gentle acupressure for caregivers.* Friday Harbor, WA: High Touch Network.

Deale, A., Chalder, T., & Wessely, S. (1998). Illness beliefs and treatment outcome in chronic fatigue syndrome. *Journal of Psychosomatic Research, 45*(1 Spec. No.), 77–83.

Fulcher, K. Y., & White, P. D. (1997). Randomised controlled trial of graded exercise in patients with the chronic fatigue syndrome. *British Medical Journal, 314,* 1647–1652.

Gherardi, R. K. (2003). Lessons from macrophagic myofasciitis: Towards definition of a vaccine adjuvant-related syndrome. *Review of Neurology, 159,* 162–164.

Griner, T., & Nunes, M. (1996). *What's really wrong with you? A revolutionary look at how muscles affect health.* Garden City Park, NY: Avery.

Landis, R. (1997). *Herbal defense.* New York: Warner Books.

Prins, J. B., Bleijenberg, G., Bazelmans, E., Elving, L. D., deBoo, T. M., Severens, J. L., et al. (2001). Cognitive behaviour therapy for chronic fatigue syndrome: A multicentre randomised controlled trial. *Lancet, 357,* 841–847.

See, D. M., Broumand, N., Sahl, L., & Tilles, J. G. (1997). In vitro effects of echinacea and ginseng on natural killer and antibody-dependent cell cytotoxicity in healthy subjects and chronic fatigue syndrome or acquired immunodeficiency syndrome patients. *Immunopharmacology, 35,* 229–235.

Simpson, M. (1997). A body with chronic fatigue syndrome as a battleground for the fight to separate from the mother. *Journal of Analytic Psychology, 42,* 201–216.

Werbach, M. R. (2000). Nutritional strategies for treating chronic fatigue syndrome. *Alternative Medical Review, 5,* 93–108.

Whiting, P., Banall, A. M., & Sowden, A. J. (2001). Interventions for the treatment and management of chronic fatigue syndrome: A systematic review. *Journal of the American Medical Association, 286,* 1360–1368

CHAPTER 9

Depression

Being pressured to be feminine and squelch their anger may place women at a greater risk for depression (Oakley, 1994). Strong feeling must go somewhere, and if it can't be expressed in aggressive games, physical fights, or verbal sparring, it can fester inside and be turned against the self, eventually developing into depression or suicidal thoughts and actions. A medical approach to depression includes antidepressants (all of which have troublesome side effects) and psychotherapy.

HOLISTIC NURSING ASSESSMENT

Study the holistic nursing assessment for Ms. B., a 45-year-old woman who smokes and was diagnosed with depression, that follows. Working in collaboration with your depressed clients, adapt the format as needed.

Client learning needs: To see the connection between her feelings and her depression.

Indicants of readiness to learn: Asking for advice about what to do.

Soul/spirituality symbol(s): Goes to church every Sunday.

Meaning of the condition to client: "My life is a mess. I can't seem to do anything right, at least according to my husband."

Relationship needs/effects as perceived by the client: "I want to do my housework, but I just can't get out of bed in the morning."

Patterns/attitudes that may create dis-ease for this client: Client uses negative affirmations (e.g., "I can't get out of bed in the morning," and "I can't do anything right").

Life purpose: Expresses hopelessness about her life.

Client strengths: Wants to be less depressed and is willing to discuss a plan of care.

Ability to participate in care: Client has periods of deep depression, but expresses interest in learning and changing mental and work patterns.

Ethical dilemmas: Client has expressed a wish to kill herself and has tried to swear the nurse to secrecy.

Nurse–client process: Client resists examining the part her feelings play in her dis-ease.

TREATMENT PLANNING: SETTING JOINTLY AGREED-UPON GOALS

In the case of the client discussed above, the following goals were agreed upon:

1. Identify feelings of anger.
2. Quit smoking.
3. Agree on a suicide prevention plan.

TREATMENT

Acceptance of condition/attitude change: To counter negative thoughts and feelings, ask the client to say or write one or more of the following affirmations daily: "I am hopeful." "I create my own life." "I go beyond fear and limitations." Client agreed to write the affirmations on 3 x 5 cards and say the words at least 20 times each day.

Facilitating the healing process/healing intention formulation: From a list of meditative statements, client agreed to meditate on the following words while in a relaxed state: "I create a life that's right for me." Nurse will use caring nonverbal and verbal communication, centering, and a meditative state to enhance client healing, will verbalize observed patterns that may be holding the client back and offer alternate approaches.

Creating a sacred space: Client asked nurse to help her organize and straighten up her work and sleep space and add wind chimes by the window.

Encouraging re-storying: Client began writing in a journal about her suicidal thoughts and feelings.

Integrative practices planned: Nurse is focusing on alternatives to suicide and how she can reach them.

Role model strategies: Showed client how to use a meditation and images to lift her out of depression.

Protection plan: Client pictures a "life angel" keeping her safe and alive.

Family strategies: Client began writing a script of how to talk to her husband about her resentment over his behavior.

Life issues/life purpose work: Client states she missed her chance to be an actress and has been feeling down ever since. Is writing in her journal about finding a life purpose.

Treatment possibilities/considerations: Other suggested treatments appear below. Most are evidence-based.

ADDITIONAL INFORMATION AND TREATMENTS FOR CLIENTS

NUTRITIONAL APPROACHES

1. *Take additional vitamin B12.* After researchers adjusted for sociodemographic characteristics and health status, participants with a vitamin B12 deficiency were found to be 2 times more likely to be severely depressed as were participants who had sufficient vitamin B12 (Penninx et al., 1998). Foods to eat to ensure a sufficient amount of this vitamin include liver, clams, oysters, sardines, mackerel, trout, herring, and eggs. Obtain nutritional yeast, sea vegetables (kombu, dulse, wakame), fermented soyfoods (tempeh, natto, and miso), and kelp at a health food store.

2. *Move toward vegetarianism.* In one study, depression was more likely to occur in nonvegetarians than in vegetarians. The researchers suggest that vegetables provide more antioxidants and thus they may protect vegetarians (Rodriguez, Rodriguez, & Gonzalez, 1998).

3. *Take additional magnesium.* A study of women in the United Kingdom found that mood swings and depressive symptoms were reduced by taking 200 milligrams of magnesium (as MgO) and 50

milligrams of vitamin B6 a day. The researchers also concluded that this form of magnesium was poorly absorbed (DeSouza, Walker, Robinson, & Bolland, 2000). Based on these findings, for greater improvement, suggest that clients take a more absorbable form of the mineral, magnesium citrate. Also suggest that clients eat foods high in magnesium and vitamin B6: whole grain breads and cereals, fresh peas, figs, soy flour, brown rice, wheat germ, nuts, Swiss chard, green leafy vegetables, citrus fruits, sunflower seeds, chicken, mackerel, salmon, tuna, bananas, peanuts, and sweet potatoes.

4. *Increase intake of sulfur.* This element is widely found in human nutrition and is the sixth most abundant macromineral in breast milk (Parcell, 2002). Sulfur-rich foods include cabbage, peas, beans, cauliflower, Brussels sprouts, eggs, horseradish, shrimp, chestnuts, mustard greens, onions, and asparagus. Sulfur supplements such as SAMe, DMSO, and taurine may also be of help (Parcell, 2002).

EXERCISE

Running or jogging is not necessary (Noreau, Martineau, Roy, & Belzile, 1995). Gardening, walking, line dancing, swimming, or any active movement will help raise mood. Encourage clients to push themselves to move even when they don't feel like it. Exercise works better than Zoloft for treating depression ("Exercise May Be as Effective," 2001).

AVOID DRUGS THAT INCREASE DEPRESSION

Many common prescription drugs can lower mood and increase depression, including antidepressants (Mindell & Hopkins, 1998; Preda et al., 2001). Avoid the following and use alternatives whenever possible: (a) amphetamines (to lose weight and stay awake, including antihistamines), (b) antibiotics, (c) anticonvulsants, (d) antidepressants, (e) barbiturates, (f) diuretics and beta-blockers, (g) hormones (estrogen, Premarin, Provera), (h) narcotics, painkillers, and sleeping pills, (i) steroids (cortisone, prednisone), (j) Tagamet and Zantac, (k) tranquilizers (Librium, Xanax, Restoril, Halcion).

A meta-analysis of 22 studies of antidepressant outcomes assessed the level of medication effects under conditions thought to be less subject to clinician bias than those in the typical double-blind drug trial. The researchers concluded that clinician outcome ratings were significantly larger than those that were based on patient ratings. When asked, patients reported no advantage for antidepressants beyond the placebo effect (Greenberg, Bornstein, Greenberg, & Fisher, 1992).

KEEP COMMUNICATION CHANNELS OPEN

Suicidal teenagers usually come from troubled families and many have experienced sexual abuse (Garnefski, Diekstra, & de Heus, 1992). Depressed teenagers show the strongest relationship with depressive symptoms and antisocial behavior when they have negative perceptions of their family. Depressive symptoms have stronger independent relationships with negative perceptions of peers, whereas antisocial behaviors have stronger relationships with negative perceptions of school (Garnefski, 2000). A study of teens who committed suicide found that they often showed signs of depression and alcohol abuse that parents missed. Parents seriously underestimated the frequency or extent of alcohol use, could not understand the depth of feelings their children were going through, did not know the extreme pessimism about the future and life in general their children held, and did not know that their children had been intoxicated at least once in the past six months before the suicide attempt (Velting, 1999). Although these findings only apply to teens, keeping communication channels open between depressed adults and their families is also crucial.

MASSAGE

When membranes around the sinus openings swell shut and pressure builds, infections and depression, among other conditions, can result (Griner & Nunes, 1996). Massage above and below the band of bone at the back of the head, working gently, but more intensely wherever pain is experienced. Follow the directions on page 43.

HERBS AND SUPPLEMENTS

1. *Take St. John's wort.* This herb can alleviate mild to moderate depression. The usual dose of St. John's wort is 300 to 450 mg twice a day of the standardized extract (Miller, 1998). Avoid taking it with nasal decongestants or hay fever and asthma medications. Amino acid supplements that contain phenylalanine and tyrosine can cause hypertension, so they should also be avoided.

2. *Take Acetyl-L-carnitine (ALCAR)*. Many major well-designed studies have shown ALCAR to be beneficial in the treatment of major depression (Pettigrew, Levine, & McClure, 2000).

3. *Try SAMe*. S-adenosylmethionine is a popular supplement synthesized from the amino acid methionine and is found throughout the body. By the end of the second week in a small trial, 66% of the SAMe participants had a reduction in depression versus 22% of participants taking imipramine (Tofranil). SAMe had no side effects whereas Tofranil has the following adverse effects: drowsiness, heart arrhythmias, low or high blood pressure, fatigue, nausea, rash, increased perspiration, headache, changes in blood sugar, sensitivity to light and sun, water retention, jaundice, muscle spasticity and uncontrollable movements, and blood cell disturbances. It must be taken with caution by many people (those with glaucoma, psychosis, diabetes, hyperthyroidism, kidney or liver disorders, asthma, and women who are pregnant or nursing, have epilepsy, heart or blood vessel disease, or urine retention). In sum, SAMe works better and has fewer adverse effects (Bell, Pion, Bunney, & Potkin, 1988.)

4. *Try Gingko biloba*. This herb may offer a significant benefit as an antidepressant on its own or in combination with standard antidepressants (Schubert & Halama, 1993).

5. *Take fish oil*. Fish oil helps stabilize the volatile moods of people suffering from manic depression ("Feeling Better with Fish Oil," 1999).

6. *Instead of Prozac, try safer 5-HTP*. This supplement is a biochemical product of the amino acid tryptophan and a direct precursor to the neurotransmitter serotonin. It may produce an upset stomach, but it subsides within three days, whereas the costly Prozac (up to $275/month as compared to $30/month for 5-HTP) may impair judgment, thinking or motor skills; produce headache, nausea and vomiting, diarrhea, anorexia, dry mouth, profuse sweating, sexual dysfunction, and blurred vision (Angelo & Miller, 2001).

MUSIC

In a study, depressed women who listened to music reported more tranquil mood states (Lai, 1999). Adding guided imagery can reduce depression, fatigue, and total mood disturbance (Penninx et al., 1998). Small group reminiscence-focused music therapy groups can help to reduce depression in older adults with dementia (Ashida, 2000).

VOLUNTEERING

Volunteering is one of the best ways to reduce depression. It removes clients from their worries and places their concentration on helping someone else. The good feelings and boost to self-esteem that result can help jog clients out of their depression. Contact the Volunteers of America, 1-800-988-0089 or National Senior Service Corps, 1-800-424-8867, or check the local newspaper for volunteer opportunities.

COGNITIVE BEHAVIOR THERAPY

Depressed clients who participated in cognitive-behavioral therapy groups improved to a considerable degree (Breslau, Peterson, Schultz, Chilcoat, & Andreski, 2000; Rief, Trenkamp, Auer, & Ficther, 2000). Even depressed participants in a nursing home (Abraham, Neundorfer, & Currie, 1992), after a stroke (Lincoln, Flannaghan, Sutcliffe, & Rother, 1997), adolescents (Albano, Marten, Holt, Heimberg, & Barlow, 1995), and young college women (Peden, Hall, Rayers, & Beebe, 2000) benefited. If you are not skilled in this method, refer clients to someone who is. In the meantime, counsel clients to avoid taking on additional responsibility, set small goals and build in a reward when each is achieved, lower expectations until depression fades, be around other people even when feeling depressed, engage in at least one "feel good" activity every day, never overdo, get plenty of rest, and refuse to get upset if results don't match expectations.

LEISURE ACTIVITIES

Staying active in leisure and productive activities has a positive effect on depression (Herzog, Franks, Markus, & Holmberg, 1998).

SOCIAL SUPPORT

Being with supportive friends can provide a buffer against depression (Hays, Steffens, Flint, Bosworth, & George, 2001).

CHURCHGOING

Frequent churchgoers were about half as likely to be depressed although private prayer and Bible reading were unrelated to depression in one study (Koenig et al., 1997).

ASSERTIVENESS TRAINING

Try assertiveness training. It has been shown to reduce depression better than traditional psychotherapy (Sanchez, Lewinsohn, & Larson, 1980).

REFRAMING

Learn to restructure negative thoughts to improve self-esteem and reduce depression (Philpot & Bamburg, 1996). Nurses can ask clients to say and/or write one or more of the following affirmations to balance the negative messages they may be giving themselves:

- I go beyond my fears and limitations.
- I create a joyous life.
- I release all anger.
- I forgive others.
- I forgive myself.

SMOKING CESSATION

Major depression has been linked to smoking. A history of daily smoking was found to significantly increase the risk of depression (Breslau et al., 1998). If you are not skilled in hypnosis, refer the client to a mental health nurse specialist or psychologist who is, or suggest the client join a quit smoking group (many are sponsored by the American Lung Association; check the white pages).

THERAPEUTIC TOUCH

Therapeutic touch has been shown to reduce depression in adults (Leb, 1998).

HOME VISITING

Home visiting for depressed women at home with young children can help. Depression lifted in mothers who were visited at home by nurses who showed them how to deal with their children, taught parenting skills, and reinforced maternal competence. The nurses also suggested resources and positive ways to cope (Gelfand, Teti, Seiner, & Jameson, 1996). If home visiting is not an option, consider providing the services yourself.

WEIGHT LIFTING

In one study, resistance training had a significant effect by lowering depression, and improving strength, morale, and quality of life (Singh, Clements, & Fiatarone, 1997).

ACUPUNCTURE

Acupuncture was found to be more effective than an antidepressant (Elavil) in reducing depression (Yang, Liu, Luo, & Jia, 1994).

GENTLE ACUPRESSURE

For sorrow, grief, sadness, shock, rejection, inability to release the past: hold top of middle of back of the hip, right hand on right side, left hand on left side, until a pulsation is felt in the index, third, and fourth fingers. For depression, obsessive behavior, worry and guilt, hold a spot on either side of the spinal cord at the top of the scapula (Dayton, 1994).

MEDITATION

Mindfulness meditation reduced depression, anxiety, and physical symptoms in participants who met for 8 weeks to learn and use mindfulness stress reduction (Prigerson et al., 2001). Meditation combined with Fordyce's Personal Happiness Enhancement Program reduced depression, too (Smith, Compton, & West, 1995).

READING

Cognitive bibliotherapy was found to work well to reduce mild to moderate depression (when combined with traditional treatment) and gains were maintained over a three-year period (Smith, Floyd, Scogin, & Jamison, 1997).

PHOTOTHERAPY

High levels of illumination have been shown to be helpful in reducing depression caused by seasonal light changes. High levels of illumination combined with antidepressant medication reduced depression. The higher the level of illumination, the greater the decrease in depression (Beauchemin & Hays, 1997).

PET THERAPY

At least one study has shown that pets can erase the stress of the death of a spouse (Bolin, 1986) and help deal with other losses, too. Other studies have shown that a pet can provide a sense of belonging and of being needed. Even a stuffed toy animal or a plant that requires attention can improve well-being.

MASSAGE AND RELAXATION THERAPIES

Field, Grizzle, Scafidi, and Schanberg (1996) found that depressed teen mothers showed diminished depression after receiving 5 weeks of massage therapy.

GO BACK TO SCHOOL

Taking a class for credit or non-credit may be a useful treatment. Educational attainment and activities are effective buffers against depression (Herzog et al., 1998).

TREATMENT EVALUATION

The client described above evaluated her level of anger after each session by rating herself as not at all angry (1) to extremely angry (10). At the end of the first session, she had a written suicide prevention plan in place and agreed to contact the nurse prior to taking any action on suicidal thoughts. After four weeks, client remained smoke free.

REFERENCES

Abraham, I. L., Neundorfer, M. M., & Currie, L. J. (1992). Effects of group interventions on cognition and depression in nursing home residents. *Nursing Research, 41,* 196–202.

Albano, A. M., Marten, P. A., Holt, C. S., Heimberg, R. G., & Barlow, D. H. (1995). Cognitive-behavioral group treatment for social phobia in adolescents. *Journal of Nervous and Mental Disease, 183,* 649–656.

Angelo, M., & Miller, A. L. (2001, November). Nature's pharmacy: Depression. *Let's Live,* 30.

Ashida, S. (2000). The effect of reminiscence music therapy sessions on changes in depressive symptoms in elderly persons with dementia. *Journal of Music Therapy, 37,* 170–182.

Beauchemin, K. M., & Hays, P. (1997). Phototherapy is a useful adjunct in the treatment of depressed in-patients. *Acta Psychiatrica Scandinavia, 95,* 424–427.

Bell, K. M., Pion, L., Bunney, W. E., Jr., & Potkin, S. G. (1988). S-adenosylmethionine treatment of depression: A controlled clinical trial. *American Journal of Psychiatry, 145,* 1110–1114.

Bolin S. (1986, August). *The role of pets in comforting the pet-owning widow.* Delta Society International Conference, Boston, MA.

Breslau, N., Peterson, E. L., Schultz, L. R., Chilcoat, H. D., & Andreski, P. (1998). Major depression and stages of smoking. *Archives of General Psychiatry, 55,* 161–166.

Dayton, B. R. (1994). *An introduction to a gentle acupressure for caregivers.* Friday Harbor, WA: High Touch Network.

DeSouza, M. C., Walker, A. F., Robinson, P. A., & Bolland, K. (2000). A synergistic effect of a daily supplement for 1 month of 200 mg magnesium plus 50 mg vitamin B6 for the relief of anxiety-related premenstrual symptoms: A randomized, double-blind, crossover study. *Journal of Womens Health and Gender Based Medicine, 9,* 131–139.

Exercise may be as effective as sertraline in the treatment of major depression. (2001). *American Journal of Nursing, 101*(2), 19.

Feeling better with fish oil. (1999). *Science News, 155,* 362

Field, T. M., Grizzle, N., Scafidi, F., & Schanberg, S. (1996). Massage and relaxation therapies' effects on depressed adolescent mothers. *Adolescence, 31,* 903–911.

Garnefski, N. (2000). Age differences in depressive symptoms, antisocial behavior, and negative perceptions of family, school, and peers among adolescents. *Journal of the American Academy of Child and Adolescent Psychiatry, 39,* 1175–1181.

Garnefski, N., Diekstra, R. F., & de Heus, P. (1992). A population-based survey of the characteristics of high school students with and without a history of suicidal behavior. *Acta Psychiatrica Scandinavia, 86,* 189–196.

Gelfand, D. M., Teti, D. M., Seiner, S. A., & Jameson, P. B. (1996). Helping mothers fight depression: Evaluation of a home-based intervention program for depressed mothers and their infants. *Journal of Clinical and Child Psychology, 25,* 406–422.

Greenberg, R. P., Bornstein, R. F., Greenberg, M. D., & Fisher, S. (1992). A meta-analysis of antidepressant outcome under "blinder" conditions. *Journal of Consulting and Clinical Psychology, 60,* 664–669.

Griner, T., & Nunes, M. (1996). *What's really wrong with you? A revolutionary look at how muscles affect health.* Garden City Park, NY: Avery.

Hays, J. C., Steffens, D. C., Flint, E. P., Bosworth, H. B., & George, L. K. (2001). Does social support buffer decline in elderly patients with unipolar depression. *American Journal of Psychiatry, 158,* 1850–1855.

Herzog, A. R., Franks, M. M., Markus, H. R., & Holmberg, D. (1998). Activities and well-being in older age: Effects of self-concept and educational attainment. *Psychology and Aging, 13,* 179–185.

Koenig, H. G., Hays, J. C., George, L. K., Blazer, D. G., Larson, D. B., & Landerman, L. R. (1997). Modeling the cross-sectional relationships between religion, physical health, social support, and depressive symptoms. *American Journal of Geriatric Psychiatry, 5,* 131–144.

Lai, Y. M. (1999). Effects of music listening on depressed women in Taiwan. *Issues in Mental Health, 3,* 229–246.

Leb, C. B. (1998, June). *The effects of healing touch on depression.* Research presentation at the American Holistic Nurses' Association Annual Conference, Tampa, FL.

Lincoln, N. B., Flannaghan, T., Sutcliffe, L., & Rother, L. (1997). Evaluation of cognitive behavioral treatment for depression after stroke: A pilot study. *Clinical Rehabilitation, 11,* 113–122.

Miller, L. G. (1998). Herbal medicinals: Selected clinical considerations focusing on known or potential drug-herb interactions. *Archives of General Medicine, 158,* 2200–2211.

Mindell, E., & Hopkins, V. (1998). *Prescription alternatives.* New Canaan, CT: Keats.

Noreau, L., Martineau, H., Roy, L., & Belzile, M. (1995). Effects of a modified dance-based exercise on cardiorespiratory fitness, psychological state and health status of persons with rheumatoid arthritis. *American Journal of Physical Medicine Rehabilitation, 74*(1), 19–27.

Oakley, I. D. (1994, Fall). Striving for "Sugar 'n Spice" may produce depression in some women. *Nursing Dimensions, 5.*

Parcell, S. (2002). Sulfur in human nutrition and applications in medicine. *Alternative Medical Review, 7*(1), 22–24.

Peden, A. R., Hall, L. A., Rayers, M. K., & Beebe, L. L. (2000). Reducing negative thinking and depressive symptoms in college women. *Journal of Nursing Scholarship, 32,* 134–151.

Penninx, B. W., van Tilburg, T., Boeke, T., Deeg, A. J. P., Kriegsman, D. J. H., & van Eijk, J. T. M. (1998). Predicting depression in the chronically ill. *Health Psychology, 17,* 551–558.

Penninx, B. W. J. H., Gurainik, J. M., Ferrucci, L., Fried, L. P., Allen, R. H., & Stabler, S. P. (2000). Vitamin B12 deficiency and depression in physically disabled older women: Epidemiologic evidence from the Women's Health and Aging Study. *American Journal of Psychiatry, 157,* 715–721.

Pettigrew, J. W., Levine, J., & McClure, R. J. (2000). Acetyl-L-carnitine physical-chemical, metabolic and therapeutic properties: Relevance for its mode of action in Alzheimer's disease and geriatric depression. *Molecular Psychiatry, 5,* 616–632.

Philpot, V. D., & Bamburg, J. W. (1996). Restructuring negative thoughts can improve self-esteem and reduce depression. *Psychological Reports, 79,* 83.

Preda, A., MacLean, R. W., Mazure, C. M., & Bowers, M. B., Jr. (2001). Antidepressant-associated mania and psychosis resulting in psychiatric admissions. *Journal of Clinical Psychiatry, 62*(1), 30–33.

Prigerson, H. G., Kasl, S. V., Reynolds, C. F. 3rd, Anderson, B., Zubenko, G. S., Houck, P. R., et al. (2001). Mindfulness-based stress reduction and health-related quality of life in a heterogeneous patient population. *General Hospital Psychiatry, 23,* 183–192.

Rief, W., Trenkamp, S., Auer, C., & Ficther, M. M. (2000). Cognitive behavior therapy in panic disorder and comorbid major depression. *Psychotherapy and Psychosomatics, 69*(2), 70–80.

Rodriguez, J. J., Rodriguez, J. R., & Gonzalez, M. J. (1998). Indicators of anxiety and depression in subjects with different kinds of diet: Vegetarians and omnivores. *Bulletin of the Medical Association of Puerto Rico, 90*(4–6), 58–68.

Sanchez, V. C., Lewinsohn, P. M., & Larson, D. W. (1980). Assertion training: Effectiveness in the treatment of depression. *Journal of Clinical Psychology, 36,* 526–529.

Schubert, H., & Halama, P. (1993). Depressive episode primarily unresponsive to therapy in elderly patients: Efficacy of Ginkgo biloba (Egb 761) in combination with antidepressants. *Geriatric Forsch, 3,* 45–53.

Singh, N. A., Clements, K. M., & Fiatarone, M. A. (1997). A randomized controlled trial of progressive resistance training in depressed elders. *Journal of Gerontology in Biological Science and Medical Science, 52*(1), M2–M35.

Smith, N. M., Floyd, M. R., Scogin, F., & Jamison, C. S. (1997). Three-year follow-up of bibliotherapy for depression. *Journal of Consulting and Clinical Psychology, 65,* 324–327.

Smith, W. P., Compton, W. C., & West, W. B. (1995). Meditation as an adjunct to a happiness enhancement program. *Journal of Clinical Psychology, 51,* 269–273.

Velting, V. (1999). Parents "clueless" about teen suicide, study shows. [Press Release.] *Ball State University News.* Muncie, IN: Ball State University.

Yang, X., Liu, X., Luo, H., & Jia, Y. (1994). Clinical observation on needling extrachannel points in treating mental depression. *Journal of Traditional Chinese Medicine, 14*(1), 14–18.

CHAPTER 10

Diabetes

Type 2 diabetes is the fastest-growing health problem in the United States. Sixteen million Americans suffer from it, including many children as young as age 10. Hispanics are two to four times more likely to have diabetes and African Americans more than twice as likely as caucasians. The increased consumption of highly refined breads, rolls, muffins, pastries, and packaged foods, and refined sugars in candy, pies, cakes, and sodas contribute to high glucose levels, as may cow's milk ("Cow's Milk Diabetes Connection Bolstered," 1999). The medical treatment includes a carefully calculated diet, planned physical activity, home blood glucose testing, and in some cases, daily oral medication or insulin injections. The oral diabetes drugs are used to block enzymes that normally break down carbohydrates. This can result in unpleasant side effects such as abdominal pain, cramps, gas and diarrhea, kidney problems, and possibly tumors. Insulin has its own problems. Even if it does help lower blood sugar, it can raise blood pressure and cholesterol levels. This is why self-care measures such as diet, supplements, and exercise are so important.

HOLISTIC NURSING ASSESSMENT

Study the holistic nursing assessment for Mr. C., a 60-year-old client diagnosed with diabetes, that follows. Working in collaboration with your clients diagnosed with diabetes, use this format to assess their holistic needs.

Client learning needs: To find a lifestyle plan that manages his diabetes well.

Indicants of readiness to learn: "The doctor gave me a diet to follow, but I don't eat any of those foods and he also told me to exercise, but I've never exercised."

Soul/spirituality symbol(s): "I was raised Lutheran, but I haven't been to church in a long time."

Meaning of the condition to client: "Ever since my son was killed in a freak accident, I haven't cared much about anything."

Relationship needs/effects as perceived by the client: "My mother-in-law lives with us and she rules the roost. My wife tells me not to get upset about her, but that's easier said than done."

Patterns/attitudes that may create dis-ease for this client: Client uses negative affirmations (e.g., "My wife cooks what she wants and I eat it," and "Since my son died, there isn't anything to look forward to").

Life purpose: Expresses lack of life purpose since son died.

Client strengths: Wants to learn how to deal with his mother-in-law and how to manage diabetes.

Ability to participate in care: Client wears soiled and moist socks and reports walking barefoot on his lawn, but expresses interest in learning and changing mental and work patterns.

Ethical dilemmas: Client requests his wife not be contacted, even though he knows what he is eating affects his nutritional status.

Nurse–client process: Client changes the subject when asked to examine the part his feelings play in his dis-ease.

TREATMENT PLANNING: SETTING JOINTLY AGREED-UPON GOALS

In the case of the client discussed above, the following goals were agreed upon:

1. Resolve grief over son's death.
2. Begin a daily walking exercise program.
3. Eat at least one wellness meal a day.

TREATMENT

Acceptance of condition/attitude change: The client chose the following affirmation to use to replace the grief he feels: "I fill each day with joy." Client agreed to write the affirmation on 3 x 5 cards and say the words at least 20 times each day.

Facilitating the healing process/healing intention formulation: From a list of meditative statements, client chose the following one to assist in the healing process: "Life is sweet." Nurse asked client to meditate on the words while in a relaxed state. Nurse will use caring nonverbal and verbal communication, centering, and a meditative state to enhance client healing, will verbalize observed patterns that may be holding the client back and offer alternate approaches.

Creating a sacred space: During client sessions, music of his choice will play in the background and peppermint oil aromatherapy will be used to open his stuffed sinuses.

Encouraging re-storying: Encouraged client to write about his personal life journey.

Integrative practices planned: Will use guided imagery, relaxation therapy, and gentle acupressure to assist in the healing process.

Role model strategies: Showed client how to use self-massage/gentle acupressure between sessions to relieve foot and leg pain.

Protection plan: Taught client to use a white light around him to protect against mother-in-law's influence on him.

Family strategies: Encouraged client to invite his wife and/or mother-in-law to a session to practice more open communication between them.

Life issues/life purpose work: Client has signed up to read to pre-schoolers at the local library.

Treatment possibilities/considerations: Other suggested treatments appear below. Most are evidence-based.

ADDITIONAL INFORMATION AND TREATMENTS FOR CLIENTS

A healthy low-calorie, low-fat diet and moderate physical activity are better protectors against the incidence of diabetes than the antihyperglycemic agent, metformin (Diabetes Prevention Program Research Group, 2000). To help clients integrate treatment recommendations into their lives, provide information about morbidity/mortality and the prevention of complications, and instill hope that enacting knowledge will enhance quality of life (Whittemore, Chase, Mandle, & Roy, 2002).

Nutritional Approaches

1. *Eliminate refined carbohydrates and high-fat foods* including white bread, pastries, cookies, candies, and cake (Brancati, Wang, Mead, Kiang, & Klag, 1999; Lukaczer, 1998; Miller, Hoenig, & Ujhelyi, 1998), *fish oil capsules* (McGrath et al., 1996), and supplements containing large amounts of *paraaminobenzoic acid* or PABA (Lukaczer, 1998). Consumption of these products can result in elevated blood sugar.

2. *Eat more whole grain products and fewer potatoes and white rice.* Whole grains reduce risk for adult diabetes (Hu et al., 2001; Salmeron, Manson, & Stampfer, 1997), and can improve insulin sensitivity in overweight and obese adults (Pereira et al., 2002). A primarily vegetarian diet can be soothing and can control diabetic neuropathy (McCarty, 2002).

3. *Eat more papaya.* It protects against and prevents diabetes complications (Savickiene, Dagilyte, Lukosius, & Zitkevicius, 2002).

4. *Add more good fats to the diet.* Use only olive oil (Garg, Bonanome, Grundy, Ahang, & Unger, 1988; Matsuda et al., 1997), and add fish, chicken, and turkey without the skin to regular eating fare (Hu et al., 2001).

5. *Eat five or more fruits and vegetables and drink tea daily.* These are correlated with reduction in risk for type 2 diabetes (Ford & Mokdad, 2001; Knekt et al., 2002), especially tomatoes (Lean et al., 1999).

6. *Eat whole fruits and stop drinking fruit juices.* Drinking fruit juice causes blood sugar to rise more rapidly than eating the fruit itself. The exception is guava juice, which can improve and maybe even prevent diabetes (Cheng & Yang, 1983).

7. *Eat foods high in vitamin C* that can protect against blood vessel changes in diabetes. Vitamin C plays a central role in the antioxidant defense system, and participates in many cellular oxidation-reduction reactions that are required for collagen production and metabolism and storage of catecholamines in neurons (Root-Bernstein, Busik, & Henry, 2002). The vitamin also inhibits the process of glycosylation, the binding of glucose (sugar) onto proteins in the blood, nerve cells, and lenses of the eyes that may be responsible for many of the long-term effects of diabetes. Vitamin C supplements may slow this process (Ting, Timini, & Boles, 1996). Because too much vitamin C can interfere with other body functions, consider eating more foods high in this vitamin, rather than taking a supplement. Green peppers, strawberries, citrus fruit, honeydew melon, cooked broccoli, Brussels sprouts or kale, cantaloupe, papaya, cooked cauliflower,

raspberries, parsley, raw cabbage, blackberries, onions, and spinach are all full of vitamin C, which may correct insulin resistance and the inflexible blood vessels characteristic of diabetes.

8. *Add onions and garlic to every meal.* To lower blood sugar, blood pressure, and cholesterol add onions (Babu & Srinivasan, 1997) and garlic to meals (Augusti, 1996; Murray, 1994). Onions also have an antithrombotic effect (Jung et al., 2002) and protect against diabetes complications (Savickiene, Dagilyte, Lukosius, & Zitkevicius, 2002).

9. *Eat more essential fatty acids* to prevent type 2 diabetes (Simopoulos, 1999). Sources include green leafy vegetables, flaxseed, and walnuts.

10. *Eat more mushrooms.* They retard the development of hypoglycemia and reduce hyperphagia, polydipsia, body weight loss, and glycated hemoglobin (Swanston-Flatt, Day, Flatt, & Bailey, 1989b).

11. *Sprinkle turmeric on food.* This spice can reduce blood sugar (Arun & Nalini, 2002; Shekhar, Achike, Kaur, Kumar, & Hashim, 2002) and ameliorate renal lesions associated with diabetes (Suresh & Srinivasan, 1998).

12. *Try coenzyme Q10* (10 mg/kg/day). This enzyme can relieve sleep disturbance, paresthesia and edema of the legs, and palpitations (Suzuki et al., 1997) and reverse diabetic effects on liver, kidneys, heart, and brain (Rauscher, Sanders, Watkins, & Pettit, 2001).

TOPICAL APPLICATIONS

Castor oil has an anti-inflammatory effect and has been used to reduce eyelid and extremity edema (Vieira et al., 2000). Topical .075% *capsaicin* may be of value in diabetic neuropathy and intractable pain (Tandan, Lewis, Krusinski, Badger, & Fries, 1992).

LOG FOOD TO CONTROL BLOOD SUGAR

Ask clients to log their last meal or snack anytime their blood sugar is above 150 mg/dL. That will allow them to discover offending foods and gain a sense of power over their blood sugar (Dockter, 2002).

AVOID DIABETES-ASSOCIATED DRUGS

Some clients on protease-inhibitor therapy have developed new-onset diabetes, and others who already had the condition have experienced loss of blood glucose control (FDA, 1997). At the least, report cases of diabetes, hypoglycemia, or any other serious signs and symptoms associated with use of protease inhibitors to MED-WATCH at 1-800-FDA-1088. Beta-blockers and diuretics promote an undesirable lipid profile that contributes to insulin resistance (Kelley, 1997).

BREAST FEEDING

To protect children from diabetes, breast feed them. Several studies provide evidence that cow's milk can trigger diabetes in children (Monetini et al., 2001; Virtanen et al., 2000;).

HERBS

1. *Aloe vera pulp* from the leaves has been shown to reduce blood glucose level (Okyar, Can, Akev, Baktir, & Sutiupinar, 2001).

2. *Golden seal, tarragon, bearberry, and mistletoe* reduce the hyperphagia and polydipsia associated with diabetes (Swanston-Flatt et al., 1989a).

3. *Fig leaf tea* has a hypoglycemic action (Serraclara et al., 1998).

4. *Use gingko and panax ginseng.* Both have been used to treat symptoms related to venous and lymphatic vessel insufficiency and digestive disorders, and to stabilize membranes through antioxidant and radical scavenging actions (Li et al., 1998; Liberti, 1985; Savickiene et al., 2002).

5. *Licorice root* ameliorates postural hypotension caused by diabetic autonomic neuropathy (Basso, Dalla, Erie, Boscarok, & Armanini, 1994).

6. *Ginseng* root can lower glucose levels (Attelle et al., 2002; Lim et al., 2002). **Caution:** Do not use this herb if you have high blood pressure.

7. *Try fenugreek seeds as a tea or powder.* Fenugreek seeds have shown significant antidiabetic effects (Murray, 1994; Sharma, Raghuram, & Rao, 1990; Shekhar et al., 2002).

8. *Take milk thistle* (silymarin), an antioxidant that enhances function of the liver, an organ that works with the pancreas to regulate glucose level. A study showed that taking 600 mg of silymarin daily reduced glucose by 9.5 to 15% over 12 months, lowered the level of sugar in the urine, lowered the amount of insulin required, and showed less glucose damage to the cells (Velussi et al., 1997). Silymarin can also decrease glucose and triglyceride plasma levels in clients with diabetes and chronic alcoholic liver disease (Lirussi et al., 2002).

9. *Mushroom and guayusa* improve the effect of insulin (Swanston-Flatt et al., 1989b).

Vitamins and Supplements

Preventing diabetes is especially important now that several studies have shown that older adults with diabetes have almost twice the risk that nondiabetic persons do of developing dementia or Alzheimer's disease, and those who take insulin for diabetes have a fourfold risk (Ott, Stolk, & van Harskamp, 1999). This notion of vascular involvement and the link to silent cerebral infarcts makes it especially important to aid circulation.

1. *Take additional vitamin E* to reduce the risk of hardening of the arteries (atherosclerosis) in people with diabetes (Fuller, Chandalia, Garg, Grundy, & Jialal, 1996). Epidemiological evidence indicates low vitamin E intake is a risk factor for the development of type 2 diabetes, and small scale human intervention studies indicate that the vitamin can improve endothelial function, retinal blood flow, and renal dysfunction (Halliwell, 2002). Ten ml of Concord grape juice may work just as well (O'Byrne, Devaraj, Grundy, & Jialal, 2002) or eat plenty of nutritional yeast, wheat germ, peanuts, outer leaf of cabbage, leafy portions of broccoli and cauliflower, raw spinach, asparagus, whole grain rice or oats, cornmeal, eggs, and sweet potatoes (Mayer-Davis, Costacou, King, Zaccaro, & Bell, 2002).

2. *Add a vitamin C supplement to protect the ocular surface milieu* (Peponis et al., 2002) or eat foods that contain vitamin C (see Nutritional Approaches above).

3. *Take 500 mg/day of vitamin C and 800 IU/day of vitamin E with 500 ml tomato juice.* This combination was shown to increase plasma lycopene levels and the intrinsic resistance of LDL to oxidation almost as effectively as supplementation with a high dose of vitamin E and may reduce risk of myocardial infarction in clients with diabetes (Upritchard, Sutherland, & Mann, 2000).

4. *Avoid taking supplements containing the amino acid cysteine (interferes with insulin absorption), and large amounts of vitamin B1 (thiamine).* Excessive amounts can inactivate insulin.

5. *Take additional chromium, aloe vera, and vanadium.* All have been shown to be useful in the treatment of diabetes (Yeh et al., 2003).

6. Chromium improves insulin binding, but many clients with type 2 diabetes have a chromium deficiency (Pettit, 2001). Elevated

intakes of supplemental chromium as chromium picolinate (100 microg two times per day) can have significant beneficial effects on glucose, insulin, and cholesterol (Anderson et al., 2001).

7. *Obtain sufficient vitamin D* as a supplement or by obtaining sufficient protected sunlight.

8. *Get extra zinc, iron, and manganese* (Shvets, Kramarenko, Vydyborets, & Gaidukova, 1994). Zinc status in clients with diabetes is significantly lower than in healthy individuals. Ho and colleagues (2001) concluded that zinc supplementation can significantly inhibit the development of type 1 diabetes. Because too much zinc can lower the immune system's function, consider instead eating foods high in the mineral, including oysters, herring, eggs, nuts, wheat germ, and organically grown liver and red meat. Iron and manganese can be found in a good multivitamin or cook food in iron pots and eat more nuts, seeds, whole grain, fruits and vegetables, dry beans and peas, and unprocessed oatmeal (Clark, 1996).

9. *Ingest additional magnesium.* Hypomagnesemia is associated with the development of neuropathy and abnormal platelet activity, both of which add to the risk for foot ulcers (Rodriguez-Moran & Guerrero-Romero, 2001). Instead of a supplement, eat more whole grain breads and cereals, fresh peas, brown rice, soy products, wheat germ, nuts, Swiss chard, figs, green leafy vegetables, and citrus fruits (Clark, 1996).

10. *Take alpha lipoic acid as a supplement* (50–200 mg a day). It greatly improves insulin function and protects against nerve damage, a complication of diabetes (Nagamatsu et al., 1995), hypertension, hyperglycemia, and the increase in heart mitochondrial superoxide production (Midaoui, Elimadi, Wu, Haddad, & de Champlain, 2003).

11. *Use evening primrose oil.* A rich source of gamma-linolenic acid, evening primrose oil helps to reduce urine calcium excretion (Tulloch, Smellie, & Buck, 1994).

DAILY EXERCISE

Nine out of 10 cases of type 2 diabetes could be prevented if clients exercised more, ate better, and adopted other healthy behaviors (Hu et al., 2001). Even postmenopausal women have a lower risk of developing diabetes if they are physically active (Agurs-Collins, Kumanyika, & Adams-Campbell, 1997; Folsom, Kushi, & Hong, 2000). Walking and a healthy diet can lead to a lessened need for oral diabetes medicines (Harper, 2002).

PRACTICE INTERNAL EXERCISES

These ancient movements are believed to filter toxins from the body, increase energy flow, and build up the relationship between the digestive organs, stomach, and liver (Chang, 1986). Here are two examples.

Sit or lie in a comfortable position and place the palm of the right hand on the base of the rib cage. Follow the ribs up toward the sternum, rubbing across and then down the left lateral side of the chest. Repeat the movement up to 26 times, using the heel of the hand. Alternate hands, beginning the next round with the left hand on the lateral left side and follow the lower ribs to the right side, completing 36 rotations.

Stand and place hands on the outside of the thighs. In a continuous motion, rub the hands down the inside of the thighs to the ankles, breathing normally and then coming back up the inside of the thighs. In the morning, upon arising, practice the upward massage only.

BIOFEEDBACK

Biofeedback-assisted relaxation has been shown to afford control of insulin-dependent diabetes (McGrady, 1993).

COUNSELING

Seven to twenty psychotherapy sessions can help clients diagnosed with diabetes to cope better and reduce medical bills (Schlesinger, 1983). If you aren't a clinical specialist in psychiatric/mental health nursing, consider referring clients to a colleague who can provide psychotherapy.

AUTOGENIC TRAINING

Autogenic training in children and adolescents with type 1 diabetes for a period of 11 weeks has resulted in a significant reduction in the need for aggressive forms of dominance behavior, emotional lability, and tendency to depend on adults, and increased self-confidence about one's own meaning, decisions and planning ability (Gehr, Ropcke, Pister, & Eggers, 1997).

ENVIRONMENTAL ACTIONS

Light exposure at night during sleep may help prevent retinopathy in diabetes by inhibiting the eyes' response to darkness. Light transmission through closed lids is sufficient (Drasdo, Chiti, Owens, & North, 2002).

MASSAGE

Massaging the suboccipital muscles can unblock the swollen sinus openings and may be helpful to clients suffering from diabetes (Griner & Nunes, 1996). Refer to page 43 for the technique.

For leg ulcers, promote healing in the ulcer by gently and carefully massaging the red center of the ulceration in a circular manner once a day. To block pain, use a mixture of 2% lidocaine or any sunburn ointment containing lidocaine. If not available, ice the area prior to massage and use an antibacterial ointment. Honey can also be used as it covers a much broader range of antibacterial, antifungal, and antiviral activity than a simple antibiotic (Williams, 1999). This method increases circulation and healing. After a few days begin to massage the area more firmly and gradually expand the massage to include the outer rim of the circle. Leave only a light covering of lubrication (vitamin E will work) and leave the wound exposed to the air (Dawson, 1998).

MAGNETS

Wearing magnet-laden socks may reduce diabetic foot pain (Weintraub, 1998). Magnets attached to auricular acupuncture points may also lower blood glucose levels and improve eye conditions (Chen, 2002). Exposing clients to impulsed magnetic fields has been shown to reduce blood sugar more quickly than conservative therapy alone (Kirillov, Suchkova, Lastushkin, Sigaev, & Nekhaeva, 1996).

YOGA

Changes in blood glucose and glucose tolerance occurred after 40 days of yoga therapy in 149 non-insulin-dependent diabetic clients (Jain, Uppal, Bhatnagar, & Talukdar, 1993).

AFFIRMATIONS

To begin to reverse negative thoughts that could be damaging, ask clients to choose one of the following statements and write or say it

20 times a day. Also write it on 3 x 5 cards and put them in prominent places around them.

- I fill each moment with joy and sweetness.
- I experience the wonder and sweetness of this day.

TREATMENT EVALUATION

The client described above evaluated his feelings about his son. For the first time, he was able to acknowledge that it wasn't his fault that his son died. He has begun a walking program and has lost 5 pounds so far. He is taking a cooking class and learning to prepare wellness meals.

REFERENCES

Agurs-Collins, T. D., Kumanyika, T. R., & Adams-Campbell, L. L. (1997). A randomized controlled trial of weight reduction and exercise for diabetes management in older African-American subjects. *Diabetes Care, 20,* 1503–1511.

Anderson, R. A., Roussel, A. M., Zouari, N., Mahjoub, S., Matheau, J. M., & Kerkeni, A. (2001). Potential antioxidant effects of zinc and chromium supplementation in people with type 2 diabetes mellitus. *Journal of the American College of Nutrition, 20,* 212–218.

Arun, N., & Nalini, N. (2002). Efficacy of turmeric on blood sugar and polyol pathway in diabetic albino rats. *Plant Foods in Human Nutrition, 57,* 41–52.

Attelle, A. S., Zhou, Y. P., Xie, J. T., Wu, J. A., Zhang, L., Dey, L., et al. (2002). Antidiabetic effects of Panax ginseng berry extract and the identification of an effective component. *Diabetes, 51,* 1851–1858.

Augusti, K. T. (1996). Therapeutic values of onion and garlic. *Indian Journal of Experimental Biology, 34,* 634–640.

Babu, P. S., & Srinivasan, K. (1997). Influence of dietary capsaicin and onion on the metabolic abnormalities associated with streptozotocin induced diabetes mellitus. *Molecular Cell Biochemistry, 175*(1–2), 49–57.

Basso, A., Dalla, P. L., Erle, G.; Boscarok M., & Armanini, D. (1994). Licorice ameliorates postural hypotension caused by diabetic autonomic neuropathy. *Diabetic Care, 17,* 1356.

Brancati, F. L., Wang, N., Mead, L. A., Kiang, K., & Klag, M. J. (1999). Body weight patterns from 20 to 49 years of age and subsequent risk for diabetes mellitus: The Johns Hopkins Precursors Study. *Archives of Internal Medicine, 159,* 957–963.

Chang, S. T. (1986). *The complete system of self-healing internal exercises.* San Francisco: Tao.

Chen, Y. (2002). Magnets on ears helped diabetics. *American Journal of Chinese Medicine, 30*(1), 183–185.

Cheng, J. T., & Yang, R. S. (1983). Hypoglycemic effect of guava juice in mice and human subjects. *American Journal of Chinese Medicine, 11*(1-4), 74–76.

Clark, C C. (1996). *Wellness practitioner: Concepts, research and strategies.* New York: Springer Publishing Co.

Cow's milk, diabetes connection bolstered. (1999). *Science News, 155,* 4044–4055.

Dawson, J. B. (1998). Massage for leg ulcers. *American Family Physician, 57,* 2628–2629.

Diabetes Prevention Program Research Group. (2002). Reduction in the incidence of Type 2 diabetes with lifestyle intervention or metformin. *New England Journal of Medicine, 346,* 393–403.

Dockter, T. (2002, March). Make diabetic diet detectives. *Clinical Advisor, 71.*

Drasdo, N., Chiti, Z., Owens, D. R., & North, R. V. (2002). Effect of darkness on inner retinal hypoxia in diabetes. *Lancet, 359,* 2251–2253.

FDA. (1997). *Public Health Advisory.* Accessed June 11, 1997, from http://www.fda.gov/ceder/proteaseletter.htm

Folsom, A. R., Kushi, L. H., & Hong, C. P. (2000). Physical activity and incident diabetes mellitus in postmenopausal women. *American Journal of Public Health, 90,* 134–138.

Ford, E. S., & Mokdad, A. H. (2001). Fruit and vegetable consumption and diabetes mellitus incidence among U.S. adults. *Preventive Medicine, 32*(1), 33–39.

Fuller, C. J., Chandalia, M., Garg, A., Grundy, S. M., & Jialal, I. (1996). RRR-Alpha-tocopherol acetate supplementation at pharmacologic dose decreases low-density lipoproprotein oxidative susceptibility but not protein glycation in patients with diabetes mellitus. *American Journal of Clinical Nutrition, 63,* 753–759.

Garg, A., Bonanome, A., Grundy, S. M., Ahang, Z., & Unger, R. H. (1988). Comparison of a high carbohydrate diet with a high monounsaturated fat diet in patients with non–insulin-dependent diabetes mellitus. *New England Journal of Medicine, 319,* 829–834.

Gehr, M., Ropcke, B., Pister, K., & Eggers, C. (1997). Autogenic training in children and adolescents with type 1 diabetes mellitus. *Prax Kinderpsychology und Kinderpsychiatry, 46,* 288–303.

Griner, T., & Nunes, M. (1996). *What's really wrong with you? A revolutionary look at how muscles affect health* Garden City Park, NY: Avery.

Halliwell, B. (2002). Vitamin E and the treatment and prevention of diabetes: A case for a controlled clinical trial. *Singapore Medicine Journal, 43,* 479–484.

Harper, P. (2002). Diet, walking replace medications for some. *Clinician Reviews, 12*(10), 96–97.

Ho, E., Quan, N., Tsai, Y. H., Lai, W., & Bray, T. M. (2001). Dietary zinc supplementation inhibits NFkappaB activation and protects against chemically induced diabetes in CD1 mice. *Experimental Biological Medicine, 226,* 103–111.

Hu, F. B., Manson, J. E., Meir, J., Stampfer, M. J., Colditz, G., Liu, S., et al. (2001). Diet, lifestyle and the risk of type 2 diabetes in women. *New England Journal of Medicine, 345,* 790–794.

Jain, S. C., Uppal, A., Bhatnagar, S. O., & Talukdar, B. (1993). A study of response pattern of non-insulin dependent diabetics to yoga therapy. *Diabetes Research in Clinical Practice, 19,* 69–74.

Jung, Y. S., Kim, M. H., Lee, S. H., Baik, E. J., Park, S. W., & Moon, C. H. (2002). Antithrombotic effect of onion in streptozotocin-induced diabetic rat. *Prostaglandins Leukot and Essential Fatty Acids, 66,* 453–458.

Kelley, C. D. P. (1997). Understanding Syndrome X. *Clinician Reviews, 7*(10), 55–63, 69–70, 73–74, 76, 78, 80.

Kirillov, I. B., Suchkova, Z. V., Lastushkin, A. V., Sigaev, A. A., & Nekhaeva, T. I. (1996). Magnetotherapy in the comprehensive treatment of vascular complications of diabetes mellitus. *Klinical Medicine (Mosk), 74*(5), 39–41.

Knekt, P., Kumpulainen, J., Jarvinen, R., Rissanen, H., Heliovaara, M., Reunanen, A., et al. (2002). Flavonoid intake and risk of chronic diseases. *American Journal of Clinical Nutrition, 76,* 560–568.

Lean, M. E., Noroozi, M., Kelly, I., Burns, J., Talwar, D., Sattar, N., & Crozier, A. (1999). Dietary flavonols protect diabetic human lymphocytes against oxidative damage to DNA. *Diabetes, 48,* 176–181.

Li, A. L., Shi, Y. D., Landsmann, B., Schanowski-Bouvier, P., Dikta, G., Bauer, U., et al. (1998). Hemorheology and walking of peripheral arterial occlusive diseases patients during treatment with Ginkgo biloba extract. *Zhongguo Yao Li Xue Bao, 19,* 417–421.

Liberti, L. E. (1985). Therapeutic uses of gingko. *Lawrence Review of Natural Products, 6*(6), 1–4.

Lim, B. V., Shin, M. C., Jang, M. H., Lee, T. H., Kim, Y. P., Kim, H. B., et al. (2002). Ginseng radix increases cell proliferation in dentate gyrus of rats with streptozotocin-induced diabetes. *Biological Pharmacy Bulletin, 25,* 1550–1554.

Lirussi, F., Beccarello, A., Zanette, G., De Monte, A., Donadon, V., Velussi, M., et al. (2002). Silybin-beta-cyclodextrin in the treatment of patients with diabetes mellitus and alcoholic liver disease: Efficacy study of a new preparation of an anti-oxidant agent. *Diabetes Nutrition and Metabolism, 15,* 222–231.

Lukaczer, D. (1998, July). Managing high insulin levels. *Health and Nutrition Breakthrough,* 36.

Matsuda, H., Murakami, T., Shimada, H., Matsummura, N., Yoshikawa, M., & Yamahara, J. (1997). Inhibitory mechanisms of oleanolic acid 3-O-monodesmosides on glucose absorption in rats. *Biological Pharmacy Bulletin, 20,* 717–719.

Mayer-Davis, E. J., Costacou, T., King, I., Zaccaro, D. J., & Bell, R. A. (2002). Plasma and dietary vitamin E in relation to incidence of type 2 diabetes: The Insulin Resistance and Atherosclerosis Study (IRAS). *Diabetes Care, 25,* 2172–2177.

McCarty, M. F. (2002). Favorable impact of a vegan diet with exercise on hemorheology: Implications for control of diabetic neuropathy. *Medical Hypotheses, 58,* 476–486.

McGrady, A. (1993). *Biofeedback assisted relaxation in control of insulin dependent diabetes.* Accessed July 21, 1997 from http://altmed.od.nih. gov/oam/cgi-bin/research/search_simple.cgi

McGrath, L. T., Brennan, G. M., Donnelly, J. P., Johnston, G. D., Hayes, J. R., & McVeigh, G. E. (1996). Effect of dietary fish oil supplementation on peroxidation of serum lipids in patients with non-insulin dependent diabetes mellitus. *Atherosclerosis, 121,* 275–283.

Midaoui, A. E., Elimadi, A., Wu, L., Haddad, P. S., & de Champlain, J. (2003). Lipoic acid prevents hypertension, hyperglycemia, and the increase in heart mitochondrial superoxide production. *American Journal of Hypertension 16,* 173–179.

Miller, A. W., Hoenig, M. E., & Ujhelyi, M. R. (1998). Mechanisms of impaired endothelial function associated with insulin resistance. *Journal of Cardiovascular Pharmacology Therapy, 3,* 125–134.

Monetini, L., Cavallo, M. G., Stefanini, L., Ferrazzoli, F., Bizzarri, C., Marietti, G., et al. (2001). Bovine beta-casein antibodies in breast- and bottle-fed infants: Their relevance in Type 1 diabetes. *Diabetes Metabolism Research Reviews, 17,* 51–54.

Murray, J. T. (1994). Are botanical medicines useful in diabetes? *American Journal of Natural Medicine, 1(3),* 5–7.

Nagamatsu, M., Nickander, K. K., Schmelzer, J. D., Raya, A., Wittrock, D. A., Tritscherl, H., et al. (1995). Lipoic acid improves nerve blood flow, reduces oxidative stress, and improves distal nerve conduction in experimental diabetic neuropathy. *Diabetes Care, 18,* 1160–1167.

Nagaraj, R. H., Kern, T. S., Sell, D. R., Fogarty, J., Engerman, R. L., & Monnier, V. M. (1996). Evidence of a glycemic threshold for the formation of pentosidine in diabetic dog lens but not in collagen. *Diabetes, 45,* 587–594.

O'Byrne, D. J., Devaraj, S., Grundy, S. M., & Jialal, I. (2002). Comparison of the antioxidant effects of Concord grape juice flavonoids alpha-tocopherol n markers of oxidative stress in healthy adults. *American Journal of Clinical Nutrition, 76,* 1367–1374.

Okyar, A., Can, A., Akev, N., Baktir, G., & Sutiupinar, N. (2001). Effect of Aloe vera leaves on blood glucose level in type I and type II diabetic rat models. *Phytotherapy Research, 15,* 157–161.

Ott, A., Stolk, R. P., & van Harskamp, F. (1999). Diabetes mellitus and the risk of dementia: The Rotterdam study. *Neurology, 53*, 1937–1942.

Peponis, V., Papathanasiou, M., Kapranou, A., Magkou, C., Tyligada, A., Melidonis, A., et al. (2002). Protective role of oral antioxidant supplementation in ocular surface of diabetic patients. *British Journal of Ophthalmology, 86*, 1369–1373.

Pereira, M. A., Jacobs, D. R., Jr., Pins, J. J., Raatz, S. K., Gross, M. D., Slavin, J. L., et al. (2002). Effect of whole grains on insulin sensitivity in overweight hyperinsulinemic adults. *American Journal of Clinical Nutrition, 75*, 848–855.

Pettit, J. L. (2001). Alternative medicine: Chromium. *Clinican Reviews, 11*(10), 66, 72.

Rauscher, F. M., Sanders, R. A., & Watkins, J. B., 3rd, & Pettit, J. L. (2001). Effects of coenzyme Q10 treatment on antioxidant pathways in normal and streptozotocin-induced diabetic rats. *Journal of Biochemical and Molecular Toxicology, 15*(1), 41–46.

Rodriguez-Moran, M., & Guerrero-Romero, F. (2001). Low serum magnesium levels and foot ulcers in subjects with type 2 diabetes. *Archives of Medical Research, 32*, 300–303.

Root-Bernstein, R., Busik, J. V., & Henry, D. N. (2002). Are diabetic neuropathy, retinopathy and nephropathy caused by hyperglycemic exclusion of dehydroascorbate uptake by glucose transporters? *Journal of Theoretical Biology, 216*, 345–359.

Salmeron, J., Manson, J. E., & Stampfer, M. J. (1997). Dietary fiber, glycemic load, and risk of non-insulin-dependent diabetes mellitus in women. *Journal of the American Medical Association, 277*, 472–477.

Savickiene, N., Dagilyte, A., Lukosius, A., & Zitkevicius, V. (2002). Importance of biologically active components and plants in the prevention of complications of diabetes mellitus. *Medicina, 38*, 970–975.

Schlesinger, R. (1983). Psychotherapy can lower medical costs. *American Journal of Public Health, 73*, 422–430.

Serraclara, A., Hawkins, F., Perez, C., Dominguez, E., Campello, J. E., & Torres, M. D. (1998). Hypoglycemic action of an oral fig leaf decoction in type-1 diabetes. *Diabetes Research in Clinical Practice, 39*(1), 19–22.

Sharma, R. D., Raghuram, T. C., & Rao, N. S. (1990). Effect of fenugreek seeds on blood glucose and serum lipids in type 1 diabetes. *European Journal of Clinical Nutrition, 44*, 301–306.

Sheela, C. G., & Augusti, K. T. (1992). Antidiabetic effects of S-ayl cysteine sulphoxide isolated garlic. *Indian Journal of Experimental Biology, 30*, 523–526.

Shekhar, K. C., Achike, F. I., Kaur, G., Kumar, P., & Hashim, R. (2002). A preliminary evaluation of the efficacy and safety of Cogent db (an Ayurvedic drug) in the glycemic control of patients with type 2 diabetes. *Journal of Alternative and Complementary Medicine, 8*(4), 445–457.

Shvets, N. V., Kramarenko, L. D., Vydyborets, S. V., & Gaidukova, S. N. (1994). Disordered trace element content of the erythrocytes in diabetes mellitus. *Likarstka Sprava, 1,* 52–55.

Simopoulos, A. P. (1999). Essential fatty acids in health and chronic disease. *American Journal of Clinical Nutrition, 70*(3, Suppl.), 560S–569S.

Suresh, B. P., & Srinivasan, K. (1998). Amelioration of renal lesions associated with diabetes by dietary curcumin in streptozotocin diabetic rats. *Molecular Cell Biochemistry, 181*(1-2), 87–96.

Suzuki, Y., Taniyama, M., Muramatsu, T., Atsumi, Y., Hosokawa, K., Asahina, T., et al. (1997). Diabetes mellitus associated with 3243 mitochondrial tRNA [Leu(UUR)] mutation: Clinical features and coenzyme Q10 treatment. *Molecular Aspects of Medicine, 18*(Suppl.), S181–S188.

Swanston-Flatt, S. K., Day, C., Bailey, C. J., & Flatt, P. R. (1989a). Evaluation of traditional plant treatments for diabetes. *Acta Diabetology Latina, 26*(1), 51–55.

Swanston-Flatt, S. K., Day, C., Flatt, P. R., & Bailey, C. J. (1989b). Glycaemic effects of traditional European plant treatments for diabetes. *Acta Diabetology Latina, 10*(2), 69–73.

Tandan, R., Lewis, G. A., Krusinski, P. B., Badger, G. B., & Fries, T. J. (1992). Topical capsaicin in painful diabetic neuropathy: Controlled study with long-term follow-up. *Diabetes Care, 15*(1), 8–14.

Ting, H. H., Timini, F. K., & Boles, K. S. (1996). Vitamin C improves endothelium-dependent vasodilation in patients with non–insulin-dependent diabetes mellitus. *Journal of Clinical Investigation, 97*(1), 22–28.

Tulloch, I., Smellie, W. S., & Buck, A. C. (1994). Evening primrose oil reduces urinary calcium excretion in both normal and hypercalciuric rats. *Urology Research, 22,* 227–230.

Upritchard, J. E., Sutherland, W. H., & Mann, J. L. (2000). Effect of supplementation with tomato juice, vitamin E, and vitamin C on LDL oxidation and products of inflammatory activity in type 2 diabetes. *Diabetes Care, 23,* 733–738.

Velussi, M., Cernigoi, A. M., De Monte, A. D., Dapas, F., Caffau, C., & Zilli, M. (1997). Long term (12 months) treatment with an antioxidant (silymarin) is effective on hyperinsulinemia, exogenous insulin and malondialdehyde levels in cirrhotic diabetic patients. *Journal of Hepatology, 16,* 871–879.

Vieira, C., Evangelista, S., Cirillo, R., Lippi, A., Maggi, C. A., & Manzini, S. (2000). Effect of ricinoleic acid in acute and subchronic experimental models of inflammation. *Mediators Inflammation, 9,* 223–228.

Vincent, J. B. (2000). Quest for the molecular mechanism of chromium action and its relationship to diabetes. *Nutrition Reviews, 58*(3, part 1), 67–72.

Virtanen, S. M., Laara, E., Hypponen, E., Reijonen, H., Rasanen, L., Aro, A., et al. (2000). Cow's milk consumption, HLA-DQB1 genotype, and type 1 diabetes: A nested case-control study of siblings of children with diabetes. Childhood Diabetes in Finland Study Group. *Diabetes, 49,* 912–917.

Vuksan, V., Stavro, M. P., Sievnenpiper, J. L., Koo, V. Y., Wong, E., Beljan-Zdravkovic, U., et al. (2000). American ginseng improves glycemia in individuals with normal glucose tolerance. *Journal of the American College of Nutrition, 19,* 738–744.

Weintraub, M. I. (1998). Chronic submaximal magnetic stimulation in peripheral neuropathy: Is there a beneficial therapeutic relationship? *American Journal of Pain Management, 8*(1), 12–16.

Whittemore, R., Chase, S. K., Mandle, C. L., & Roy, C. (2002). Lifestyle change in type 2 diabetes. *Nursing Research, 51*(1), 18–25.

Williams, D. G. (1999). Massage technique for diabetic ulcers. *American Family Physician, 57,* 2628–2629.

CHAPTER 11

Digestive Problems

Digestive problems run the gamut from constipation, diarrhea, and flatulence to Crohn's disease, colitis, diverticular disease, irritable bowel syndrome, ulcers, leaky gut syndrome, and esophageal reflux disease. Many digestive conditions have similar symptoms. Medical care includes a wide variety of medications, depending on the most prominent symptoms. For example, antacids and acid-blocking drugs such as Tagamet and Zantac may be used for heartburn or ulcers. Both can make it difficult for the body to absorb necessary nutrients from food.

HOLISTIC NURSING ASSESSMENT

Study the holistic nursing assessment for Ms. K., a 26-year-old client diagnosed with digestive problems, that follows. Working in collaboration with clients diagnosed with digestive disorders, use the format that follows to assess them.

Client learning needs: To find a way to manage inflammation and lack of digestion.

Indicants of readiness to learn: "I want to feel more comfortable after I eat."

Soul/spirituality symbol(s): "I wear this cross to protect me."

Meaning of the condition to client: "I started a new job and my new boss expects too much of me. When we moved, I had to leave my friends. I really miss them."

155

Relationship needs/effects as perceived by the client: "My boss is a dictator, but I can't afford to quit. I have to support my daughter, but since we moved closer to my job, my daughter has been doing poorly in her new school."

Patterns/attitudes that may create dis-ease for this client: Client uses negative affirmations (e.g., "I'll never get the hang of this job and no one else will hire me").

Life purpose: Expresses no life purpose.

Client strengths: Wants to learn how to deal with her boss, how to manage her new job, and find new friends.

Ability to participate in care: Client can participate fully in care.

Ethical dilemmas: None identified.

Nurse–client process: Client denies any part in her digestive disease and searches for a "medical" reason to explain it.

TREATMENT PLANNING: SETTING JOINTLY AGREED-UPON GOALS

In the case of the client discussed above, the following goals were agreed upon:

1. Find new friends.
2. Use a symptom/mood diary to track the connection between her feelings and digestive symptoms.
3. Ask boss for tips on doing a good job at work.
4. Assist daughter to adjust to new school.

TREATMENT

Acceptance of condition/attitude change: The client chose the following affirmation to use to replace the upset she feels: "What I take in I assimilate easily and eliminate what isn't needed." Client agreed to write the affirmation on 3 x 5 cards and say the words at least 20 times each day.

Facilitating the healing process/healing intention formulation: From a list of meditative statements, client chose the following one to assist in the healing process: "I am at peace with my life." Asked client to meditate on the words while in a relaxed state. Nurse will use caring nonverbal and verbal communication, centering, and a meditative state to enhance client healing, will verbalize observed patterns that may be holding the client back and offer alternate approaches.

Creating a sacred space: During client sessions, music of her choice will play in the background and lavender aromatherapy will assist with the relaxation process.

Encouraging re-storying: Encouraged client to recall an upsetting situation with her new boss and choose an ending that inspires her.

Integrative practices planned: Will use therapeutic touch and guided imagery to assist client in the healing process.

Role model strategies: Showed client how to role play problematic interchanges with her boss and daughter.

Protection plan: Requested client use an image of the cross to protect her when she feels fear or doubt.

Family strategies: Encouraged client to invite her daughter to a session with nurse to practice more open communication between them.

Life issues/life purpose work: Client has agreed to write in her journal about life purpose.

Treatment possibilities/considerations: Other suggested treatments appear below. Most are evidence-based.

ADDITIONAL INFORMATION AND TREATMENT FOR CLIENTS

APPROACHES FOR ALL DIGESTIVE CONDITIONS

1. *Chew well before swallowing.* This will trigger acid in the stomach and enzymes that aid in digestion. This action will also put less stress on the rest of the digestive system.

2. *Move toward a vegetarian diet.* Vegetarians have lower cholesterol and may also have a lower risk for constipation, diverticular disease, appendicitis, and gallstones (Key, Davey, & Appleby, 1999).

3. *To have healthy digestive enzymes, eat foods rich in B-vitamins, zinc, magnesium, pantothenic acid, biotin, molybdenum, manganese, copper, iron, and selenium.* Each plays the role of digestive enzyme cofactor. Foods rich in these nutrients include seeds (pumpkin and sunflower), whole grains, rolled oats, green peas, seafood (crabmeat,

salmon, tuna, mackerel, sardines, trout, herring, lobster, oysters), brown rice, raisins, wheat germ, chicken, nuts (hazelnuts, hickory nuts, walnuts, almonds), spinach, kale, peas, prunes, lentils, turkey, rabbit, bananas, sweet potatoes, cooked cabbage, sea vegetables (kombu, dulse, kelp, wakame), fermented soy products (tempeh, natto, miso), turnips, cantaloupe, buckwheat, broccoli, cauliflower, figs, green leafy vegetables especially dandelion greens, citrus fruits, liver, eggs, nutritional yeast, mushrooms, yogurt, beans (kidney beans, white beans, lima beans, soybeans), dark green leafy vegetables, avocados, barley, lentils, asparagus, and garlic.

4. *Avoid drinking fluids, especially cold ones, when eating.* They can suppress stomach acid (Mindell & Hopkins, 1998). A large percentage of people over 50 make too little stomach acid and so they aren't able to thoroughly digest their food. Taking antacids, Tagamet, and Zantac can alleviate symptoms for a while, but they can aggravate the underlying problem. Long-term use of these drugs can compromise digestion and decrease the uptake of needed vitamins and minerals.

5. *Drink a teacupful of hot water 1 hour before each meal.* Alternately, squeeze a lemon into the cup of hot water and drink.

6. *Test to see if the amount of stomach acid is appropriate.* Take a tablespoon of apple cider vinegar or lemon juice at heartburn. If the heartburn goes away, more acid, not less is needed. If symptoms worsen, take enzyme products or supplements that contain HCL. Find them at any health food store (Williams, 1995).

6. *Drink fresh vegetable juices daily.* Extra vitamin A can promote healing of the intestines. Buy a juicer at a health food store and combine 12 ounces of carrot juice with 2 ounces of kale, watercress, beet, spinach, or dandelion juice.

7. *Eat papaya or fresh pineapple, pears, blackberries, strawberries, or tangerines to aid digestion* (Davis, 1980).

8. *Drink 2–3 ounces of aloe vera juice after each meal.* (Do not use an aloe plant; buy the juice from a health food store.)

9. *Take probiotics such as acidophilus and bifidus ("good" bacteria) to restore the normal flora of the intestinal tract.*

10. *Use extra virgin olive oil for salads, cooking, baked potatoes, bread, and noodles.* A review of studies of olive oil reported that patients with ulcerative colitis and Crohn's disease generate high quantities of reactive oxygen species. Antioxidant compounds present in olive oil inhibit this free radical generation and enhance healthy tissue (Owen et al., 2000). Take a teaspoonful when digestive tract is irritated; it will soothe and coat inflamed tissue.

11. *Massage ileocecal valve points.* A lazy ileocecal valve can make it difficult for the body to process food properly, resulting in food backing up or moving too quickly through the body. Massaging some points on the body could help. These points may be extremely sore at first. If too weak to complete the massage, use a vibrator (available in health food and department stores). Massage with firm pressure for no longer than 10–20 seconds (a) the inside and outside of the thighs, (b) angling across the top of the left arm, (c) beneath the bony ridge that runs across the back of the head on the right side, and (d) the outside of the right calf about a third of the way down from the knee. Massaging longer than 20 seconds is not beneficial and could negate the effect. For "backed up" conditions, detoxify the body by taking chlorophyll tablets or liquid, eliminating spicy foods for a week or ten days, and totally eliminating alcohol, cocoa, chocolate, and caffeine products (Williams, 1990).

12. *Gently hold the following points* with the 2nd, 3rd, and 4th fingers of each hand on its own side of the body until a pulsation is felt in each finger, then move on to the next spot: inside of knees, two inches outside of spinal cord just above the scapula, bottom of big toe, behind knees, and 1½ inches on either side of the spinal cord just below the scapula (Dayton, 1994).

13. *Unless allergic to these flowers, sip chamomile tea.* The dried flowers of this plant have sedative and spasmolytic effects (Avallone et al., 2000).

COLITIS

1. *Take acidophilus* (health food store) daily to restore the overgrowth of *Clostridia difficile,* an organism that can cause relentless colitis.

2. *Eliminate sweets, alcohol, and caffeine.* All can irritate the intestinal lining ("Fructose Linked to GI Distress," 2002).

3. *Avoid dairy products for a lactase deficiency.* These can trigger an inflammation in the intestine.

4. *Eat foods high in essential fatty acids.* These substances can prevent ulcerative colitis and are found in green leafy vegetables, flaxseed, rapeseed, and walnuts (Simopoulos, 1999).

5. *Take silymarin.* Milk thistle has been shown to be effective in animal studies of colitis (Cruz, Galvez, Crespo, Ocete, & Zarzuelo, 2001) and humans (Savickiene, Dagilyte, Lukosius, & Zitkevicius, 2002).

6. *Try chlorella.* This supplement may prove useful (Merchant & Andre, 2001).

7. *Explore hypnosis and meditation.* There is a strong association between atittude, stress, and flares of inflammatory bowel diseases (Anton, 1999).

8. *Use extravirgin olive oil.* Previous studies have shown that the colon mucosa of those suffering from ulcerative colitis generates appreciably higher quantities of reactive oxygen species compared with normal tissue. Extravirgin olive oil contains an abundance of phenolic antioxidants, potent inhibitors of reactive oxygen species (Owen et al., 2000).

CONSTIPATION

1. *Slowly move to a vegetarian eating style.* Vegetarians have a lower incidence of constipation (Key et al., 1999; Nair & Mayberry, 1994). Constipation is a result of a low-fiber diet. Eating vegetables, fruits, and grains increases fiber (McDougall, 1999).

2. *Drink at least 10 glasses of water every day.* Water is used by many digestive processes, and for them to work correctly, sufficient water must be supplied daily. Drink a glass of warm water with a little fresh lemon juice in it upon arising to stimulate the bowels (Williams, 1991).

3. *Avoid aluminum-containing antacids.* They cause constipation, intestinal blockage and dangerously high levels of aluminum (Mindell & Hopkins, 1998).

4. *Try psyllium.* Place a teaspoon in a full glass of water before breakfast and drink it down before it gels.

5. *Eat more fresh vegetables, fruits, legumes (dry beans, peas, and peanuts) and prunes.* Eating guava, plum, mango, and quince can also prevent Escherichia coli infections (Coutino-Rodriguez, Hernandez-Cruz, & Giles-Rios, 2001).

6. *Exercise every day.* Gradually build up to walking 20 minutes a day at a brisk clip. This will massage the digestive system and aid its function.

7. *Find alternatives to medicines that cause constipation* including diuretics, painkillers (especially nonsteroidal anti-inflammatory agents like aspirin), tranquilizers, calcium channel blockers, calcium supplements, 5HT3 antagonists, antihistamines, narcotics, decongestants, antidepressants, iron supplements, antiparkinsonian agents, and the overuse of laxatives (Mindell & Hopkins, 1998; Schiller, 2001). Beverley and Travis (1992) found a mixture of prune juice blended with raisins, currants, prunes, figs, and dates was as effective a laxative as drugs, enemas, or suppositories.

8. *Use acidophilus.* The culture taken with a little milk (for better absorption) or as plain yogurt with active cultures may also help. It builds up "good" bacteria, which help digest stagnating food and increase the movement of the intestine in a day or two.

9. *Take the herb silymarin (milk thistle).* It can reduce colon damage and has an anti-inflammatory activity (Cruz et al., 2001).

10. *Improve toileting habits.* Make a trip to the bathroom 10 to 60 minutes after eating and use a low step-stool under the feet when sitting on the toilet (Wolfsen, 1993).

11. *Use self-massage.*

A. Lie on the back, bend the head well forward. This tenses the abdominal muscles. Let the head fall back to the normal position and feel the muscles relax. While simultaneously raising and lowering the head, gently thump fists against the abdomen three to four times. As abdominal muscles strengthen, hit harder. This will enhance circulation and strengthen digestive organs. Finish by massaging the abdomen and then rest (Davis, 1980).

B. *The Crane.* Lie on a mat on the floor or on a bed. Place the hands palms down on the lower abdomen. Keep the mouth closed and inhale easily through the nostrils, exhaling slowly while pressing the hands down lightly on the abdomen. Slowly inhale and extend the abdomen outward like a balloon, keeping the chest still. Work up to 12 rounds of inhaling and exhaling (Chang, 1986).

C. Hold index, third, and fourth fingers on each spot until a steady pulse is felt in each finger: inside of each knee, bottom of both big toes, middle back of hip bone, either side of chest (Dayton, 1994).

12. *Consider biofeedback.* Constipation showed significant improvement after biofeedback treatment (Aldoori et al., 1995).

13. *Try acupuncture.* The procedure works for children with constipation (Broide et al., 2001).

14. *Use affirmations:* "I release the past," or "I allow life to flow through me" (Hay, 2000).

CROHN'S DISEASE

1. *Increase intake of fatty acids.* They have been shown to be helpful in Crohn's disease (Geerling, Houeligen, Badart-Smook, Stockbrugger, & Brummer, 2000; Simopoulos, 1999). Eat plenty of fish, green leafy vegetables, flaxseed, and walnuts to get sufficient fatty acids.

2. *Take extra beta-carotene, vitamin E, and gluthathione peroxidase.* Individuals with Crohn's disease have lower levels of these antioxidants (Geerling et al., 1999; Girodon et al., 1997).

3. *Add more vegetables and soy products and eliminate milk and cheese.* Capristo and colleagues (2000) found that a vegetable, soy, and lactose- (milk) free diet improved the nutritional status of participants with Crohn's disease.

4. *Take more zinc.* This mineral helped heal the gut in patients with Crohn's disease and could help reduce the risk of relapse (Sturniolo, DeLeo, Ferronato, D'Idorico, & D'Inca, 2001). Foods rich in zinc include oysters, herring, liver, eggs, nuts, wheat germ, and red meats. Reduce substances that lead to insufficient zinc intake, including foods containing phytate (beans, whole grains, and peanut butter), dairy foods (calcium interferes), fast foods, white bread, fried potatoes, rich desserts, alcohol, birth control pills, exposure to lead in gasoline or paint, and lead.

5. *Explore hypnosis and meditation.* There is a strong association between atittude, stress, and flares of inflammatory bowel diseases (Anton, 1999).

6. *Use extravirgin olive oil.* Previous studies have shown that the colon mucosa of those suffering from Crohn's disease generates appreciably higher quantities of reactive oxygen species compared with normal tissue. Extravirgin olive oil contains an abundance of phenolic antioxidants that can inhibit reactive oxygen species (Owen et al., 2000).

Diarrhea

1. *Drink at least 10 glasses of water every day* to reduce the risk of dehydration.

2. *Try carob powder.* Mix 1 heaping teaspoonful of the substance with ¼ to ½ cup of water and drink 1–3 times a day.

3. *Avoid magnesium-containing antacids.* (Check the label.) These antacids can worsen diarrhea.

4. *Eat guavas.* This fruit has lectins that interfere with bacterial adhesion, preventing E. coli from adhering to epithelial intestinal cells (Coutino-Rodriguez et al., 2001).

5. *Take a zinc and vitamin A supplement.* These two supplements lower the prevalence of diarrhea (Al-Sonboli, Gurgel, Shenkin, Hart, & Cuevas, 2003; Rahman et al., 2001).

6. *Avoid caffeine, soft drinks, and sugary foods that exacerbate the condition* (Dennison, 1996).

7. *Eat rice, cereal, bananas, and potatoes.* They are rich in carbohydrates and gentle to the stomach.

8. *Fill up on acidophilus or plain yogurt* to restore the good bacteria lost through diarrhea (Boudraa et al., 2001; Montalto et al., 2002) or antibiotic administration (Cremonini, DiCaro, & Nista, 2002).

9. *To restore lost electrolytes, take a mineral supplement that includes potassium and magnesium.*

10. *Avoid sorbitol, mannitol, and xylitol.* These sugar alcohols are associated with diarrhea. They are used as sweeteners and vehicles for liquid drugs taken orally, so they're omnipresent, found in everything from diabetic and dietetic foods to cough medicines and chewing gum.

11. *Take 10,000–50,000 I.U. of vitamin A, zinc, and folate* temporarily for persistent diarrhea and dysentery (Mahalanabis & Bhan, 2001).

12. *Try dietary fiber found in psyllium for fecal incontinence.* Psyllium was associated with a decrease in the percentage of incontinent stools (Bliss et al., 2001).

13. *Use gentle acupressure.* Hold the index, third, and fourth fingers of the left hand on the middle back of the hip bone and the same three fingers of the right hand on the back of the right knee. Hold until a steady, even pulsation is felt in all six fingers, then move the right hand to the spot to the right side of the spinal column at the top of the shoulder (Dayton, 1994).

14. *Use affirmations:* "I am at peace with life," or "I take in, assimilate, and eliminate in perfect order" (Hay, 2000).

DIVERTICULOSIS

1. *Avoid nuts, seeds, corn, and popcorn if they irritate.*

2. *Avoid meat.* Frequent meat consumption is correlated with diverticulosis (Lin et al., 2000).

3. *Gradually eat more fruits, vegetables, and whole grains.* A high-fiber diet seems to completely relieve symptoms and may prevent further diverticular formation (Field, 2001). A total vegetarian diet may be best. Vegetarians were found to have a lower incidence of diverticular disease than nonvegetarians (Key et al., 1999; Nair & Mayberry, 1994).

4. *Take 1–3 teaspoons of psyllium* in a glass of water an hour before breakfast (Bliss et al., 2001).

5. *Avoid antibiotics without a diagnosed infection.*

6. *Exercise.* Physical activity, especially jogging and running, along with a high fiber diet, can prevent the symptoms of diverticular

disease (Aldoori et al., 1995). If unable to jog or run, start walking, building up gradually to a brisk rhythm.

7. *Use gentle acupressure.* Use the index, third, and fourth fingers of each hand and hold them on the following spots until a steady, even pulsation is felt in all fingers: inside of knee, two inches to the side of the spine at the top of shoulder blades, bottom of big toes, back of knees, and bottom of shoulder blades about two inches out from the spine (Dayton, 1994).

GAS AND UPSET STOMACH

1. *Take 3–4 charcoal capsules* after meals for one to two days. **Caution:** Don't take for more than three days in a row because it will retard the body's ability to absorb needed nutrients. Do not take charcoal with other medicines or nutritional supplements. Charcoal can turn stools black.

2. *Avoid eating melons with other foods.* Eat them separately at least 2 hours between other foods.

3. *Start a food/gas diary.* See what foods, what combinations of foods, and at what time of day result in gas. Avoid eating those foods and those combinations. Foods that often cause gas are oat bran, high fiber cereals, beans, onions, apples, and broccoli, but you may have your own set of foods that creates gas for you. Consider trying Beano (for gas from beans, or add cider vinegar to beans). Lactaid may reduce gas from milk and dairy products.

4. *Drink peppermint tea.* It has been used for centuries in Europe to quell stomach and liver ailments. Peppermint oils treat functional dyspepsia and can reduce gastroduodenal motility (Micklefield, Jung, Greving, & May, 2003) and gastric spasm (Hiki et al., 2003).

5. *Drink chamomile tea.* This tea is made from the dried flower-heads of Roman chamomile. If allergic to those flowers, don't use this beverage. The tea releases an almost hypnotic odor that may exert a calming effect on the brain and nervous system. A cup of it can neutralize gas and reduce muscle spasms (Avallone et al., 2000).

6. *Eat more papaya.* The unripe fruit, leaves, and trunk yield a milky substance rich in papain, an enzyme that assists with digestion (Savickiene et al., 2002). Papaya can also be taken in tablet form, but many of the products have sugar and other questionable substances in them. Consider eating a slice of ripe papaya or drinking a glass of papaya juice with meals.

7. *Use clove or sage as a spice.* Both effectively treat gas (Landis & Khalsa, 1997).

8. *Use gentle acupressure.* Hold the index, third, and fourth fingers of each hand on the following points until a steady, even pulsation is felt in all fingers: bottom of big toes, back of knees, at height of the middle of shoulder blade about two inches away from the spine, and middle of chest on each side (Dayton, 1994).

9. *Use affirmations:* "I relax and let life flow through me."

HEARTBURN (GERD OR GASTROESOPHAGEL REFLUX)

1. *Eliminate caffeinated foods and drinks* (coffee, tea, cola, and chocolate), esophageal irritants (citrus fruits, vinegar, spicy foods, tomatoes), lower esophageal sphincter relaxants (onions, garlic, mint, alcoholic beverages), high-fat foods such as fried foods, cheese, meat, cakes and pies, and processed foods that contain oil and high fat content (Hubbard, 2002).

2. *Don't drink fluids while eating.* Drink before meals or 2 hours later so as not to dilute digestive enzymes.

3. *To aid digestion, eat up to six small meals a day and don't eat within 3 hours of bedtime* (Hubbard, 2002).

4. *Eat a dark green salad or raw vegetables at least once a day.* Add sprouted beans, peanuts, and seeds.

5. *Only eat when feeling relaxed,* and then concentrate on chewing food thoroughly.

6. *Chew gum for half an hour after eating.* Chewing sugarless gum (Peelu and Sylifresh NF are both all natural and sugar-free) after meals increases saliva production, which helps clear away the gastric acids that cause heartburn ("Chewing Away Heartburn," 1996).

7. *If over age 50 and low on stomach acid, add a teaspoon to a tablespoon of cider vinegar to a glass of water and drink it half an hour before meals.*

8. *Try deglycyrrhizinated licorice.* It increases the production of protective mucus in the stomach (Borrelli & Izzo, 2000).

9. *Drink a glass of raw cabbage or potato juice.* Both are known for their anti-inflammatory properties (Landis, 1997).

10. *Try an herbal tea.* A cup of fennel, fenugreek, slippery elm, or licorice tea, or three spoonfuls of angelica-root tea morning and evening may produce desired results (Davis, 1980).

11. *Eat fresh papaya* (Savickiene et al., 2002).

12. *Avoid lying down for 3 hours after eating* (Hubbard, 2002).

13. *Avoid drugs that can cause heartburn:* (antacids, antibiotics, antidepressants, antihistamines, aspirin (take the herb white willow instead; it is the basis of aspirin, but doesn't upset your digestion),

transdermal nicotine (to stop smoking), anticholinergics, adrenergic antagonists, benzodiazepines, calcium channel blockers, cholecystokinin, levodopa, narcotics, nitrates, ibuprofen, asthma drugs, chemotherapy drugs, prednisone, beta-blockers, cholesterol-lowering and blood-pressure–lowering drugs, painkillers/narcotics, Premarin, Provera, tranquilizers/barbiturates, and ulcer drugs (sulfasalazine, sucralfate, misoprostol). Stop taking the over-the-counter drugs and find alternatives (Mindell & Hopkins, 1998).

14. *Eat artichokes or take artichoke-leaf extract.* Artichoke stimulates the formation and flow of bile to and from the liver and reduces dyspepsia (Marakis et al., 2002).

15. *Learn stress reduction techniques* such as relaxation therapy, guided imagery, meditation, and/or self-hypnosis. Adapt the relaxation script on pps. 97–98. A relaxation tape can also be purchased and listened to at least twice a day. It is suggested that it play softly in the background the rest of the day. The subconscious mind will hear it and relax. Relaxation training reduced the symptom reports of patients with gastroesophageal reflux disease (GERD), including gas production (McDonald-Hail, Bradley, Bailey, Schan, & Richter, 1994).

16. *Avoid wearing tight-fitting clothing.*

17. *Stop smoking* (Hubbard, 2002).

18. *Take an herbal preparation of chamomile, peppermint, and licorice root.* The combination has been shown to improve symptoms of upset stomach ("Dyspepsia Patients Respond to Herbal Formulation," 1999).

19. *Avoid alcohol.* It irritates the digestive tract (Hubbard, 2002).

20. *Elevate the head of the bed* (Hubbard, 2002).

21. *Begin an exercise program.*

22. *Lose weight if overweight.*

IRRITABLE BOWEL SYNDROME

1. *Start a food diary and identify foods that make the bowel act up.* Digestive disturbances, minor aches and pains, rashes, and vague health complaints are often due to food allergies from wheat, corn, dairy products, soy, citrus fruit, tomatoes, potatoes, eggplant, red and green peppers, cayenne pepper, peanuts (especially if not organically grown), eggs, beef, or coffee. Almost any food can create a sensitivity if eaten every day. Food additives and colorings such as BHT, BHA, MSG, benzoates, nitrates, red and yellow food dyes, sulfites, antibiotics, ibuprofen, and aspirin can also cause reactions.

If unable to identify the culprit, avoid eating the same food more often than once every four days to give the body time to clear the irritating substance.

Read all cans and bottles, looking for hidden allergens. Eliminate those foods, too. Avoid getting into the habit of eating new foods every day. In severe cases of IBS, restrict the diet to chicken, lamb, potatoes, rice, and fruit. Gradually add other foods one at a time, keeping track of reactions as each food is added. Keep drinking 8–10 glasses of water and take a good multivitamin and multimineral every day. The lining of the intestine is shed and regenerated every three days, so it's possible to heal quite rapidly as long as irritating substances are not ingested. When reintroducing a food once sensitive to, symptoms may occur. Stop eating that food and wait another two months before reintroducing it. If the symptoms return when trying to reintroduce the food, wait another six months before trying to eat it again. Eventually it will be possible to eat those foods again, but only occasionally (Williams, 1995).

2. *Take ⅓ to ½ cup of aloe vera juice two to three times a day after meals* (Williams, 1995).

3. *Try enteric-coated peppermint/caraway oil* to produce smooth muscle relaxation (Avallone et al., 2000; Micklefield et al., 2003). Peppermint oil alone will work, even with children (Kline, Kline, DiPalma, & Barbero, 2001). Adult participants who took the capsules were pain free and reported less flatulence, reduced stool frequency, and reduced bloating (Liu et al., 1997). Try taking peppermint capsules unless diagnosed with gallstones, severe liver damage, gallbladder inflammation, or gastroesophageal reflux disease (GERD).

4. *Obtain sufficient fiber and drink at least 8 glasses of water every day.* Wait until all signs of diarrhea are gone before gradually reintroducing fiber. Wheat bran and cereals aren't the best source of fiber because those with IBS are often sensitive or allergic to them. Instead, select water-soluble fibers that promote the formation of protective gel and mucus in the bowel, including oat bran, flax seeds, fruits, vegetables, and legumes (dried beans and peas). Because most of these fiber sources are binding agents or absorbents, they need water to soften, swell, and increase in volume, creating the extra bulk necessary to stimulate the cleansing movement through the colon. This means a minimum of eight glasses of water a day (Bonis & Norton, 1996; Williams, 1995).

5. *Investigate the use of Sialex.* It contains mucin, the compound of mucus, and can help reestablish the protective mucus layer and provide a lubricating action in the lower bowel (Williams, 1995).

6. *If IBS is the result of radiation therapy,* take 1–2 grams of glutamine a day to stimulate the formation of the intestinal villi that are responsible for the absorption and transport of nutrients (Williams, 1995).

7. *If heavy metals like mercury are present,* take 500 mg of the amino acid L-cysteine twice a day with meals to help remove the toxic substance, and avoid eating canned tuna, salt-water fish, and fish from lakes contaminated from acid rain, all of which may contain mercury (Williams, 1995).

8. *Try hypnosis.* Psychological treatments, including hypnotherapy, are not widely available but may play an important role in the relief of pain for IBS (Camilleri, 1999). One study found that symptoms of abdominal pain, constipation, and gas improved significantly with hypnosis (Galovski & Blanchard, 1998).

9. *Use red chili powder* to accelerate gut transit and increase rectal threshold for pain (Agarwal, Bhatia, Desai, Bhure, & Melgiri, 2002).

10. *Avoid using laxatives* (Mindell & Hopkins, 1998).

11. *Take a zinc supplement.* It tightens "leaky gut" in Crohn's disease (Sturniolo et al., 2001).

12. *Exercise daily* (Bonis & Norton, 1996). Start with a short walk and work up to a longer walk with a more brisk rate.

13. *Learn relaxation therapy.* A group of participants who attended a six-week relaxation response meditation class showed significant improvement in gas, belching, bloating, diarrhea, and constipation (Keefer & Blanchard, 2001).

14. *Try cognitive-focused group therapy* (Heitkemper & Jarrett, 2001). It is especially useful for IBS (van Dulmen, 1996).

ULCERS

1. *Eat fruits and vegetables daily.* They protect against duodenal ulcer (Aldoori et al., 1997), helicobacter pylori (Brown, 2000), and aspirin-induced gastric ulcer (Dehpour, Zolfaghari, Samadian, & Vahedi, 1994).

2. *Try deglycyrrhizinated licorice.* It increases the production of protective mucus in the stomach (Borrelli & Izzo, 2000).

3. *Use unripe banana extract* (150 mg 4–6 times a day) or plantain banana (Goel, Sairam, Rao, Keefer, & Blanchard, 2001).

4. *Take enteric-coated peppermint capsules* (Pettit, 2001).

5. *Drink the juice of raw cabbage.* This vegetable contains sulfur compounds and the amino acid glutamine that heal and soothe inflamed tissues (Landis, 1997).

6. *Try 3 ounces of aloe gel after eating.*

7. *Use capsicum or red chiles* to accelerate gut transit time and increase threshold for pain (Agarwal et al., 2002; Kang et al., 1995).

8. *Eat garlic and onions every day.* They exhibit a broad antibiotic spectrum against all kinds of bacteria, including *H. pylori* bacteria (Cellini, Di Campli, Masulli, Di Bartolomeo, & Allocati, 1996; Sivam, 2001).

9. *Take zinc, selenium, and vitamins A, B, and C daily.* Zinc and selenium alone or associated with these vitamins protect against infectious events (Girodon et al., 1997). Vitamin A protects against duodenal ulcer (Aldoori et al., 1997).

10. *Try flax seed.* Place 3 cups of cold water and 3 tablespoons of flax seed (available at a health food store) in a pot and heat on the stove until the water bubbles. Let simmer for 10 minutes, then cool for 7–10 minutes. Strain and put the thick liquid in the refrigerator. Thirty minutes before each meal pour ¼ cup of liquid in a cup, add ¼ cup of water, and drink between meals when stomach feels uncomfortable.

11. *Take probiotics* to block the invasion of human intestinal cells by enteroinvasive bacteria (Montalto et al., 2002). Find them in the health food store, or, if necessary, eat plain yogurt with active cultures.

12. *Try affirmations:* "I am calm. All is well" (Hay, 2000).

TREATMENT EVALUATION

The client described above self-evaluated her progress toward her wellness goals. "I've made a new friend at work and invited him to dinner twice." "My symptom/mood diary shows my digestion is getting better now that I'm on a vegetarian food plan." "I made an appointment with the boss to ask him for tips about my job, but we haven't met yet." "Sophie has a new friend at school and she seems a lot more relaxed. That makes me more relaxed."

REFERENCES

Agarwal, M. K., Bhatia, S. J., Desai, S. A., Bhure, U., & Melgiri, S. (2002). Effect of red chilies on small bowel and colonic transit and rectal sensitivity in men with irritable bowel syndrome. *Indian Journal of Gastroenterology, 21,* 179–182.

Aldoori, W. H., Giovannucci, E. L., Rimm, E. B., Ascherio, A., Stampfer, M. J., Colditz, G. A., et al. (1995). Prospective study of physical activity and the risk of symptomatic diverticular disease in men. *Gut, 36,* 276–282.

Aldoori, W. H., Giovannucci, E. L., Stampfer, M. J., Rimme, E. G., Wing, A. L., & Willett, W. C. (1997). Prospective study of diet and the risk of duodenal ulcer in men. *American Journal of Epidemiology, 145*(1), 42–50.

Al-Sonboli, N., Gurgel, R. Q., Shenkin, A., Hart, C. A., & Cuevas, L. E. (2003). Zinc supplementation in Brazilian children with acute diarrhoea. *Annals of Tropical Paediatrics, 23,* 3–8.

Anton, P. A. (1999). Stress and mind-body impact on the course of inflammatory bowel disease. *Seminars in Gastrointestinal Disease, 10,* 14–19.

Avallone, R., Zanoli, P., Puia, G., Kleinschnitz, M., Schreier, P., & Baraldi, M. (2000). Pharmacological profile of apigenin, a flavonoid isolated from Matricaria chamomilla. *Biochemical Pharmacology, 59,* 1387–1394.

Beverley, L., & Travis, I. (1992). Constipation: Are natural laxatives better? *Journal of Gerontological Nursing, 18,* 6.

Bliss, D. Z., Jung, H. J., Savik, K., Lowry, A., LeMoine, M., Jensen, L., et al. (2001). Supplementation with dietary fiber improves fecal incontinence. *Nursing Research 50,* 203–213.

Bonis, P. A. L., & Norton, R. A. (1996). Irritable bowel syndrome. *American Family Physician, 53,* 1229.

Borrelli, F., & Izzo, A. A. (2000). The plant kingdom as a source of anti-ulcer remedies. *Phytotherapy Research, 14,* 581–591.

Boudraa, G., Benbouabdellah, M., Hachelaf, W., Boisset, M., Desjeux, J. F., & Touhami, M. (2001). Effect of feeding yogurt versus milk in children with acute diarrhea and carbohydrate malabsorption. *Journal of Pediatric Gastroenterology and Nutrition, 33,* 307–313.

Broide, E., Pintov, S., Portnoy, S., Barg, J., Klinowski, E., & Scapa, E. (2001). Effectiveness of acupuncture for treatment of childhood constipation. *Digestive Diseases and Science, 46,* 1270–1275.

Brown, L. M. (2000). Heliocoter pylori: Epidemiology and routes of transmission. *Epidemiology Review, 22,* 283–297.

Camilleri, M. (1999). Therapeutic approach to the patient with irritable bowel syndrome. *American Journal of Medicine 107,* 27S–32S.

Capristo, E., Mingrone, G., Addolorato, G., Green, A. V., & Gasbarrini, G. (2000). Effect of a vegetable-protein-rich polymeric diet treatment on body composition and energy metabolism in inactive Crohn's disease. *European Journal of Gastroenterology and Hepatology, 12*(1), 5–11.

Cellini, L., Di Campli, E., Masulli, M., Di Bartolomeo, S., & Allocati, N. (1996). Inhibition of Helicobacter pylori by garlic extract (Allium sativum). *FEMS Immunological Medical Microbiology, 13,* 273–277.

Chang, S. T. (1986). *The complete system of self-healing internal exercises.* San Francisco CA: Tao.

Chewing away heartburn. (1996). *Psychology & Health Update, 6*(2), 4.

Coutino-Rodriguez, R., Hernandez-Cruz, P., & Giles-Rios, H. (2001). Lectins in fruits having gastrointestinal activity: Their participation in the hemagglutinating property of Escherichia coli O157:H7. *Archives of Medical Research, 32,* 251–257.

Cremonini, F. DiCaro, S., & Nista, E. C. (2002). Meta-analysis: The effect of probiotic administration on antibiotic-associated diarrhoea. *Alimentary and Pharmcological Therapy, 16,* 1461–1467.

Cruz, T., Galvez, J., Crespo, E., Ocete, M. A., & Zarzuelo, A. (2001). Effects of silymarin on the acute stage of the trinitrobenzenesulphonic acid model of rat colitis. *Planta Medica, 67*(1), 94–96.

Davis, B. (1980). *Rapid healing foods.* West Nyack, NY: Parker.

Dayton, B. R. (1994). *An introduction to a gentle acupressure for caregivers.* Friday Harbor, WA: High Touch Network.

Dehpour, A. R., Zolfaghari, M. E., Samadian, T., & Vahedi, Y. (1994). The protective effect of liquorice components and their derivatives against gastric ulcer induced by aspirin in rats. *Journal of Pharmacy and Pharmacology, 46,* 148–149.

Dennison, B. A. (1996). Fruit juice consumption by infants and children: A review. *Journal of the American College of Nutrition, 15*(5, Suppl.), 4S–411.

Dyspepsia patients respond to herbal formulation. (1999). *Clinician Reviews, 9,* 123–124.

Fructose linked to GI distress. (2002). *Clinician Reviews, 12,* 126–127.

Field, S. (2001, September). Approaches to diverticular disease. *Clinical Advisor,* pp. 25–31.

Galovski, T. E., & Blanchard, E. B. (1998). The treatment of irritable bowel syndrome with hypnotherapy. *Applied Psychophysiology and Biofeedback, 23,* 219–232.

Geerling, B. J., Houeligen, A. C., Badart-Smook, A., Stockbrugger, R. W., & Brummer, R. J. (1999). The relation between antioxidant status and alterations in fatty acid profile in patients with Crohn's disease and controls. *Scandinavian Journal of Gastroenterology, 34,* 1108–1116.

Girodon, F., Lombard, M., Galan, P., Brunet-Lecomte, P., Monget, A. L., Arnaud, J., Preziosi, P., & Hercber, S. (1997). Effect of micronutrient supplementation on infection in institutionalized elderly subjects: A controlled trial. *Annals of Nutrition and Metabolism, 41,* 98–107.

Goel, R. K., Sairam, K., Rao, C. V., Keefer, L., & Blanchard, E. B. (2001). The effects of relaxation response meditation on the symptoms of irritable bowel syndrome: Results of a controlled treatment study. *Behavior Research and Therapy, 39*(7), 801–811.

Hay, L. (2000). *Heal your body.* Carlsbad, CA: Hay House, Inc.

Heitkemper, M., & Jarrett, M. (2001). Irritable bowel syndrome. *American Journal of Nursing, 101,* 26–33.

Hiki, N., Kurosaka, H., Tatsutomi, Y., Shimoyama, S., Tsuji, E., Kojima, J., et al. (2003). Peppermint oil reduces gastric spasm during upper endoscopy: A randomized, double-blind, double-dummy controlled trial. *Gastrointestinal Endoscopy, 57,* 475–482.

Hubbard, P. M. (2002, February). Update on gastroesophageal reflux disease. *American Journal for Nurse Practitioners*, pp. 9–16.

Kang, J. Y., Yeoh, K. G., Chia, H. P., Lee, H. P., Chia, Y. W., Guan, R., et al. (1995). Chili—Protective factor against peptic ulcer? *Digestive Diseases and Science, 40*, 576–579.

Keefer, L., & Blanchard, E. B. (2001). The effects of relaxation response meditation on the symptoms of irritable bowel syndrome: Results of a controlled treatment study. *Behavior Research Therapy, 39*, 801–811.

Key, T. J., Davey, G. K., & Appleby, P. N. (1999). Health benefits of a vegetarian diet. *Proceedings of the Nutrition Society, 58*, 271–275.

Kline, R. M., Kline, J. J., DiPalma, J., & Barbero, G. J. (2001). Enteric-coated, pH-dependent peppermint oil capsules for the treatment of irritable bowel syndrome in children. *Journal of Pediatrics, 138*(1), 125–128.

Landis, R., & Rhalso, K. P. (1997). *Herbal defense*. New York: Warner.

Lin, O. S., Soon, M. S., Wu, S. S., Chen, Y. Y., Hwang, I. L., & Triadafilopoulos, G. (2000). Dietary habits and right-sided colonic diverticulosis. *Diseases of the Colon and Rectum, 43*, 1412–1418.

Liu, J. H., Chen, G. H., Yeh, H. A., Huang, C. K., & Poon, S. K. (1997). Enteric-coated peppermint-oil capsules in the treatment of irritable bowel syndrome: A prospective, randomized trial. *Journal of Gastroenterology, 32*, 765–768.

Mahalanabis, D., & Bhan, M. K. (2001). Micronutrients as adjunct therapy of acute illness in children: Impact on the episode outcome and policy implications of current findings. *British Journal of Nutrition, 85*(Suppl. 2), S151–S158.

Marakis, G., Walker, A. F., Middleton, R. W., Booth, J. C., Wright, J., & Pike, D. J. (2002). Artichoke leaf extract reduces mild dyspepsia in an open study. *Phytomedicine, 9*, 694–699.

McDonald-Hail, J., Bradley, L. A., Bailey, M. A., Schan, C. A., & Richter, J. E. (1994). Relaxation training reduces symptom reports and acid exposure in patients with gastroesophageal reflux disease. *Gastroenterology 107*, 61–69.

McDougall, J. A. (1999, October). Relief for diverticulosis. *To your health*, 8.

Merchant, R. E, & Andre, C. A. (2001). A review of recent clinical trials of the nutritional supplement Chlorella pyrenoidosa in the treatment of fibromyalgia, hypertension, and ulcerative colitis. *Alternative Therapies in Health and Medicine, 7*(3), 79–81.

Micklefield, G., Jung, O., Greving, I., & May, B. (2003). Effects of intraduodenal application of peppermint oil and caraway oil on gastroduodenal motility in healthy volunteers. Phytotherapy Research, 17, 135–130.

Mindell, E., & Hopkins, V. (1998). Drugs for the digestive tract and their natural alternatives. In *Prescription alternatives* (pp. 184–223). New Canaan, CT: Keats.

Montalto, M., Arancio, F., Izzi, D., Cuoco, L., Curigliano, V., Manna, R., & Basbarrini, G. (2002). Probiotics: History, definition, requirements and possible therapeutic applications. *Annals of Italian Medicine International, 17,* 157–163.

Murphy, J. (2001). *Nurse Practitioners' Prescribing Reference, 8,* 135-153.

Nair, P., & Mayberry, J. F. (1994). Vegetarianism, dietary fibre and gastrointestinal disease. *Digestive Diseases, 12,* 177–185.

Owen, R. W., Giacosa, A., Hull, W. E., Haubner, R., Spiegelhalder, B., & Bartsch, H. (2000). The anti-oxidant/anticancer potential of phenolic compounds isolated from olive oil. *European Journal of Cancer, 36,* 1235–1247.

Pettit, J. L. (2001). Peppermint. *Clinician Reviews, 11*(3), 71–73.

Rahman, M. M., Vermund, S. H., Wahed, M. A., Fuchs, G. J., Baqui, A. H., & Alvarez, J. O. (2001). Simultaneous zinc and vitamin A supplementation in Bangladeshi children: Randomised double blind controlled trial. *British Journal of Medicine, 323,* 314–318.

Savickiene, N., Dagilyte, A., Lukosius, A., & Zitkevicius, V. (2002). Importance of biologically active components and plants in the prevention of complications of diabetes mellitus. *Medicina, 38,* 970–975.

Schiller, L. (2001). *New paradigm in the treatment of constipation.* Proceedings from an educational symposium. Atlanta, GA.

Simopoulos, A. P. (1999). Essential fatty acids in health and chronic disease. *American Journal of Clinical Nutrition, 70*(3, Suppl.), 560S–569S.

Sivam, G. P. (2001). Protection against Helicobacter pylori and other bacterial infections by garlic. *Journal of Nutrition, 131*(3, Suppl.), 1106S–1108S.

Sturniolo, G. C., De Leo, V., Ferronato, A., D'Idorico, A., & D'Inca, R. (2001). Zinc supplementation tightens "leaky gut" in Crohn's Disease. *Inflammatory Bowel Disease, 7*(2), 94–98.

van Dulmen, A. M. (1996). Cognitive-behavioral group therapy for irritable bowel syndrome effects and long-term followup. *Psychosomatic Medicine, 58,* 508–514.

Williams, D. G. (1990). What and where is this (ileocecal) valve? *Alternatives, 1*(3), 1–4.

Williams, D. G. (1991). Correct constipation or headaches by just drinking 6 to 8 glasses of water a day. *Alternatives, 1*(14), 1.

Williams, D. G. (1995). Irritable bowel syndrome. *Alternatives, 5*(21), 161–166.

Wolfsen, C. R. (1993). Constipation: Medication isn't the solution. *Archives of Family Medicine, 2,* 853.

CHAPTER 12

Fibromyalgia

Fibromyalgia is a chronic disorder of unknown origin characterized by widespread pain in the bones and muscles, fatigue, and multiple tender points in the neck, spine, shoulders, and hips. Fibromyalgia is often found in conjunction with anxiety, irritable bowel syndrome, sleep disturbances, depression, malabsorption problems, and morning stiffness. Medical treatment may include antidepressants that can lead to dry mouth, dizziness, weight gain, and drowsiness. The benefit from antidepressants decreases to the level of a placebo after 6 months. Muscle relaxants and pain medication may also be prescribed, but most are ineffective.

HOLISTIC NURSING ASSESSMENT

Study the holistic nursing assessment for Mrs. Y., a 40-year-old client diagnosed with fibromyalgia. Working in collaboration with clients diagnosed with fibromyalgia, use the format presented to conduct a holistic nursing assessment.

Client learning needs: "To find a way out of this pain, a reason to get up every morning."

Indicants of readiness to learn: "The pills the doctor gave me don't work anymore."

Soul/spirituality symbol(s): "I go to church when I can get out of bed."

Meaning of the condition to client: "I read someplace that what I have may be due to a food or chemical sensitivity, but I think it's a punishment."

Relationship needs/effects as perceived by the client: "My husband didn't want me to come to see you. I can't stay for a whole hour. If he finds out I'm here, he's going to be really mad. He's a lot like my daddy. He used to drink and then come home and take everything out on my mother."

Patterns/attitudes that may create dis-ease for this client: Client uses negative affirmations (e.g., "I'm just too tired to work anymore," and "I can't sleep," and "My body punishes me for every move I make").

Life purpose: Expresses no life purpose except to relieve pain.

Client strengths: Wants to learn how to deal with her condition.

Ability to participate in care: Client cancels every other appointment due to "fatigue."

Ethical dilemmas: Client hints that husband may be abusive, but denies it when questioned.

Nurse–client process: Client tries to set up a dependent relationship, asking nurse to make all decisions about care.

TREATMENT PLANNING: SETTING JOINTLY AGREED-UPON GOALS

In the case of the client discussed above, the following goals were agreed upon:

1. Use a symptom/mood/food/chemical diary to track the connection between her feelings and body symptoms.
2. Reduce intake of foods and chemicals that are related to body symptoms.
3. Begin an exercise program. -

TREATMENT

Acceptance of condition/attitude change: To counter negative thoughts and feelings, nurse asked the client to say or write one or more of the following affirmations daily: "I can handle this." "I am getting more hopeful." "Energy abounds in me." Client agreed to write the affirmation on 3 x 5 cards and say the words at least 20 times each day.

Facilitating the healing process/healing intention formulation: From a list of meditative statements, client chose the following one to assist in the healing process: "I trust the flow of life." Client was asked to meditate on the words while in a relaxed state. Nurse will use caring nonverbal and verbal communication, centering, and a meditative state to enhance client healing, will verbalize observed patterns that may be holding the client back and offer alternate approaches.

Creating a sacred space: During client sessions, music of her choice will play in the background and guided imagery will assist with the relaxation process.

Encouraging re-storying: Encouraged client to recall an upsetting situation with her husband and choose an ending that inspires her.

Integrative practices planned: Will use massage and acupressure to assist client in the healing process.

Role model strategies: Showed client how to role play problematic interchanges with her husband.

Protection plan: Requested client use an image of white light around her when she feels fear or pain.

Family strategies: Encouraged client to invite her husband to a session with nurse to practice more open communication between them.

Life issues/life purpose work: Client has agreed to write in her journal about life purpose.

Treatment possibilities/considerations: Other suggested treatments appear below. Most are evidence-based.

ADDITIONAL INFORMATION AND TREATMENTS FOR CLIENTS

NUTRITIONAL AND ENVIRONMENTAL APPROACHES

1. *Keep a food/environmental stress diary for at least two weeks.* Write down everything eaten and all environmental exposures to dust, mold, pollen, cleaning materials, pesticides, and so on. For

each, note body symptoms for up to an hour afterward. Begin to notice patterns. If no patterns are noted, keep the diary for another 2 weeks. Eliminate each stressor as identified (Smith, Terpening, Schmidt, & Gums, 2001).

2. *Read labels* of all foods, drinks, and drugs and make sure they do not contain aspartate or monosodium glutamate (MSG); both are excitotoxins that can induce fibromyalgia symptoms. Glutamic acid, the main component of MSG, can be found listed by any of the following names: autolyzed yeast, calcium caseinate, hydrolyzed protein, hydrolyzed oat flour, hydrolyzed plant protein, hydrolyzed vegetable protein, monosodium glutamate, plant protein extract, sodium caseinate, textured protein, yeast extract, bouillon, broth, flavoring, malt extract, malt flavoring, natural beef flavoring, natural chicken flavoring, natural flavoring, seasoning, spices, carrageenan, enzymes, soy protein concentrate, soy protein isolate, or whey protein concentrate. Try eliminating all products with any of these ingredients for two months and see if symptoms are relieved. Forego eating in restaurants during this time period (Smith et al., 2001).

3. *Eat a diet rich in whole, fresh foods* (Saputo, 1998), including fresh fruits and vegetables, raw nuts and seeds, whole grains (if tolerated), dry beans and peas, soy products, and fish. Once in a while, eat skinless turkey or chicken. This kind of regime will help the body neutralize dangerous free radicals. Try to eat 50% raw foods and fresh juices. Buy a juicer and drink at least 12 ounces of carrot juice (diluted with water) a day. Add up to 2 ounces of spinach juice and/or 2 ounces of beet or 2 ounces of cucumber juice.

4. *If other dietary interventions don't work, try a raw vegetarian diet.* One study showed that food plan of raw fruits, salads, carrot juice, tubers, grain products, nuts, seeds, and dehydrated barley grass juice resulted in significant reduction in shoulder pain, range of motion, flexibility, and ability to walk (Donaldson, Speight, & Loomis, 2001).

5. *Eat foods rich in magnesium and vitamin B6.* Magnesium depletion occurs in fibromyalgia due to a dysregulating biorhythm (Durlach et al., 2002). In a trial of 12 clients at the Pain & Stress Center who were diagnosed with fibromyalgia and chronic pain syndrome, all participants reported a remarkable improvement in overall feeling after taking 1200 mg of magnesium combined with 600 mg of malic acid (morning and evening) and vitamin B6. They reported less stiffness and soreness and fewer trigger points. About 50% required fewer trigger point injections after 2 weeks. After 90 days, all participants returned to normal activities and regular exercise, such as walking

and swimming (Mazzio & Soliman, 2003; Sahley, 1995). Foods rich in magnesium include whole grain breads and cereals, fresh peas, brown rice, soy flour, wheat germ, nuts, Swiss chard, figs, green leafy vegetables, and citrus fruit. Foods rich in vitamin B6 include sunflower seeds, toasted wheat germ, brown rice, soybeans, white beans, liver, chicken, mackerel, salmon, tuna, bananas, walnuts, peanuts, sweet potatoes, and cooked cabbage.

6. *Eat foods high in manganese.* Manganese is important to thyroid hormone metabolism. As fatigue is one of the chief complaints of fibromyalgia, hypometabolism due to secondary hypothyroidism may be one of the sources of the condition (Eder, Kralik, & Kirchgessner, 1996; McIntosh, Hong, & Sapolsky, 1998; Sahley, 1995). Foods rich in manganese include nuts, seeds, whole grains, fruits and vegetables, dry beans and peas, and oatmeal.

7. *Avoid green peppers, eggplant, tomatoes, and white potatoes.* These foods contain solanine, which interferes with enzymes in muscles and may cause pain and discomfort.

8. *Avoid meat, dairy products, or any other foods high in saturated fats* that can raise cholesterol levels and interfere with circulation. They can also promote inflammation and pain. Avoid fried foods, processed foods (in cans, bottles, bakeries, and fast food restaurants), shellfish, and white flour products such as bread and pasta.

9. *Avoid sugar in candy, cake, pies, ice cream, and even yogurt unless it's plain.* Sweet processed foods can promote fatigue, distress, depression, decreased energy and pain (Bell, Baldwin, Stoltz, Walsh, & Schwartz, 2001; Christensen, 1993; Christensen & Burrows, 1990; Reid & Hammersley, 1995).

10. *Avoid caffeine and alcohol.*

11. *Eat four to five small meals daily* to keep a steady supply of protein and carbohydrates available.

12. *Never skip breakfast and never eat after 7 p.m.* This will ensure hunger at breakfast time and is a natural way to lose weight.

13. *Don't eat junk foods, but carry a snack at all times.* A small bag of fresh nuts (no oil or salt added) and raisins or an apple are good choices.

14. *Eat plain low-fat yogurt or take acidophilus and related "good" bacteria* that can balance the flora in the intestine, aid in healthy digestion, and help prevent yeast infections (Reid, 2002; Reid et al., 2003).

15. *Drink at least 10 glasses of distilled water a day* or purchase a reverse osmosis water filtration system to avoid taking in parasites. Infection by these creatures can mimic fibromyalgia symptoms (Leav, Mackay, & Ward, 2003).

SUPPLEMENTS

1. *Take SAMe to alleviate depression and pain and promote healing.* SAMe or S-adenosylmethionine is synthesized from the amino acid methionine and is found throughout the body. SAMe protects your chondrocytes, the cells that manufacture the main components of cartilage, against wear and tear on the joints. SAMe worked just as well as naproxen (Naprosyn), ibuprofen (Motrin, Advil, Midol IB, Bayer Select Pain Relief, Nuprin, IBU) and indomethacin (Indocin) for pain relief, but had fewer side effects. It also worked faster and produced more significant improvements than antidepressants and had fewer reported adverse effects. No studies have shown any reason not to use SAMe, as long as the normal daily dose recommended (1,200 to 1,600 mg divided in several doses for 21 days, then reduced to 400 mg a day) is followed (Bell, Plon, Bunney, & Potkin, 1988).

2. *Other supplements that have been reported to be helpful* include 300–900 mg/day of magnesium malate, 25 mg twice a day of pycnogenol, chromium picolinate, vitamin C, 50–100 mg three times a day of CoQ10, 400–800 IU a day of vitamin E, 150 mg three times a day of glutathione, and 250 mg three times a day of acetyl carnitine (Durlach et al., 2002; Ruiz et al., 1998; Sahley, 1995). These supplements can reduce oxidative stress due to free radicals that cause severe inflammation and destruction. Borage oil or evening primrose oil capsules may help with inflammation and pain.

HERBS

Investigate the use of herbs. Buy a book with research-based references or find a health care professional with expertise in the use of herbs. Some herbs that have provided relief from fibromyalgia include the Chinese herb combination Tuo Li Xiao and Gui Pi Tang. St. John's wort taken with Bach Rescue Remedy at the first sign of a FMS flare-up can be an emergency relief. St. John's wort decreases pain and is an antidepressant and a muscle relaxer. Devil's claw is a muscle and joint anti-inflammatory. Skullcap decreases pain and is a nerve sedative and muscle relaxant. Milk thistle can help protect the liver. Skullcap and valerian root improve sleep, and Ginkgo biloba improves circulation and brain function. Topical applications of 1 part cayenne powder mixed with 3 parts wintergreen oil can help relieve muscle pain. Teas brewed from dandelion and red clover can promote healing by cleansing the bloodstream and enhancing immune function. Parasites can be a problem in fibromyalgia. Black walnut and garlic can help remove them (Covan,1996).

HOMEOPATHIC REMEDIES

Pulsatilla is a homeopathic remedy used to decrease tension, anxiety, and emotional agitation. Arnica removes blood from congested areas; is an analgesic, muscle relaxant, and warmer; and can reduce stress (Covin, 1996).

EXERCISE

Pain and fatigue from fibromyalgia encourage physical inactivity. This fuels a hopeless cycle of pain, physical inactivity, and more pain. Low-level aerobic exercise such as swimming, walking, low-impact aerobic dancing, and bicycling can reduce FMS pain and stress. Inactive individuals should begin with just 5 minutes a day. Warm water pool exercises may be the easiest way to start, but must be performed under the water, and begun slowly, using only a few maneuvers and short repetitions. Walking up a single flight of stairs instead of taking the elevator is another easy exercise. Use isometrics for gradual stretching. Fast floor aerobics are contraindicated. Moist heat may be helpful, but stay out of drafts (Clark, 1994; Marlowe, 1998). Also obtain a stretching video or text and follow it.

MASSAGE

Connective tissue massage may help. A random study of 48 individuals diagnosed with fibromyalgia (23 in the treatment group and 25 in the reference group) showed that a series of 15 treatments with connective tissue massage evoked a pain-relieving effect of 37%, reduced depression and the use of analgesics, and enhanced quality of life. After three months, 30% of the pain was relieved and 6 months after treatment, period pain was back to 90% of the basic value (Bennett, Burckhardt, & Brattberg, 1999).

PACE DAILY ACTIVITIES

Overexertion, even with the most minimal movement, can exacerbate aches and fatigue. Pace activities. For example, plan one day for washing clothes, another for cleaning bathrooms, another for paying bills or cooking and freezing meals (Marlowe, 1998).

COGNITIVE-BEHAVIORAL TRAINING

Benefits of a cognitive-behavioral program have been shown to last up to $2\frac{1}{2}$ years (Bennett et al., 1996; Sandstrom & Keefe, 1998;

Vlaeyen et al., 1996; White & Nielson, 1995). Find a skilled mental health nurse-clinician to teach prioritization skills, ways to change self-critical attitudes when tasks take longer than they used to, ways to deal with daily hassles without feeling stressed, and ways to reduce attention spent on symptoms while increasing focus on accomplishments.

RELAXATION STRATEGIES

1. *Relaxation strategies, meditation-based stress reduction techniques, self-hypnosis, and guided imagery techniques can help restructure negative thoughts* that lead to feeling helpless and hopeless.

2. *Consider a support group.* It may be beneficial to meet with other individuals suffering from fibromyalgia. It may be easier to listen to peer ideas than to take advice from a therapist.

3. *Purchase or develop a relaxation, hypnosis, and/or fibromyalgia healing tape* and listen to it at least twice a day. When the body is relaxed, less pain will be perceived. Listen to the tape upon awakening to relax and energize. Listen to it before sleep, and play it softly in the background during the day.

4. *Use relaxation with guided imagery to reduce pain.* In a controlled trial, the use of pleasant imagery showed the most significant decline in pain, but amitriptyline had no significant advantage over placebo during a 28-day study period (Fors, Sexton, & Gotestam, 2002). See pages 97–98, this volume.

SELF-STATEMENTS

Individuals diagnosed with fibromyalgia tend to catastrophize (make situations sound worse than they really are) and make depressive self-statements. Both of these behaviors may have a role in exacerbating pain (Hassett, Cone, Patella, & Sigal, 2000).

OBTAIN PSYCHOTHERAPY FOR ABUSE

Clients who develop chronic fatigue syndrome and fibromyalgia have a tendency to come from a life of neglect and physical abuse; a considerable subgroup experiences lifelong victimization. Family and/or a current partner were the most frequent abusers according to one study (Van Houdenhove et al., 2001). Refer clients to a mental health nurse-clinical specialist to help them overcome the victim role.

Gentle Touch Acupressure

1. Hold the 2nd, 3rd, and 4th fingers of the right hand in the spot on the right side of the body where the neck meets the shoulder, and the same fingers of the left hand on the left side of the body on the spot where the neck meets the shoulder. Hold gently until pulsation is felt in all fingers.
2. Move both hands and hold the back of the knees.
3. When pulsation is felt in all fingers, hold the inside of each knee, then the instep.
4. When pulsation is felt in all fingers, hold the left and right outside of the middle of the heel.
5. When pulsation is felt, hold one hand on either side of the spine just above the scapula (Dayton, 1994).

Postural Retraining

Common postural distortions in individuals with chronic pain conditions such as FMS include a forward positioned head, rounded shoulders with a locked chest, and inefficient mouth breathing. Postural retraining can help correct improper use of muscles for long-term relief.

1. *Listen to a relaxation tape prior to trying the following exercises.*

A. Stand against a wall with your hands at your sides and your buttocks, head, and back touching the wall. While inhaling from your abdomen, slowly raise the arms up along the wall until they touch over the head. While exhaling, slide your arms down the wall until they are at the sides again. Repeat several times, building up to ten times a day.

B. Stand against a wall with arms bent and knuckles touching each other at nipple level. Slowly inhale from the abdomen while pulling the hands apart and letting the elbows move toward the wall until they touch it. Hold the breath for several seconds, then slowly exhale, returning bent arms to nipple level. Repeat several times, building up to ten times a day

2. *Avoid staying in the same position for long periods of time.* Shuffle the feet, slowly reach out in front of the body with arms, slowly stretch arms overhead, or touch the knees and then the buttocks several times. When driving, pull over at least every hour, get out, walk around the car, stretch up to the sky, take a deep breath, and find at least one thing to enjoy in the surroundings.

3. *Sit in a rocker and rock when watching television or sitting and relaxing.* This will prevent the back muscles from locking and build up strength in knees and ankles.

4. *When standing up, lean forward and let gravity help.* Avoid pushing up with the arms only.

5. *Sleep with a small soft pillow between the knees* to keep the back in alignment. Never sleep on the stomach.

6. *When turning in bed, roll with head down and float gently,* using the arms to help turn. Relieve stress on your neck by not lifting the head or leading with it to roll over.

7. *Avoid sitting in drafts or cold rooms.* Both can tighten muscles, especially in the neck and shoulders, and increase pain. Put a small towel or scarf around shoulders and neck to keep them warm.

MAGNET THERAPY

One study investigated the effect of magnets on the prevention of musculoskeletal disorders. The results showed that the magnets prevented muscle contractures that arose due to sitting in one position for a prolonged period of time (Capodaglio & Vicenzi, 2000). Another report found that two-thirds of participants who slept on mattresses with magnets reported substantial pain relief, decreased fatigue, and an improved sense of well-being (Rosch, 1998).

MEDITATION

Participants with fibromyalgia in a meditation-based stress reduction program showed moderate to marked improvement (Kaplan, Goldenberg, & Galvin-Nadeau, 1992). Another study, presented at a meeting of the American Psychosomatic Society, found that women with fibromyalgia who meditated six days a week slept better, improved their quality of life, and alleviated their depressive symptoms (Sephton, Lynch, Weissbecker, Ho, & Saimen, 2001).

PARTNER SUPPORT

A woman's fibromyalgia has a great impact on her partner's life. The whole family is influenced and limited by fibromyalgia. The partner's role changes, and the responsibilities and workload within the family change as well as the need for information and knowledge about fibromyalgia (Soderberg, Strand, Haapala, & Lundman, 2003). Partners often lack information so share your thoughts and feelings.

TREATMENT EVALUATION

The client described above made the following comments in evaluating treatment: "I've learned I'm not a victim. I am not being acted upon. I can make myself feel better. I have!" "I don't eat meat any more and I feel a lot better. I've also cut down on junk food. Sure I miss ice cream and cake, but you only taste it for a minute or two. A ripe apple is just as good and much better for me." "I swim 4 days a week and exercise in the pool."

For more ideas, see: arthritis, chronic fatigue syndrome, digestive problems.

REFERENCES

Bell, I. R., Baldwin, C. M., Stoltz, E., Walsh, B. T.,& Schwartz, G. E. (2001). EEG beta 1 oscillation and sucrose sensitization in fibromyalgia with chemical intolerance. *International Journal of Neuroscience, 108*(1–2), 31–42.

Bell, K. M., Plon, L, Bunney, W. E. Jr, & Potkin, S. G. (1988). S-adenosylmethionine treatment of depression: A controlled clinical trial. *American Journal of Psychiatry, 145,* 1110–1114.

Bennett, R. M., Burckhardt, C. S., & Brattberg, G. (1999). Connective tissue massage in the treatment of fibromyalgia. *European Journal of Pain, 3,* 235–244.

Capodaglio, P., & Vicenzi, G. (2000). Efficacy of a chair with magnets in the prevention of musculo-skeletal disorders caused by prolonged sitting. *Journal Italian Medical Laboratory of Ergonomics, 22,* 332–225.

Caruso, I., & Petrogrande, V. (1987). Italian double-blind multicenter study comparing S-adenosylmethionine, naproxen, and placebo in the treatment of degenerative joint disease. *American Journal of Medicine, 83*(5A), 66–71.

Christensen, L. (1993). Effects of eating behavior on mood: A review of the literature. *International Journal of Eating Disorders, 14,* 171–183.

Christensen, L., & Burrows, R. (1990). Dietary treatment of depression. *Behavior Therapy, 21,* 183–194.

Clark, S. R. (1994). Prescribing exercise for fibromyalgia patients. *Arthritis Care and Research, 7,* 221–225.

Clark, S. R., et al. (1996). Group treatment of fibromyalgia: A 6-month outpatient program. *Journal of Rheumatology, 23,* 521–528.

Covan, M. (1996). Herbal medicine for fibromyalgia. *Massage Therapy Journal, Summer,* 100–104.

Dayton, B. R. (1994). *An introduction to a gentle acupressure for caregivers.* Friday Harbor, WA: High Touch Network.

Donaldson, M. S., Speight, N., & Loomis, S. (2001). Fibromyalgia syndrome improved using a mostly raw vegetarian diet: An observational study. *BMC Complementary and Alternative Medicine, 1*(1), 7.

Durlach, J., Pages, N., Bac, P., Bara, M., Guiet-Bara, A., & Agrapart, C. (2002). Chronopathological forms of magnesium depletion with hypofunction or with hyperfunction of the biological clock. *Magnesium Research, 15*(3–4), 263–268.

Eder, K., Kralik, A., & Kirchgessner, M. (1996). The effect of manganese supply on thyroid hormone metabolism in the offspring of manganese-depleted dams. *Biology Trace Element Research, 55*(1–2), 137–145.

Fors, E. A., Sexton, H., & Gotestam, K. G. (2002). The effect of guided imagery and amitriptyline on daily fibromyalgia pain: A prospective, randomized, controlled trial. *Journal of Psychiatric Research, 36,* 179–187.

Hassett, A. L., Cone, J. D., Patella, S. J., & Sigal, L. H. (2000). The role of catastrophizing in the pain and depression of women with fibromyalgia syndrome. *Arthritis and Rheumatism, 43,* 2493–2500.

Kaplan, K. H., Goldenberg, D. L., & Galvin-Nadeau, M. (1992). The impact of a meditation-based stress reduction program on fibromyalgia. *General Hospital Psychiatry, 15,* 284–289.

Leav, B. A., Mackay, M., & Ward, H. D. (2003). Cryptosporidium species: New insights and old challenges. *Clinical Infectious Diseases, 36,* 903–908.

Marlowe, S. M. (1998, January). Calming the fire of fibromyalgia. *Advance for Nurse Practitioners,* 51–55.

Mazzio, E., & Soliman, K. F. (2003). The role of glycolysis and gluconeogenesis in the cytoprotection of neuroblastoma cells against 1-methyl 4-phenylpyridinium ion toxicity. *Neurotoxicology, 24*(1), 137–147.

McIntosh, L. J., Hong, K. E., & Sapolsky, R. M. (1998). Glucocorticoids may alter antioxidant enzyme capacity in the brain: Baseline studies. *Brain Research, 791*(1–2), 209–214.

Reid, G. (2002). Probiotics for urogenital health. *Nutrition in Clinical Care, 5*(1), 3–8.

Reid, G., Charbonneau, D., Erb, J., Kochanowski, B., Beurerman, D., Pochner, R., & Bruce, A. W. (2003). Oral use of Lactobacillus rhamnosus GR-1 and L. fermentum RC-14 significantly alters vaginal flora: Randomized, placebo-controlled trial in 64 healthy women. *FEMS Immunology and Medical Microbiology, 35,* 131–134.

Reid, M., & Hammersley, R. (1995). Effects of carbohydrate intake on subsequent food intake and mood state. *Physiology and Behavior, 58,* 421–427.

Rosch, P. (1998). The amazing power of magnets. *Newsletter of the American Institute of Stress, 2,* 7–8.

Ruiz, F., Alvarez, G., Pereira, R., Hernandez, M., Villalba, M., Cruz, F., et al. (1998). Protection by pyruvate and malate against glutamate-mediated neurotoxicity. *Neuroreport, 9,* 1277–1282.

Sahley, B. J. (1995). *Malic acid and magnesium for fibromyalgia and chronic pain syndrome: Understanding why you hurt all over and what you can take naturally to stop the pain.* San Antonio TX: Pain & Stress Therapy Center Publications.

Sandstrom, M. J., & Keefe, F. J. (1998). Self-management of fibromyalgia: The role of formal coping skills training and physical exercise training programs. *Arthritis Care Research, 11,* 432–447.

Saputo, L. (1998, April). Drug-free relief from fibromyalgia. *Greatlife,* pp. 28–31.

Sephton, S. E., Lynch, G., Weissbecker, I., Ho, I., & Saimen, P. (2001, March). *Effects of a meditation program on symptoms of illness and neuroendocrine responses in women with fibromyalgia.* Presented at the 59th Annual Scientific Meeting of the American Psychosomatic Society, Monterey, CA.

Smith, J. D., Terpening, C. M., Schmidt, S., & Gums, J. G. (2001, July/August). Relief of fibromyalgia symptoms following dietary excitotoxins. *American Journal for Nurse Practitioners,* 51–59.

Soderberg, S., Strand, M., Haapala, M., & Lundman, B. (2003). Living with a woman with fibromyalgia from the perspective of the husband. *Journal of Advanced Nursing, 42,* 143–150.

Van Houdenhove, B., Neerinck, E., Lysens, R., Vertommen, H., Van Houdenhove, L., Onghena, P., et al. (2001). Victimization in chronic fatigue syndrome and fibromyalgia in tertiary care: A controlled study on prevalence and characteristics. *Psychosomatics, 42*(1),21–28.

Vlaeyen, J. W., Teeken-Gruben, N. J., Goossens, M. E., et al. (1996). Cognitive-educational treatment of fibromyalgia: A randomized clinical trial 1. Clinical effects. *Journal of Rheumatology, 23,* 1237–1245.

White, K. P., & Nielson, W. R. (1995). Cognitive behavioral treatment of fibromyalgia syndrome: A followup assessment. *Journal of Rheumatology, 22,* 717–721.

CHAPTER 13

Heart and Blood Vessel Disorders

Heart and blood vessel disorders include many conditions from myocardial infarct to stroke, rheumatic heart disease, high blood pressure, congestive heart failure, arteriosclerosis, coronary artery disease, hemorrhoids, and varicose veins. Diuretics, beta-blockers, calcium-channel blockers, angina pain-reducing drugs, blood-thinning drugs, and surgical procedures are some of the medical approaches used.

HOLISTIC NURSING ASSESSMENT

Study the holistic nursing assessment for Mr. A., a 50-year-old husband and father diagnosed with myocardial infarction. Working in collaboration with clients diagnosed with heart-related conditions use the format that follows to perform a holistic nursing assessment.

Client learning needs: "I don't want to have another heart attack."

Indicants of readiness to learn: "I've been reading everything I can find about the heart and heart attacks."

Soul/spirituality symbol(s): "I go to church and tithe."

Meaning of the condition to client: "I've been overdoing it. My aunt said this is my heart's way of slowing me down."

Relationship needs/effects as perceived by the client: "I haven't spent much time with my wife and children. I've been so busy making money."

187

Patterns/attitudes that may create dis-ease for this client: Client uses negative affirmations (e.g., "I'll never forgive my father for abandoning me and my mother").

Life purpose: Expresses no life purpose except to get back at his father.

Client strengths: Wants to learn better eating habits and how to plot out more time to spend with his family.

Ability to participate in care: Client can participate fully in care, but is fearful about having sex or engaging in exercise because "I might have another attack."

Ethical dilemmas: "My partner is stealing from our customers, but he's been a good friend for many years."

Nurse–client process: Client orders nurse around and continually asks to talk to the doctor.

TREATMENT PLANNING: SETTING JOINTLY AGREED-UPON GOALS

In the case of the client discussed above, the following goals were agreed upon:

1. Find a healthy meal plan he can live with.
2. Resolve resentment toward his father.
3. Learn relaxation measures.
4. Find a way to spend more time with his family.

TREATMENT

Acceptance of condition/attitude change: The client chose the following affirmation to use to replace the upset he feels: "I bring joy back to the center of my heart." Client agreed to write the affirmation on 3 x 5 cards and say the words at least 20 times each day.

Facilitating the healing process/healing intention formulation: From a list of meditative statements, client chose the following one to assist in the healing process: "I express love and understanding." Asked client to meditate on the words while in a relaxed state. Nurse will use caring nonverbal and verbal communication, centering, and a meditative state to enhance client healing, will verbalize observed patterns that may be holding the client back and offer alternate approaches.

Creating a sacred space: During client sessions, music of his choice will play in the background and jointly produced relaxation tapes will assist with relaxing sleep.

Encouraging re-storying: Encouraged client to recall an upsetting situation with his family and choose an ending that inspires him.

Integrative practices planned: Will use therapeutic touch and guided imagery to assist in the healing process.

Role model strategies: Nurse showed client how to role play problematic interchanges with his wife and children.

Protection plan: Requested client use an image of his church to protect him when he feels stressed.

Family strategies: Encourage client to invite his family to a session with nurse to practice more open communication between them.

Life issues/life purpose work: Client has agreed to write in his journal about his father.

Treatment possibilities/considerations: Other suggested treatments appear below. Most are evidence-based.

ADDITIONAL INFORMATION AND TREATMENTS TO SHARE WITH CLIENTS

NUTRITIONAL APPROACHES

1. *Move toward a vegetarian diet.* It can lower blood pressure and correct lipid metabolism (Appleby, Davey, & Key, 2002; Lvanov, Medkova, & Mosiagina, 2002; Robinson, Hackett, Billington, & Stratton, 2002).

2. *Eat foods high in antioxidants, flavonoids, lycopene, carotenoids, and sulfur, which protect the heart* (Kris-Etherton et al., 2002). Some foods to concentrate on are soy, flaxseed oil, whole grains, fruits and vegetables (especially cherries, papaya, grapes and grape juice, onions, cabbage, peas, beans, cauliflower, Brussels sprouts, mustard greens, hot peppers, tomatoes, and asparagus), shrimp, chestnuts, leafy greens, legumes, bananas, olives and olive oil, nuts, and garlic (Knekt et al., 2002; Kris-Etherton et al., 2002; O'Byrne, Devaraj, Grundy, & Jialal, 2002; Parcell, 2002; Rao, 2002; Rosa et al., 2002; Savickiene, Dagilyte, Lukosius, & Zitkevicius, 2002). Foods to concentrate on for lowering blood pressure are fresh apricots,

peaches, cherries, pineapples, oranges, and grapefruits. The best juices are citrus, black currant, and grape. To prevent clots, use garlic, onions, and wheat germ. For angina, focus on mangos and papaya. For edema, watercress, pears, peaches, nectarines, and watermelon can start diuresis. Place a small cube of watermelon in the mouth every fifteen minutes and let it dissolve. For leg ulcers, add onion and garlic to carrot juice. Citrus and apple juices may also prove helpful. For valve problems eat apples, apricots, fresh artichokes, asparagus, string beans, beet tops, celery, cucumbers, eggplant, endive, figs, kale, mustard greens, parsley, prunes, spinach, summer squash, Swiss chard, tomatoes, turnip tops, wheat germ, zucchini, and drink lemon juice (Davis, 1980; Kris-Etherton et al., 2002).

3. *Eat less or no meat, dairy products (milk, cheese, butter, eggs), fried foods, desserts (except for a piece of fruit), chips, French fries, and sugar.* Saturated (animal) fats and sugar raise triglycerides, now linked with an increased risk of heart attack (Stampfer et al., 1997). Sugar is also linked with exacerbation of the inflammatory process. A high intake of rapidly digested and absorbed carbohydrates increases the risk of ischemic heart disease, especially in overweight women prone to insulin resistance (Liu et al., 2002), while honey may be protective (Busserolles, Gueux, Rock, Mazur, & Rayssigiguier, 2002).

4. *Avoid eating salty foods or adding salt to food* if hypertensive. To reduce blood pressure, follow the DASH Diet (Moore, Conlin, Ard, & Svetkey, 2001). The food plan includes eating many fruits, vegetables, low-fat dairy products, whole grains, poultry, fish, and nuts, and reduced fat, red meat, and refined sugars.

5. *Eat potassium-rich foods* (bananas, cantaloupes, orange juice, baked potatoes, and low-fat yogurt) to lower blood pressure (Whelton et al., 1997).

6. *Stop drinking coffee.* It is correlated (Nygard et al., 1997) with homocysteine, a blood risk factor for heart and blood vessel disease.

7. *Eat an apple a day.* Apples are especially good for the heart. Drinking 12 ounces of apple juice or eating 2 apples a day can dramatically reduce the amount of LDL ("bad" cholesterol) in the blood and enhance the lag time for cholesterol to oxidize (which is associated with a reduced risk of heart disease). Persimmons may be even better (Gorenstein et al., 2001).

8. *Eat at least one green salad a day.* Forget about iceburg lettuce. It doesn't have enough nutrients. Try kale, arugula, escarole, spinach, parsley, romaine, and/or endive. Top it off with a tablespoon of olive oil and some cider or plum vinegar. Olive oil is heart healthy, so use it for salads and cooking.

9. *Eat more fish,* the oilier, the better. Mackerel, salmon, and sardines are best. They all contain Coenzyme Q10, a vital heart nutrient, and protect against high cholesterol and irregular heartbeat. They also contain omega-3 fatty acids that can improve blood pressure control (Holm et al., 2001).

10. *Drink fresh juices daily.* Get a juicer. Use fresh and, if possible, organic vegetables. Studies show organic fruits and vegetables have fewer toxic minerals and pesticides (Carl, Fenske, & Elgethun, 2003; Karavoltsos, Sakellari, Dimopoulos, Dasenakis, & Scoulios, 2002), fewer bacteria (Pascual, Garcia, Hernandez, Lerma, & Lynch, 2002), and more beneficial minerals in them (Ginocchio, Rodriguez, Badilla-Ohlibaum, Allen, & Lagos, 2002). Cut the tops and bottoms off carrots and beets. Have several glasses of one or more of the following to help heal heart and blood vessel conditions. Sip the juices slowly and enjoy their fresh taste: (a) carrot juice with 2 ounces of spinach juice, (b) carrot juice with 2 ounces of spinach, celery and an ounce of parsley, or (c) carrot juice with 2 ounces each of cucumber and beet juice. *Note:* Because all fiber is removed from the vegetables, they are easy to digest.

11. *Obtain sufficient fiber* from whole grain breads, cereals, and whole fruits and vegetables because it can help reduce cholesterol (Maxson, 2002).

12. *Eat food rich in B-vitamins.* They can enhance heart health. Eat the following foods to increase B-vitamin intake: lentils, chicken, peanuts, sunflower seeds, tuna, turkey, brown rice, bananas, walnuts, sweet potatoes, cooked cabbage, sesame seeds, cauliflower, mushrooms, lima beans, prunes, green peas, asparagus, raisins, liver, and spinach. Niacin can help lower cholesterol and protect against heart and blood vessel conditions (Ito, 2002; Symons, Mullick, Ensunsa, Maj, & Rutledge, 2002). Foods rich in niacin include wheat germ, wheat bran, brewer's yeast, salmon, prunes, lentils, chicken, peanuts, sunflower seeds, tuna, turkey, and rabbit.

13. *Eat rice bran products.* Phytonutrients from rice bran have shown promise in preventing heart disease and providing health benefits (Jariwalla, 2001).

SUPPLEMENTS

1. *Take lecithin.* This derivative of soy can increase stress tolerance (Kumar, Divekar, Gupta, & Srivastava, 2002).

2. *Try alpha-lipoic acid.* This supplement prevents development of hypertension and hyperglycemia and prevents an increase in heart

mitochondrial superoxide anion production in the aorta (Midaoui, Elimadi, Wu, Haddad, & de Champlain, 2003).

3. *Use essential thyme oil.* It is a strong antioxidant that reduces the superoxide dismutase activities in the heart (Youdim & Deans, 1999).

4. *Take grape seed extract.* This supplement can improve cardiac functional assessments including post-ischemic left ventricular function, reduced myocardial infarct size, reduced ventricular fibrillation, and tachycardia (Bagchi et al., 2003).

5. *Consider taking vitamins C and E.* They can retard arteriosclerosis (Liu & Meydani, 2002), reduce blood pressure in mild hypertension (Boshtam, Rafiei, Sadeghi, & Sarraf-Zadegan, 2002), reduce risk of cardiovascular diseases (Baydas, Yilmaz, Celkik, Yasar, & Gursu, 2002), dilate constricted blood vessels (Drossos et al., 2003), and protect against plaque progression (Nakata & Maeda, 2002).

6. *Try additional vitamin D.* If food sources or exposure to sunlight do not provide sufficient vitamin D, a supplement may be needed to assist with intracellular calcium metabolism (Zittermann et al., 2003).

7. *Take arginine.* This semi-essential amino acid is involved in numerous areas of human biochemistry and can be utilized in therapeutic regimens for angina pectoris, congestive heart failure, hypertension, coronary heart disease, and intermittent claudication (Appleton, 2002).

TOUCH

1. *Obtain sufficient touch every day.* Hugs and massage can help. If necessary, provide hugs for clients and/or teach them how to give a foot or hand massage to a spouse or others in return for a massage themselves. Touch can reduce or normalize blood pressure and enhance the immune response (Wardell & Engebretson, 2001; Weiss, 1992).

2. *Use gentle acupressure to strengthen the heart.* Hold the little finger of the left hand with the index, middle, and fourth fingers of the right hand. Hold it gently until a steady, strong, and comforting pulse is felt in each finger of the right hand. It may take a few minutes. Experiment with tightening and loosening the grip until the pulses are felt, allowing blockages to open. Persevere. After pulses in all the left fingers emerge, repeat with the right hand.

EXERCISE

Exercise daily. Intensity doesn't matter, but regularity does. Walking is best, as running or jogging may be too stressful. Walk at a comfortable rate, one that allows conversation with a partner, and not in the heat of the day, slowly building up distance and pace. Even clients diagnosed with heart failure should exercise, but be carefully monitored (Pina, Apstein, & Balady, 2003).

RELATIONSHIPS

1. *Open the heart.*

A. Lie on the back on a bed, carpet, or pad. Breathe in through the nose and then breathe out naturally. Hold one hand over the abdomen and feel the abdomen rise, pushing the hand out on inhalation, and feeling the abdomen retract on exhalation.

B. Focus on breathing, exhaling and inhaling three times naturally. As the air moves in through the nose and back down the throat, say "one." Feel the air moving back out of the lungs and say "two." As the next breath begins to fill the lungs, say "three." Feel the air moving back out and say "four." Repeat these four actions three more times.

C. Lie on the floor or on a bed and slowly massage the chest. Start anywhere and gently and tenderly massage. Massage sore or tight spots a little more until each feels better. Keep breathing evenly and deeply while massaging. After massaging the whole chest, take an internal reading on how the heart is feeling. Let one hand rest over the heart as if ready to say the "Pledge of Allegiance." Feel the heart beat. Tell it to beat calmly and peacefully. Picture it filling up with peace and love.

D. Picture the heart healthy and happy. See the heart cells looking healthy and joyful. Fill the heart with a joyful and relaxed color. Feel the positive energy flowing through it. Let a healing color expand, filling the heart, chest, and whole body with soothing light. Give the color a voice. What does it say to you? Make it a joyful sound. Ask the color to provide a sign, to tell what it feels. Tell the heart it's healing, and that it will be cared for and protected. Repeat as often as necessary until the image and sounds are clear.

E. Place several stiff pillows on the floor in a pile or fold a blanket and lie down on it, arching the back over the hump. Surrender, letting the shoulders relax and the head relax back into the softness of the pillows or blanket. Let breathing slowly and naturally drop lower in the body all the way down to the abdomen. Hum or groan, releasing the tension in the throat and jaw. Take time. Settle in. Feel any sadness or anger in the throat and shoulders. Let it dissolve or come out as a sound or color. Replace it with forgiveness and joy.

F. Stand up and reach toward the ceiling. Feel the fingertips pulsating with energy. Open eyes and mouth wide and feel the tension in the face. Then close eyes and mouth and feel the relaxation. Bend over at the waist, letting gravity pull the head and arms down toward the floor. Feel the energy flowing up through the feet and into the pelvis. Let the head bob like a flower in the breeze. Inhale and let the oxygen flow through the body and into body tissues. Make soft sounds through the lips, recalling any sadness or loss of a loved one.

G. Stand up or sit down on the floor and look at the hands. Picture the face of a lost loved one in the palm. Let any feelings come. Crying is healing. Let the tears flow.

H. Put one hand over the heart and listen for any feelings inside. Feel the comfort that a beating heart provides. Feel any sadness or anger, then let it flow away like a quiet river.

I. Hold a tennis racket or both fists over the head. Propel the arms forward with a hitting motion picturing angry feelings toward a person. Let any sounds, words, or feelings come out while making hitting movements.

J. Lie on the back on the floor on a carpet or pad. Do a scissors kick, building up to 200 times. Shake the head back and forth crying out, "No!" or "Why?"

K. Rent a sad movie and cry while watching it. Crying cleanses the eyes and produces chemicals that help body cells relax.

L. Rent a funny movie. Watch it and laugh out loud. Really enjoy the movie, saying, "Go ahead, you deserve it."

2. *Use the relaxation script on pages 97–98 to relax, heal the heart, and reduce stress.* This is especially important if anger is the reaction when getting cut off in traffic, the person ahead in the express checkout lane has too many items, or someone else is late or doesn't perform up to standards.

3. *Mend troubled relationships,* starting with father. Practice forgiveness and invite him to lunch. Only talk about neutral topics or things he likes, getting to know him as a person, asking questions, and then listening to his answers without judging. Ask, "What are your hobbies?" and "What do you like to do with your spare time?" and "What are the best things in your life?" and "What was it like when you were growing up?" and "How did you get along with your

father?" and "What suggestions does he have for you to get along better with him?" If an argument occurs, or if being with the father touches off unhappy remembrances, before saying good-bye, say, "I'm sorry." Those may be the two most healing words to say to mend a broken heart. If he's dead or otherwise unavailable, write a letter to him. Pour out your heart. There is no need to actually send the letter; just use it to help get out feelings. Forgiveness is a major issue for heart and blood vessel conditions. Complete the same process for any other relationship that requires mending. Read and take to heart at least one of the following books: *The Self-Forgiveness Handbook* (Thom Rutledge, New Harbinger, 5674 Shattuck Avenue, Oakland, CA 94609), *When to Forgive* (Mona Gustafson Affinito, New Harbinger), *The Art of Forgiveness* (Virginia Sara Fair, POB 328, Monongahela PA 15063).

4. *Learn to play again.* Remember what it is was to be a 5-year-old, chasing a butterfly or picking up shells on the seashore and being delighted at the shapes and colors. Swing on a swing. Finger paint. Play catch with someone, maybe your father. Get on the floor with a dog or cat and roll a ball, scratch behind its ears, and snuggle up to it. Run in a field of wild flowers. Pick berries. Sit by the ocean or a lake and just watch the water for half an hour. Run in the sand and pretend to be a bird. Play has no outcome, no directions. Just enjoy (Sinatra, 1996).

HERBS

1. *Ginger* has been shown to significantly reduce plaque and clotting in arteries (Srivastava, 1984).

2. *Chinese herbs* can be beneficial. In one study in China, 90% of participants with coronary artery problems were able to stop using nitroglycerin on a regular basis after taking safflower and other herbs (Bensky & Gamble, 1993).

3. *Gingko biloba* has been shown to lower blood pressure and improve circulation (Garg, Nag, & Agrawal, 1995; McKenna, Jones, & Hughes, 2001). Gingko may affect the performance of Prozac and other antidepressants by reducing antidepressant sexual dysfunction and improving sleep. Consider using more natural methods of reducing depression (Hemmeter, Annen, Bischof, Bruderlin, Hatzinger et al., 2001; Kang, Lee, Kim, & Cho, 2002), such as enlisting the assistance of a cognitive nurse-psychotherapist and taking a B-vitamin supplement.

4. *Black cohosh* may help if depression and sleeplessness are due to perimenopause.

5. *Garlic* can enhance heart and blood vessel health. Certain herbs can increase the effect of blood thinners and aspirin so you may want to talk to your physician about switching to gingko and garlic and getting off blood thinners and aspirin, which have side effects.

6. *Make a dressing of cabbage leaves and yellow onions* for leg ulcers (Davis, 1980).

Yoga and/or Dance

Learn yogic breathing technique. Find a local yoga instructor who can help you learn the technique. Unilateral forced nostril breathing can positively affect heart function (Shannahoff-Khalsa & Kennedy, 1993). Yoga and/or dance can put clients in touch with their body and feelings.

Environmental Considerations

1. *Get involved with nature.* Spend time hiking, watching birds in the trees, and noticing flowers and animals. Take a family member or friend and share the thrill of the outdoors and each other (Sinatra, 1996).

2. *Go fishing.* Concentrate on the rhythmic motion of casting. Enjoy the fresh air and sunshine. Focus on being, not on doing (Sinatra, 1996).

3. *Avoid going outside during times of high air pollution* and/or move to an area that is less polluted. Heart attack symptoms have been correlated with times of high daily air pollution (Frankish, 2001).

4. *Sleep on the back.* Any nightmares associated with this position usually disappear in time. The next best position is on the right side. Lying on the left side puts additional weight and strain on the heart (Chang, 1986).

Meditation

Meditating for twenty minutes a day can decrease carotid arteriosclerosis (Castillo-Richmond et al., 2001), and can reduce blood pressure (Shannahoff-Khalsa & Kennedy, 1993). Ask clients to contemplate the words that follow and explain the meaning they have:

"In the greater scheme of things, how much does this current stressful situation matter?" and "I have all the time in the world to accomplish what I want to accomplish," and "To heal my heart, I must grant forgiveness to the people I feel have hurt me."

AFFIRMATIONS

Recite or write the following affirmations 20 times a day to counteract negative thoughts and feelings. Also, write them on 3 x 5 cards and put them in prominent places around your home and workplace so they will be read frequently. Suggested places include refrigerator, medicine chest, mirrors, desk, and computer or television set.

- My heart beats to the rhythm of love and understanding.
- I bring joy to the center of my being.
- I express love to all.
- Joy. Joy. Joy.
- Joy is circulating through me now and forever.

HEMORRHOIDS AND/OR VARICOSE VEINS

1. *Eat plenty of high fiber foods every day* (nuts, seeds, vegetables, fruits, and whole grains).

2. *Elevate feet on a slant board or facsimile twice a day* (at least 2 hours after eating). Start with a few minutes and work up to 15–30 minutes a day. *Warning:* avoid slant-boarding if you have had retinal detachments, glaucoma, or other conditions where increased pressure in your head is dangerous, or if you have an irritated hiatal hernia.

3. *Avoid wearing tight clothes, and don't sit or stand in one position too long.* Walk around for a minute or two at least every hour, and do some stretches: reach for the ceiling with your right hand, and for the floor with your left, keeping your body straight. Separate your fingers and gently stretch them, stretching some more until you feel them tingle.

4. *Squeeze the juice of ¼ of a lemon in a glass of warm water and drink it first thing in the morning* when constipated.

5. *Oil the anus with olive or castor oil prior to having a bowel movement* to protect it from pain and bleeding. Never strain. Breathe deep in your abdomen while you are sitting on the toilet. Never sit on the toilet to do your reading. Focus on staying calm and breathing. See "4" above. Elevate your feet on two or three bricks when

you sit on the toilet to reduce abdominal pressure. After a bowel movement, gently dry with cotton balls soaked in castor oil, and apply vitamin E to your anus (to help heal and reduce pain), alternating with witch hazel (to shrink the hemorrhoid and reduce itching).

6. *Take 2 ounces of aloe vera juice after each meal.* **Caution:** Do not use the juice from an aloe vera plant. Purchase aloe vera juice from a health food store.

7. *Massage the feet, lower legs, and hands daily* unless there are contraindications. Use olive or castor oil. Place one hand on the umbilicus. For constipation, massage clockwise out in larger and larger circles and then massage in until you reach your umbilicus again. Massage counterclockwise for diarrhea. For neither, first massage clockwise and then counterclockwise to maintain a healthy colon. Massage along the Achilles tendon gently. Massage the feet, especially the middle of the bottom of each foot, pressing in with the pads of the thumb or index finger. Work gently with sore or tight spots. Massage on the inside of the palm in a line down from the area between thumb and index finger.

8. *Use gentle acupressure.* Put three fingers (index, middle, and fourth) within two inches of the hemorrhoid and the same three fingers of the other hand on the middle of the calf of the corresponding leg. Hold both points until a gentle, open, and strong pulse is felt in all three fingers of both hands, then relax and focus on breathing in the abdomen. (This could take a while if there are energy blockages. At first you may not feel anything; then a pulse may begin, but it may come and go in one or more fingers. Some bursts of pulsation in one or more fingers may be experienced until the pulse evens out and balances in a smooth, even flow in all three fingers (Dayton, 1995).

9. *Use psyllium.* Between two meals, put 1 teaspoon of psyllium husks (available from the health food store) in a glass of water or juice, stir quickly and drink before it thickens. If this stabilizes bowel movements and reduces pressure in the hemorrhoid, continue; otherwise stop.

10. *Sleep with a small soft pillow between the knees* and sleep on the right side to take the pressure off the hemorrhoid.

11. *Try supplements.* To improve vein elasticity and strength, take vitamin C (1,000 mg 2–3 times a day with a full glass of water each time), vitamin E (400–800 IU/day), and zinc (up to 30 mg/day). Take bioflavonoids or vitamin C with added bioflavonoids. Also try horse chestnut capsules (Drossos et al., 2003; Nakata & Maeda, 2002; Symons et al., 2002).

12. *Get plenty of exercise, especially walking.* Even walking 10,000 steps a day can reduce blood pressure that may be causing hemorrhoids or varicose veins (Iwane et al., 2000).

13. *Do leg and abdomen exercises.* Lie on the back on a soft carpet or bed. Bring knees to abdomen, then stretch them out straight (lying flat), then bring legs back up to abdomen. Repeat, working up to 20 times/day. Remember to breathe with each cycle.

14. *Take milk thistle capsules* (follow directions on bottle) to cleanse the liver.

EVALUATION OF TREATMENT

The client mentioned earlier made this self-evaluation of treatment goals: "I'm eating a big meal at 1 P.M. and having plenty of pasta or potatoes, vegetables, salads, and fish. That fills me up pretty well, so with a piece or two of fruit in the late afternoon, I can get by on a sandwich or soup and salad for dinner. I've lost 3 inches off my waist and that makes me feel good. I still resent my father, but I'm working on it. I listen to my relaxation tape at least twice a day and I don't get so hot under the collar anymore. Our family has been on two camping trips together in the past month. I didn't realize how much my kids are growing."

REFERENCES

Appleby, P. N., Davey, G. K., & Key, T. J. (2002). Hypertension and blood pressure among meat eaters, fish eaters, vegetarians and vegans in EPIC-Oxfort. *Public Health Nutrition, 5,* 645–654.

Appleton, J. (2002). Arginine: Clinical potential of semi-essential amino. *Alternative Medicine Review, 7,* 512–522.

Bagchi, D., Sen, C. K., Ray, S. D., Das, D. K., Bagchi, M., Preuss, H. G., & Vinson, J. A. (2003). Molecular mechanisms of cardioprotection by a novel grape seed proanthocyanidin extract. *Mutation Research, February, 523*(4), 87–97.

Baydas, G., Yilmaz, O., Celkik, S., Yasar, A., & Gursu, M. F. (2002). Effects of certain micronutrients and malatonin on plasma lipid, lipid peroxidation, and homocysteine levels in rats. *Archives of Medical Research, 33,* 515–519.

Bensky D., & Gamble, A. (1993). *Chinese herbal medicine, materia medica* (pp. 279–280). Seattle, WA: Eastland.

Boshtam, M., Rafiei, M., Sadeghi, K., & Sarraf-Zadegan, N. (2002). Vitamin E can reduce blood pressure in mild hypertensives. *International Journal of Vitamin and Nutrition Research, 72,* 309–314.

Busserolles, J., Gueux, E., Rock, E., Mazur, A., & Rayssigiguier, Y. (2002). Substituting honey for refined carbohydrates protects rats from hypertriglyceridemic and prooxidative effects of fructose. *Journal of Nutrition, 132,* 3379.

Carl, C. L., Fenske, R. A., & Elgethun, K. (2003). Organophosphorus pesticide exposure of urban and suburban preschool children with organic and conventional diets. *Environmental Health Perspectives, 111,* 377–382.

Castillo-Richmond, A., Schneider, R. H., Alexander, C. N., Cook, R., Myers, H., Nidich, S., Haney, C., Rainforth, M., & Salerno, J. (2001). Effects of stress reduction on carotid arteriosclerosis in hypertensive African Americans. *Stroke, 31,* 568–573.

Davis, B. (1980). *Rapid healing foods.* West Nyack, NY: Parker.

Drossos, G. E., Toumpoulis, I. K., Katritsis, D. G., Ioannidis, J. P., Kontogiorgi, P., & Anagnostopoulos, C. E. (2003). Is vitamin C superior to diltiazem for radial artery vasodilation in patients awaiting coronary artery bypass grafting? *Journal of Thoracic Cardiovascular Surgery, 125,* 330–335.

Frankish, H. (2001). Air pollutants can trigger heart attacks. *Lancet, 357,* 1952.

Garg, R. K., Nag, D., & Agrawal, A. (1995). A double blind placebo controlled trial of ginkgo biloba extract in acute cerebral ischaemia. *Journal of Association Physicians (India), 43,* 760–763.

Ginocchio, R., Rodriguez, P. H., Badilla-Ohibaum, R., Allen, H. E., & Lagos, G. E. (2002). Effect of soil copper content and pH on copper uptake of selected vegetables grown under controlled conditions. *Environmental Toxicology Chemistry, 21,* 1736–1744.

Gorenstein, S., Zachwieja, Z., Folta, M., Barton, H., Piotrowicz, J., Zenser, M., et al. (2001). Dietary fiber, total phenolics and minerals in persimmons and apples. *Journal of Agricultural and Food Chemistry, 49,* 952–957.

Halpin, L. S., Speir, A. M., CapoBianco, P., & Barnett, S. D. (2002). Guided imagery in cardiac surgery. *Outcomes Management, 6,* 132–137.

Hemmeter, U., Annen, B., Bischof, R., Bruderlin, U., Hatzinger, U., Rose, U., & Holsboer-Trachsler, E. (2001). Polysomnographic effects of adjuvant ginkgo biloba therapy in patients with major depression medicated with trumipramine. *Pharmacopsychiatry, 34*(2), 50–59.

Holm, T., Andreassen, A. K., Aukrust, P., Andersen, K., Geiran, O. R., Kjekshus, J., Simonsen, S., & Gullestad, L. (2001). Omega-3 fatty acids improve blood pressure control and preserve renal function in hypertensive heart transplant recipients. *European Heart Journal, 22,* 428–436.

Ito, M. K. (2002). Niacin-based therapy for dysclipidemia: Past evidence and future advances. *American Journal of Managed Care, 8*(12, Suppl.), S315–S322.

Ivanov, A. N., Medkova, I. L., & Mosiagina, L. I. (2002). Vegetarian diet in treating elderly patients with ischemic heart disease (clinico-hemodynamic, biochemical, and hemorrheological effects. *Vopr Pitan, 71*(3), 11–14.

Iwane, M., Arita, M., Tomimoto, S., Satani, O., Matsumoto, M., Miyashita, K., & Nishio, I. (2000). Walking 10,000 steps a day or more reduces blood pressure and sympathetic nerve activity in mild essential hypertension. *Hypertension Research, 23,* 573–580.

Jariwalla, R. J. (2001). Rice-bran products: Phytonutrients with potential applications in preventive and clinical medicine. *Drugs in Experimental and Clinical Research, 27*(1), 17–26.

Kang, B. J., Lee, S. J., Kim, M. D., & Cho, M. J. (2002). A placebo-controlled, double-blind trial of Gingko biloba for antidepressant-induced sexual dysfunction. *Human Psychopharmacology, 17,* 279–284.

Karavoltsos, S., Sakellari, A., Dimopoulos, M., Dasenakis, M., & Scoulios, M. (2002). Cadmium content in foodstuffs from the Greek market. *Food Additives and Contamination, 19,* 954–962.

Kim, J., Oberman, A., Fletcher, G. F., & Lee, J. Y. (2001). Effect of exercise intensity and frequency on lipid levels in men with coronary heart disease: Training level comparison trial. *American Journal of Cardiology, 87,* 942–946.

Knekt, P., Kumpulainen, J., Jarvinen, R., Rissanen, H., Heliovaara, M., Reunanen, A., et al. (2002). Flavonoid intake and risk of chronic diseases. *American Journal of Clinical Nutrition, 3,* 560–568.

Kris-Etherton, P. M., Hecker, K. D., Bonanome, A., Coval, S. M., Binkoski, A. E., Hilpert, K. F., et al. (2002). Bioactive compounds in foods: Their role in the prevention of cardiovascular disease and cancer. *American Journal of Medicine, 113*(Suppl. 9B), 71S–88S.

Kumar, R., Divekar, H. M., Gupta, V., & Srivastava, K. K. (2002). Antistress and adaptogenic activity of lecithin supplementation. *Journal of Alternative & Complementary Medicine, 8,* 487–492.

Liu, L., & Meydani, M. (2002). Combined vitamin C and E supplementation retards early progression of arteriosclerosis in heart transplant patients. *Nutrition Reviews, 60,* 368–371.

Liu, S., Manson, J. E., Buring, J. E., Stampfer, M. J., Willett, W. C., & Ridker, P. M. (2002). Relation between a diet with a high glycemic load and plasma concentrations of high-sensitivity C-reactive protein in middle-aged women. *American Journal of Clinical Nutrition, 75,* 492–498.

Maxson, J. (2002). Remedying dyslipidemia NCEP-ATP III strategies to slow CVD. *Clinician Reviews, 12*(10), 54–60.

McKenna, D. J., Jones, K., & Hughes, K. (2001). Efficacy, safety, and use of ginkgo biloba in clinical and preclinical applications. *Alternative Therapies in Health and Medicine, 7*(5), 70–86, 88–90.

Midaoui, A. E., Elimadi, A., Wu, L., Haddad, P. S., & de Champlain, J. (2003). Lipoic acid prevents hypertension, hyperglycemia, and the increase in heart mitochondrial superoxide production. *American Journal of Hypertension, 16,* 173–179.

Moore, T. J., Conlin, P. R., Ard, J., & Svetkey, L. P. (2001). DASH (Dietary Approaches to Stop Hypertension) diet is effective treatment for stage 1 isolated systolic hypertension. *Hypertension, 38,* 155–158.

Nakata, Y., & Maeda, N. (2002). Vulnerable atherosclerotic plaque morphology in apolipoprotein E-deficient mice unable to make ascorbic acid. *Circulation, 105,* 1485–1490.

Nygard, O., Refsum, H., Ueland, P. M., Stensvold, I., Nordrehoug, J. E., Kvale, G., et al. (1997). Coffee consumption and plasma total homocysteine: The Hordaland Homocysteine Study. *American Journal of Clinical Nutrition, 65,* 136–141.

O'Byrne, D. J., Devaraj, S., Grundy, S. M., & Jialal, I. (2002). Comparison of the antioxidant effects of Concord grape juice flavonoids alpha-tocopherol n markers of oxidative stress in healthy adults. *American Journal of Clinical Nutrition, 76,* 1367–1374.

Parcell, S. (2002). Sulfur in human nutrition and applications in medicine. *Alternative Medicine Review, 7*(1), 22–44.

Pascual, J. A., Garcia, C., Hernandez, T., Lerma, S., & Lynch, J. M. (2002). Effectiveness of municipal waste compost and its humic fraction in suppressing Pythium ultimatum. *Microbiology and Ecology, 44*(1), 58–68.

Pina, I. T., Apstein, C. S., & Balady, G. I. (2003). Exercise and heart failure: A statement from the American Heart Association Committee on Exercise, Rehabilitation and Prevention. *Circulation, 107,* 1210–1225.

Rao, A. V. (2002). Lycopene, tomatoes, and the prevention of coronary heart disease. *Experimental Biological Medicine, 227,* 908–913.

Robinson, F., Hackett, A. F., Billington, D., & Stratton, G. (2002). Changing from a mixed to self-selected vegetarian diet—influence on blood lipids. *Journal of Human Nutrition and Diet, 15,* 323–329.

Rosa, A., Deiana, M., Casu, V., Paccagnini, S., Appendino, G., Ballero, M., & Dessi, M. A. (2002). Antioxidant activity of capsinoids. *Journal of Agriculture and Food Chemistry, 50,* 7396–7401.

Savickiene, N., Dagilyte, A., Lukosius, A., & Zitkevicius, V. (2002). Importance of biologically active components and plants in the prevention of complications of diabetes mellitus. *Medicina, 38,* 970–975.

Shannahoff-Khalsa, D. S., & Kennedy, B. (1993). The effects of unilateral forced breathing on the heart. *International Journal of Neuroscience, 73*(1–2), 47–60.

Sinatra, S. T. (1996). *Heartbreak and heart disease.* New Canaan, CT: Keats.

Srivastava, K. (1984). Aqueous extracts of onion, garlic and ginger inhibit platelet aggregation and alter arachidonic acid metabolism. *Biomedical Biochemistry Acta, 43,* 335–336.

Stampfer, M. J., Krauss, R. M., Ma, J., Blanche, P. J., Holl, L. G., Sacks, F. M., et al. (1997). A prospective study of triglyceride level, low-density lipoprotein particle diameter, and risk of myocardial infarction. *Journal of the American Medical Association, 276,* 882–888.

Symons, J. D., Mullick, A. E., Ensunsa, J. L., Ma, A. A., & Rutledge, J. C. (2002). Hyperhomocysteinemia evoked by folate depletion: Effects on coronary and carotid arterial function. *Arteriosclerotic Thrombotic and Vascular Biology, 22,* 772–780.

Wardell, D. W., & Engebretson, J. (2001). Biological correlates of Reiki Touch healing. *Journal of Advanced Nursing, 33,* 439–445.

Weiss, S. J. (1992). Psychophysiologic and behavioral effects of tactile stimulation on infants with congenital heart disease. *Research in Nursing and Health, 15,* 93–101.

Wenneberg, S. R., Schneider, R. H., Walton, K. G., Maclean, C. R., Levitsky, D. K., Salerno, J. W., et al. (1997). A controlled study of the effects of the Transcendental Meditation program on cardiovascular reactivity and ambulatory blood pressure. *International Journal of Neuroscience, 89*(1–2), 15–28.

Whelton, P. K., He, J., Culter, J. A., Bransatu, F. L., Appel, L. J., Fallmann, D., & Klag, M. J. (1997). Effects of oral potassium on blood pressure: Meta-analysis of randomized controlled clinical trials. *Journal of the American Medical Association, 277,* 1624–1632.

Youdim, K. A., & Deans, S. G. (1999). Dietary supplementation of thyme (Thymus vulgaris L.) essential oil during the lifetime of the rat: Its effects on the antioxidant status in liver, kidney and heart tissues. *Mechanics of Ageing and Development, 109,*163–175.

Zittermann, A., Schleithoff, S. S., Tenderich, G., Berthold, H. K., Korfer, R., & Stehle, P. (2003). Low vitamin D status: A contributing factor in the pathogenesis of congestive heart failure? *Journal of the American College of Cardiology, 41,* 105–112.

CHAPTER 14

Kidney Disease

Some of the afflictions that can affect the kidney include urinary tract infection, glomerulonephritis, polycystic kidney disease, and kidney stones. A kidney infection is usually treated with gentamicin, cephalosporin, or cotrimoxazole. The majority of kidney stones will pass spontaneously. If they don't, the medical treatment might include extracorporeal shock wave lithotripsy, or hypocitraturic calcium.

HOLISTIC NURSING ASSESSMENT

Study the holistic nursing assessment for Mr. D., a 49-year-old man, diagnosed with kidney problems. Working in collaboration with clients diagnosed with kidney conditions, use the format to perform a holistic nursing assessment.

Client learning needs: "My wife calls me a failure."

Indicants of readiness to learn: "I want to feel better about myself, but I'm not sure how to go about it."

Soul/spirituality symbol(s): "I have a cross my mother gave me that I pray to."

Meaning of the condition to client: "I've never taken care of myself. I drank too much and took drugs. I guess it's catching up with me."

Relationship needs/effects as perceived by the client: "My wife is divorcing me and I want her back."

Patterns/attitudes that may create dis-ease for this client: Client uses negative affirmations (e.g., "I never achieved what I could have. I've had one second-rate job after another").

Life purpose: Expresses no life purpose except to get his wife back.

Client strengths: Has articulated two goals.

Ability to participate in care: Client is malnourished and weak, but verbalizes the wish to change.

Ethical dilemmas: None identified.

Nurse–client process: Client cries and asks the nurse to decide for him.

TREATMENT PLANNING: SETTING JOINTLY AGREED-UPON GOALS

In the case of the client discussed above, the following goals were agreed upon:

1. Commence vegetarian meal plan.
2. Complete counseling sessions with estranged wife.
3. Find a job he likes.

TREATMENT

Acceptance of condition/attitude change: The client chose the following affirmation to use to replace the upset he feels: "Only good comes from each experience." Client agreed to write the affirmation on 3 x 5 cards and say the words at least 20 times each day.

Facilitating the healing process/healing intention formulation: From a list of meditative statements, client chose the following one to assist in the healing process: "I can grow to my full potential." Client was asked to meditate on the words while in a relaxed state. Nurse will use caring nonverbal and verbal communication, centering, and a meditative state to enhance client healing, will verbalize observed patterns that may be holding the client back and offer alternate approaches.

Creating a sacred space: During client sessions, a soft lamp light will burn in the room and Mozart will play in the background.

Encouraging re-storying: Encouraged client to recall an upsetting situation with his family and choose an ending that inspires him.

Integrative practices planned: Will use soft touch acupressure and hypnosis to assist client in the healing process.

Role model strategies: Showed client how to role play problematic interchanges with his wife.

Protection plan: Client plans to use a white light image around him for protection.

Family strategies: Encouraged client to invite his wife to a session with nurse to practice more open communication between them.

Life issues/life purpose work: Client has agreed to meditate on his life purpose.

Treatment possibilities/considerations: Other suggested treatments appear below. Most are evidence-based.

ADDITIONAL INFORMATION AND TREATMENTS TO SHARE WITH CLIENTS

FOR ANY KIDNEY CONDITION

1. Either stand up or sit in a chair behind client.
2. Rub the hands together vigorously, until energy is felt flowing in the palms and fingers.
3. Place palms on the small of the back on each side of spine, feeling the heat and energy flowing in. Keep the upper body tilted slightly forward.
4. Rub up and down the back and then massage in a circular motion.

Teach client to:

1. Use both fists to pummel the small of the back for several seconds. Repeat two more times (Chang, 1986).
2. Hold index, third, and fourth fingers on the following spots until a steady quiet pulsation is felt in all three fingers: (a) both little toes, (b) middle of pubic bone, (c) coccyx, (d) spot on either side of the spinal column where the neck meets the shoulder (Dayton, 1995).
3. Avoid over-the-counter pain medicines including NSAIDs (ibuprofen, Advil, Nuprin, etc.) and aspirin, which can damage the kidneys and liver (Wallace, 1996; Wolfe, 1994).

URINARY TRACT INFECTIONS

1. Drink plenty of fluids every day, including a large glass of cranberry juice to prevent bacteria from attaching to urinary cells.
2. Always urinate immediately at the first sign of an urge.
3. Empty the bladder completely each time during urination.
4. Wipe from front to back after going to the bathroom.
5. Clean the area around the vagina (first) and (then) rectum daily and before sex, using warm soapy water.
6. Say or write at least one of the following affirmations 20 or more times every day:

   - I am safe and secure.
   - I release old angers and disappointments.
   - I welcome the new into my life.

7. Take ginkgo biloba to reduce toxicity if taking Gentamicin (Naidu, Shifow, Kumar, & Ratnakar, 2000).

KIDNEY STONES

1. *Drink 10 glasses of water daily.* Water flushes toxins out of the body, and not drinking enough water is a frequent cause of kidney stones (Borghi et al., 1999).

2. *Eat more foods rich in essential fatty acids.* Not eating enough essential fatty acids may be a cause of some kidney conditions (Simopoulos, 1999). The benefits of polyunsaturated fatty acids have been shown in the prevention of some renal diseases. Some foods to eat include fatty fish (tuna, salmon, mackerel, herring, whitefish), green leafy vegetables, flaxseed (add to salads, soups, yogurt, cereals, baked goods, or fresh juices), olive oil, seeds, and nuts.

Eat foods rich in magnesium. This mineral is an effective inhibitor of the formation and growth of calcium oxalate kidney stones. Eating an ovo-lacto-vegetarian diet (vegetables, fruits, whole grains, milk and milk products, and eggs) is a good way to get and keep the magnesium the body needs to ward off kidney stones (Siener & Hesse, 1995). Consider taking a magnesium supplement. One study demonstrated that oral supplementation of magnesium in adults with kidney stones resulted in a reduced risk for stone formation (DeSwart, Sokole, & Wilmink, 1998).

3. *Drink reconstituted lemonade.* This drink increased urinary citrate levels and lowered urinary calcium levels, two things that will reduce kidney stones (Seltzer, Low, McDonald, Shami, & Stoller, 1996).

4. *Reduce consumption of protein, salt, and foods high in oxalates* such as peanuts, cocoa, and chocolate, and the following cooked vegetables: beets, spinach, collards, rhubarb, and chard. The heat from cooking turns the calcium they contain into calcium oxalate, and stone formation can occur (Parivar, Low, & Stoller, 1996).

5. *Avoid drinking apple juice and possibly grapefruit juice.* Both were correlated with stone formation (Curhan, Willett, Rimm, Spiegelman, & Stampfer, 1996), although grapefruit juice was not correlated with stone formation in another study (Goldfarb & Asplin, 2001).

6. *Eat more foods high in calcium* (dairy foods, broccoli, green leafy vegetables, tomatoes, whole wheat bread, canned sardines, almonds, soy milk, tofu). It may be difficult to get the full 1200–1500 mg of calcium necessary every day, so consider a calcium citrate supplement. There is no need to restrict dairy products in those prone to form kidney stones (Hall, 2002; Trinchieri et al., 1997) or calcium intake (Hall, 2002), unless sufficient water, potassium, and magnesium are not ingested (Heller, Doerner, Brinkley, Adams-Huet, & Pak, 2003).

7. *Avoid sugar and salt.* Kidney stones are correlated with sucrose and sodium intake (Curhan, Willett, Speizer, Spiegelman, & Stampfer, 1997).

8. *Lower intake of animal protein,* including meat, chicken, eggs, milk, and cheese (Parivar et al., 1996). Chronic high protein intake can produce structural change in the glomerulus and tubules of the kidneys (Brandle, Sieberth, & Hautmann, 1996).

9. *Eat more foods high in vitamin B6,* including brewer's yeast, sunflower seeds, toasted wheat germ, brown rice, soybeans, white beans, liver, chicken, mackerel, salmon, tuna, bananas, walnuts, sweet potatoes and cooked cabbage. High intake of vitamin B6 through food or supplements has been shown to protect against kidney stone formation, and vitamin C need not be restricted because it is not associated with risk for kidney stones (Curhan, Willett, Speizer, & Stampfer, 1999).

10. *Avoid colas, even sugar-free ones.* In one study, individuals who completely eliminated phosphoric acid-containing colas reduced their risk of recurring kidney stones (Shuster et al., 1992).

11. *Eat rice bran products.* Phytonutrients from rice bran have shown promise in preventing kidney stones (Jariwalla, 2001).

12. *Eat more foods high in potassium,* including shredded raw cabbage, bananas, turkey, apples, fresh apricots, cooked broccoli, baked potato, wheat germ, spinach, dried fruit, and fresh fruits to prevent stone growth (Pierratos et al., 2000).

13. *Try a kidney flush to pass a painful kidney stone.* Take 2 alfalfa tablets every hour. For the first day, take the juice of 6 lemons in a gallon of distilled water. Drink all of this the first day. If the stone hasn't passed, on the next days, only use water with the alfalfa tablets. Continue to eat lightly during this time.

14. *Vitamin A and C can protect the kidney against oxidative stress* (Curhan et al., 1999; Patra, Swarup, & Dwivedi, 2001).

Say or write one of the following affirmations at least 20 times daily:

- I let go of all anger
- I easily dissolve my past problems

PROGRESSIVE KIDNEY DISEASE/CHRONIC RENAL FAILURE

1. *Eat polyunsaturated fatty acid foods* (Holm et al., 2001; Simopoulos, 1999; Sulikowska, Manitus, Nieweglowski, Szydlowska-Lysiak, & Rutkowski, 2002). Foods to include are fatty fish (tuna, salmon, mackerel, herring, whitefish), green leafy vegetables, flaxseed (add to salads, soups, yogurt, cereals, baked goods, or fresh juices), olive oil, seeds, and nuts.

2. *Fish oil may reduce high blood pressure, prevent the development of proteinuria, and minimize lesions* (Donadio, Holman, Johnson, Bibas, & Spencer, 1994; Hobbs, Rayner, & Howe, 1996). Fish oil is available in capsules at a health food store.

3. *Eat a high soy (especially tofu) and vegetarian diet and include flaxseeds* (Velasquez & Bhathena, 2001).

4. *Increase intake of garlic.* It can protect the kidney cortex (Pedraza-Chaverri et al., 2000b), stop kidney damage in chronic kidney syndrome (Pedraza-Chaverri et al., 2000a), and protect the kidney from toxicity (Pedraza-Chaverri et al., 2000a, 2000b) and amebic virulence (Ankri, Miron, Rabinkov, Wilchek, & Mirelman, 1997).

5. *Take a vitamin B6 supplement.* It can improve tingling, numbness, and burning pain in fingers and toes that sometimes accompany chronic kidney failure (Okada et al., 2000).

6. *Take 400 IU vitamin E daily* (Mydlik et al., 2002).

7. *Reduce intake of protein and eat that amount consistently* (Brandle et al., 1996).

8. *Try thymus essential oil as a supplement to protect against kidney damage due to aging* (Youdim & Deans, 1999).

9. *Try Chinese herbs.* A Chinese herbal recipe called Yishen Huanshuai markedly retarded the rate of progression of chronic kidney disease when combined with a low protein diet and controlled blood pressure (Yin, Dai, & Rao, 1998).

10. *Drink a pint of raw carrot juice mixed with a pint of raw spinach juice daily.* It would be best to purchase a juicer because the juice must be made fresh daily and drunk immediately. To juice spinach, wash the vegetable carefully in filtered water and vinegar. Roll several leaves up, then put them, including the stems, in the juicer stems first. Use a blender to blend the vegetables very finely, adding a small amount of distilled water to dilute it. After blending, strain and drink immediately (Williams, 1998).

11. *Eat Chinese medicine kidney tonics,* including beef kidney, chestnuts, cinnamon, cloves, dill, fennel, fenugreek, lobster, pistachios, raspberries, and strawberries.

12. *Balance negative thoughts by saying or writing affirmations* 20 times every day. Choose one of more of the following:

- It is safe to grow and be joyful.
- The right action is always taking place in my life.
- All things good come into my life.

13. *Try an herbal tea.* Parsley, corn silk, watermelon seed, or juniper berry tea may help.

14. *Exercise training can reduce blood pressure and increase muscular strength and functional aerobic capacity* (Boyce et al., 1997).

TREATMENT EVALUATION

The client described above reported the following movement toward his goals: "I'm a vegetarian now and my wife and I have had three counseling sessions. She still wants a divorce, but at least I understand more about what bothers her. I'm having three job interviews this week."

REFERENCES

Ankri S., Miron, T., Rabinkov, A., Wilchek, M. & Mirelman, D. (1997). Allicin from garlic strongly inhibits cysteine proteinases and cytopathic effects of *Entamoeba histolytica. Antimicrobial Agents and Chemotherapy, 41,* 2286–2288.

Borghi, L., Meschi, T., Schianchi, T., Briganti, A., Guerra, A., Allegri, F., & Novarini, A. (1999). Urine volume: Stone risk factor and preventive measures. *Nephron, 81*(Suppl. 1), 31–37.

Boyce, M. I., Robergs, R. A., Avasthi, P. S., Roldan, C., Foster, A., Montner, P., et al. (1997). Exercise training by individuals with predialysis renal failure: Cardiorespiratory endurance, hypertension, and renal function. *American Journal of Kidney Disease, 30,* 180–192.

Brandle, E., Sieberth, H. G., & Hautmann, R. E. (1996). Effect of chronic dietary protein intake on the renal function in healthy subjects. *European Journal of Clinical Nutrition, 50,* 734–740.

Chang, S. T. (1986). *The complete system of self-healing internal exercises.* San Francisco: Tao.

Curhan, G. C., Willett, W. C., Rimm, E. B., Spiegelman, D., & Stampfer, M. J. (1996). Prospective study of beverage use and the risk of kidney stones. *American Journal of Epidemiology, 143,* 240–247.

Curhan, G. C., Willett, W. C., Speizer, F. E., Spiegelman, D., & Stampfer, M. J. (1997). Comparison of dietary calcium with supplemental calcium and other nutrients as factors affecting the risk for kidney stones in women. *Annals of Internal Medicine 126,* 497–450.

Curhan, G. C., Willett, W. C., Speizer, F. E., & Stampfer, M. J. (1999). Intake of vitamins B6 and C and the risk of kidney stones in women. *Journal of the American Society of Nephrology, 10,* 840–848.

Dayton, B. R. (1995). *An introduction to a gentle acupressure for caregivers.* Friday Harbor, WA: High Touch Network.

DeSwart, P. M., Sokole, E. B., & Wilmink, J. M. (1998). The interrelationship of calcium and magnesium absorption in idiopathic hypercalciuria and renal calcium stone disease. *Journal of Urology, 159,* 669–672.

Donadio, J. V., Holman, R. T., Johnson, S. B., Bibas, D., & Spencer, D. C. (1994). Essential fatty acid deficiency profiles in idiopathic immunoglobin A nephropathy. *American Journal of Kidney Disease 23,* 648–654.

Goldfarb, D. S., & Asplin, J. R. (2001). Effect of grapefruit juice on urinary lithogenicity. *Journal of Urology, 166,* 263–267.

Hall, P. M. (2002). Preventing kidney stones: Calcium restriction not warranted. *Cleveland Clinical Journal of Medicine, 69,* 885–888.

Heller, H. J., Doerner, M. F., Brinkley, I. J., Adams-Huet, B., & Pak, C. Y. (2003). Effect of dietary calcium on stone forming propensity. *Journal of Urology, 169,* 470–474.

Hobbs, L. M., Rayner, T. E., & Howe, P. R. (1996). Dietary fish oil prevents the development of renal damage in salt-loaded stroke-prone spontaneously hypertensive rats. *Clinical & Experimental Pharmacology & Physiology, 23,* 508–513.

Holm, T., Andreassen, A. K., Aukrust, P., Andersen, K., Geiran, O. R., Kjekshus, J., et al. (2001). Omega-3 fatty acids improve blood pressure control and preserve renal function in hypertensive heart transplant recipients. *European Heart Journal, 22,* 428–436.

Jariwalla, R. J. (2001). Rice-bran products: Phytonutrients with potential applications in preventive and clinical medicine. *Drugs in Experimental and Clinical Research, 27,* 17–26.

Mydlik, M., Derzsiova, K., Racz, O., Sipulova, A., Boldizsar, J., Lovasova, E., & Hribikova, M. (2002). Vitamin E as an antioxidant agent in CAPD patients. *International Journal of Artificial Organs, 25,* 373–378.

Naidu, M. U., Shifow, A. A., Kumar, K. V., & Ratnakar, K. S. (2000). Ginkgo biloba extract ameliorates gentamicin-induced nephrotoxicity in rats. *Phytomedicine, 7,* 191–197.

Okada, H., Moriwaki, K., Kianno, Y., Sugahara, S., Nakamoto, H., Yoshizawa, M., & Suzuki, H. (2000). Vitamin B6 supplementation can improve peripheral polyneuropathy in patients with chronic renal failure on high-flux haemodialysis and human recombinant erythropoietin. *Nephrology, Dialysis and Transplants, 15,* 1410–1313.

Parivar, F., Low, R. K., & Stoller, M. L. (1996). The influence of diet on urinary stone disease. *Journal of Urology, 155,* 432–440.

Patra, R. C., Swarup, D., & Dwivedi, S. K. (2001). Antioxidant effects of alpha tocopherol, ascorbic acid and L-methionine on lead induced oxidative stress to the liver, kidney and brain in rats. *Toxicology, 162,* 81–88.

Pedraza-Chaverri, J., Maldonado, P. D., Medina-Campos, O. N., Olivares-Corichi, I. M., Granados-Silvestre, M. A., Hernandez-Pando, R., et al. (2000a). Garlic ameliorates gentamicin nephrotoxicity: Relation to antioxidant enzymes. *Free Radical Biological Medicine, 29,* 602–611.

Pedraza-Chaverri, J., Medina-Campos, O. N., Granados-Silvestre, M. A., Maldonado, P. D., Olivares-Corichi, I. M., & Hernandez-Pando, R. (2000b). Garlic ameliorates hyperlipidemia in chronic aminonucleoside nephrosis. *Molecular and Cell Biochemistry, 211*(1–2), 69–77.

Pierratos, A., Dharamsi, N., Carr, L. K., Ibanez, D., Jewett, M. A. S., Honey, R., & John, D. A. (2000). Higher urinary potassium is associated with decreased stone growth after shock wave lithotripsy. *Journal of Urology, 164,* 1486–1489.

Seltzer, M. A., Low, R. K., McDonald, M., Shami, G. S., & Stoller, M. L. (1996). Dietary manipulation with lemonade to treat hypocitraturic calcium nephrolithiasis. *Journal of Urology, 156,* 907–909.

Shuster, J., Jenkins, A., Logan, C., Barnett, T., Richle, R., Zackson, D., et al. (1992). Soft drink consumption and urinary stone recurrence: A randomized prevention trial. *Journal of Clinical Epidemiology, 45,* 911–916.

Siener, R., & Hesse, A. (1995). Influence of a mixed and a vegetarian diet on urinary magnesium excretion and concentration. *British Journal of Nutrition, 73,* 783–790.

Simopoulos, A. P. (1999). Essential fatty acids in health and chronic disease. *American Journal of Clinical Nutrition, 70*(3 Suppl.), 560S–569S.

Sulikowska, B., Manitus, J., Nieweglowski, T., Szydlowska-Lysiak, W., & Rutkowski, B. (2002). The effect of therapy with small doses of mega-3 polyunsaturated fatty acid on renal reserve and metabolic disturbances in patients with primary IGA glomerulopathy. *Polish Archives of Medicine, 108,* 753–760.

Trinchieri, A., Nespoli, R., Ostini, F., Rovera, F., Zanetti, G., & Pisani, E. (1998). A study of dietary calcium and other nutrients in idiopathic renal calcium stone formers with low bone mineral content. *Journal of Urology, 159,* 654–657.

Velasquez, M. T., & Bhathena, S. J. (2001). Dietary phytoestrogens: a possible role in renal disease protection. *American Journal of Kidney Disease, 37,* 1056–1068.

Wallace, K. (1996). National kidney foundation warns against heavy use of over-the-counter painkillers. Press Release, February 19, Orlando, FL (800) 927-9659.

Williams, D. G. (1998). How to protect yourself from one of the next big epidemics. *Alternatives for the Health Conscious Individual, 7*(10), 73–75.

Wolfe, S. (1994). Two over-the-counter pain pills lack important warnings about kidney damage. *Public Citizen's Health Research Group Health Letter, 10*(8), 3.

Yin, D., Dai, X., & Rao, X. (1998). Yishen huanshuai recipe retards progression of chronic renal failure. *Zhongguo Zhong Xi Yi Jie He Za Zhi, 18,* 402–404.

Youdim, K. A., & Deans, S. G. (1999). Dietary supplementation of thyme (*Thymus vulgaris L.*) essential oil during the lifetime of the rat: Its effects on the antioxidant status in liver, kidney and heart tissues. *Mechanics of Ageing and Development, 109,* 163–175.

CHAPTER 15

Liver Disease

All drugs stress the liver to some extent, but those that are hardest on this body organ are INH (isoniazid, a treatment for tuberculosis), chemotherapy drugs, methyldopa (Aldomet and Aldoril, used to lower blood pressure), and monoamine oxide inhibitors (Mindell & Hopkins, 1998). Diagnostic tools include an enzyme immunoassay, used as the initial test in patients with liver disease. However, false positive reactions can occur, making it look as if there is liver disease when it doesn't exist (Hubbard, 1998). The remedy for that is to have a second immunoassay completed by a different doctor using another laboratory.

HOLISTIC NURSING ASSESSMENT

Study the holistic nursing assessment for Mrs. T., a 54-year-old woman diagnosed with chronic liver disease. Working in collaboration with clients diagnosed with liver and gall bladder conditions, adapt the following holistic nursing assessment form.

Client learning needs: "I want to find out how I got this."

Indicants of readiness to learn: "I've been talking to people about my condition and I'm confused."

Soul/spirituality symbol(s): "I was raised Lutheran, but I haven't been to church since high school."

Meaning of the condition to client: "This liver thing is ruining my life."

Relationship needs/effects as perceived by the client: "Since I was diagnosed with this condition, my husband has been ignoring me."

Patterns/attitudes that may create dis-ease for this client: Client uses negative affirmations (e.g., "This is all my fault" and "I always feel so bad").

Life purpose: Expresses no life purpose except to feel better.

Client strengths: Wants to learn more about her condition.

Ability to participate in care: Client is in a weakened condition, but can discuss priorities and problem solve.

Ethical dilemmas: Client has been lying to her husband about her condition.

Nurse–client process: Client complains about every aspect of care.

TREATMENT PLANNING: SETTING JOINTLY AGREED-UPON GOALS

In the case of the client discussed above, the following goals were agreed upon:

1. Be honest with her husband about her condition.
2. Eat more wellness foods.
3. Cleanse her liver.

TREATMENT

Acceptance of condition/attitude change: The client chose the following affirmation to use to replace the anger and bitterness she feels: "Love prevails." Client agreed to write the affirmation on 3 x 5 cards and say the words at least 20 times each day.

Facilitating the healing process/healing intention formulation: From a list of meditative statements, client chose the following one to assist in the healing process: "My life is filled with joy and wonder." Asked client to meditate on the words while in a relaxed state. Will use caring nonverbal and verbal communication, centering, and a meditative state to enhance client healing, will verbalize observed patterns that may be holding the client back and offer alternative approaches.

Creating a sacred space: During client sessions, music of her choice will play in the background and peppermint aromatherapy will assist with the healing process.

Encouraging re-storying: Encouraged client to recall an upsetting situation with her husband and choose an ending that inspires her.

Integrative practices planned: Will use guided imagery and relaxation therapy to assist client in the healing process.

Role model strategies: Showed client how to role play problematic interchanges with her husband.

Protection plan: Client will use an image of stained glass windows from her childhood church.

Family strategies: Encouraged client to invite her husband to a session with nurse to practice more open communication between them.

Life issues/life purpose work: Client has agreed to write in her journal about life purpose.

Treatment possibilities/considerations: Other suggested treatments appear below. Most are evidence-based.

ADDITIONAL INFORMATION AND TREATMENTS TO SHARE WITH CLIENTS

1. *Use a breakfast drink to cleanse liver.* Mix the juice of 1 to 2 grapefruit or 2 oranges, 1 clove of garlic, 1 tablespoon of olive oil, and the juice of two fresh lemons. A sprinkle of cayenne pepper is optional. Follow with two glasses of warm water or herbal tea (dandelion leaf or root, oatstraw, peppermint, yarrow, chickweed, or red clover). Eat nothing solid until lunch.

2. *Eat the following foods to cleanse the liver:* artichokes, watercress, fresh lemon juice, celery, pineapple, parsley, fresh grapes, and papaya.

3. *Take milk thistle* (Luper, 1998).

4. *Switch to a vegetarian diet* (Key, Davey, & Appleby, 1999) or, at the least, avoid all meats and eat more fresh fruits and vegetables. Eat only fish and chicken. No sugar, alcohol, coffee, or tea (except herbal), fried foods, processed foods or flours, salt, strong spices, preservatives, additives, or synthetic vitamins. Eat pickles, sauerkraut and other fermented vegetables to stimulate the healthy function of the liver. Eat a lot of steamed vegetable and tofu meals, concentrating on green vegetables. With lunch and dinner have 2 tablespoons of grated beets with 1 tablespoon of olive oil and a teaspoon of fresh

lemon juice. Eat bland foods, avoiding onion, garlic (except in the liver flush drink), radishes, and spices. Avocados are good.

5. *Ingest Aloe vera daily (3 ounces after each meal) to protect against liver damage* (Ikeno, Hubbard, Lee, Yu, & Herlihy, 2002).

6. *Take SAMe for pain.* This popular supplement works as well as ibuprofen and other pain killers, but has fewer adverse effects (Holst, 2001). It may also help relieve liver condition symptoms.

7. *For infectious hepatitis,* take 1,000 mg of vitamin C every 2–4 hours with a full glass of water and a calcium citrate-magnesium capsule; take a B complex capsule, vitamin E, and lecithin (Worden, 1981).

8. *For cirrhosis, take zinc as a supplement.* Individuals who were given zinc considerably improved after 30 days (Badulici, Chirulescu, Chirila, Chirila, & Rosca, 1994).

9. *Use rice bran products.* They have been shown to provide preventive and/or nutraceutical effects for fatty liver (Jariwalla, 2001).

10. *Use licorice abstract* (not the candy). In Chinese medicine, this herb has been used for thousands of years as a treatment for liver dysfunction (Mehta, 1994). Licorice (glycyrrhiza root) is a substance that prevents disease progression in hepatitis C (Yamashiki, Nishimura, Suzuki, Sakaguchi, & Kosaka, 1997). Licorice extract was also effective in preventing liver cancer in individuals with chronic hepatitis C (Arase et al., 1997).

11. *Use black pepper.* This substance was shown to be a potent liver detoxifier (Singh & Rao, 1993).

12. *Use lemon myrtle to counteract microbial activity* (Hayes & Markovic, 2002).

13. *Use nutmeg to protect the liver* (Morita et al., 2003).

14. *Use thyme essential oil to detoxify* (Youdim & Deans, 1999).

15. *Complete the following exercises morning and night, working up to three to four times a day.*

A. Stand with arms hanging freely. Twist vigorously from side to side, inhaling deeply while twisting to the left and exhaling when twisting to the right. Repeat up to 20 times.

B. Inhale and reach up with the arms, clasping hands above the head. Bend to the left while exhaling and hold for 5 slow counts. Inhale slowly, bringing the arms back up above the head. Bend to the right while exhaling and hold for 5 slow counts. Repeat up to 5 times.

C. Kneel on the floor, extending the left leg to the side and stretching the right arm up and over the head while sliding the left arm down the leg toward the left foot. Keep elbows and unbent knee straight. Hold while inhaling and exhaling slowly for ten breaths. Picture the liver releasing toxins on each exhalation and cleansing itself in inhalation (Berkson, 1977).

D. Sit or lie down in a quiet, comfortable place. Place the palm of the right hand on the side of the body next to the bottom of the rib cage. Rub hand across the bottom of the rib cage up to the sternum (center of your rib cage). Rub up and back 36 times (Chang, 1986).

E. Hold index, third, and fourth fingers of left hand gently on each of the following points until a steady but quiet pulsation is felt in all fingers, then move on to the next point: (1) left fingers on the right side of the spinal column where the shoulder begins, (2) right fingers on the middle bottom of the right buttocks, (3) left fingers on the right middle top of the hip bone, (4) right fingers on the back of the knee.

16. *Avoid taking over-the-counter pain medicines.* Acetaminophen (Tylenol) is associated with liver toxicity (Whitcomb & Block, 1994), and so are ibuprofen, Advil, Nuprin, and aspirin (Wallace, 1996; Wolfe, 1994). Use SAMe instead (see # 6 above).

17. *Use affirmations to heal the liver.* Say or write at least one of the following statements 20 times each day to counter negative thoughts:

- I feel only peace.
- I feel only love.
- I feel only joy.

EVALUATION OF TREATMENT

Client self-evaluated treatment concluded, "I'm working on being more honest with my husband, but it's tough. In my family, we had a lot of secrets. I've been drinking the liver flush and I take milk thistle every day. I cut out all meat and am eating 5–6 vegetables and fruits every day."

REFERENCES

Arase, Y., Ikeda, K., Murashima, N., Chayama, K., Tsubota, A., Koida, I., et al. (1997). The long term efficacy of glycyrrhizin in chronic hepatitis C patients. *Cancer, 79,* 1494–1500.
Badulici, S., Chirulescu, Z., Chirila, P., Chirila, M., & Rosca, A. (1994).

Treatment with zincum metallicum CH5 in patients with liver cirrhosis. *Romanian Journal of Internal Medicine, 32,* 215–219.

Berkson, D. (1977). *The foot book: Healing the body through reflexology.* New York: Harper.

Chang, S. T. (1986). *The complete system of self-healing internal exercises.* San Francisco: Tao.

Hayes, A. J., & Markovic, B. (2002). Toxicity of Australian essential oil Backhousia citriodora (Lemon myrtle). Part 1: Antimicrobial activity and in vitro cytotoxicity. *Food Chemistry and Toxicology, 40,* 535–543.

Holst, B. (2001). Managing viral hepatitis. *Clinician Reviews, 11*(1), 51–66.

Hubbard, P. (1998). Hepatitis C. *American Journal for Nurse Practitioners, 2*(11), 17–31.

Ikeno, Y., Hubbard, G. B., Lee, S., Yu, B. P., & Herlihy, J. T. (2002). The influence of long-term Aloe vera ingestion on age-related disease in male Fischer 344 rats. *Phytotherapy Research, 16,* 712–718.

Jariwalla, R. J. (2001). Rice-bran products: Phytonutrients with potential applications in preventive and clinical medicine. *Drugs in Experimental and Clinical Research, 27,* 17–26.

Key, T. J., Davey, G. K., & Appleby, P. N. (1999). Health benefits of a vegetarian diet. *Proceedings of Nutrition Society, 58,* 271–275.

Luper, S. (1998). A review of plants used in the treatment of liver disease: Part 1. *Alternative/Medical Review, 3,* 410–421.

Mehta, R. (1994, May). *Phytopharmacology of licorice food forms.* Designer Foods III, Proceedings. Washington, DC.

Mindell, E., & Hopkins, V. (1998). *Prescription alternatives.* New Canaan CT: Keats.

Morita, T., Jinno, K., Kawagishi, H., Armimoto, Y., Suganuma, H., Inakuma, T., et al. (2003). Hepatoprotective effect of Myristicin from nutmeg on lipopolysaccharide/d-Galactosamine-induced liver injury. *Journal of Agriculture and Food Chemistry, 51*(6), 1560–1565.

Pettit, J. L. (2000). Alternative medicine: SAMe. *Clinician Reviews, 10,* 124–128.

Singh, A., & Rao, A. R. (1993). Evaluation of the modulatory influence of black pepper on the hepatic detoxification system. *Cancer Letters, 72,* 5–9.

Wallace, K. (1996). National Kidney Foundation warns against heavy use of over-the-counter painkillers. Press Release, February 19, Orlando, FL.

Whitcomb, D. C., & Block, G. (1994). Association of acetaminophen-induced liver toxicity with fasting and ethanol use. *Journal of the American Medical Association, 272,* 1845–1850.

Wolfe, S. (1994). Two over-the-counter pain pills lack important warnings about kidney damage. *Public Citizen's Health Research Group Health Letter, 10*(8), 3.

Worden, B. (1981). Treating hepatitis. *Vegetarian Times/Well Being, 46,* 52–53.

Yamashiki, M., Nishimura, A., Suzuki, H., Sakaguchi, S., & Kosaka, Y. (1997). Effects of the Japanese herbal medicine "Sho-saiko-to" (TH-9) on in vitro interleukin-10 production by peripheral blood mononuclear cells of patients with chronic hepatitis C. *Hepatology, 25,* 1390–1397.

Youdim, K. A., & Deans, S. G. (1999). Dietary supplementation of thyme (Thymus vulgaris L.) essential oil during the lifetime of the rat: Its effects on the antioxidant status in liver, kidney and heart tissues. *Mechanics of Ageing and Development, 109,* 163–175.

CHAPTER 16

Multiple Sclerosis

Multiple sclerosis (MS) is a progressive, degenerative disorder affecting the white (and occasionally the gray) matter of the central nervous system. The result is abnormal nerve conduction. The cause is unknown, but may be due to a virus, pesticides, industrial chemicals, heavy metals, or even eating too many saturated fats, chocolate, and drinking alcohol. A medical approach includes the use of Novantrone, which works by suppressing the T cells, B cells, and macrophages believed to attack the myelin sheath. There are other drugs being used, but they have numerous adverse reactions.

HOLISTIC NURSING ASSESSMENT

Read the holistic nursing assessment that follows. It was developed based on an interview with a holistic nurse and a 60-year-old man diagnosed with multiple sclerosis. Study it for ways to conduct holistic nursing assessments with clients suffering from multiple sclerosis.

Client learning needs: Client is losing muscle mass and strength.

Indicants of readiness to learn: "I read in a magazine that some people with multiple sclerosis exercise."

Soul/spirituality symbol(s): "I don't believe in God. If He existed, why would He give me this disease?"

Meaning of the condition to client: "I've lived a good life, worked hard, always brought home my paycheck. Why am I being punished with this?"

Relationship needs/effects as perceived by the client: "My kids want me to change my will, but I'm not going to do it. They don't deserve a cent."

Patterns/attitudes that may create dis-ease for this client: Client uses negative affirmations (e.g., "I'm stuck in this wheelchair for the rest of my life").

Life purpose: Expresses no life purpose except to make sure his children never inherit his money.

Client strengths: Is very sure of his decisions and wants to learn wheelchair exercises.

Ability to participate in care: Client gets around in his wheelchair, but needs to build upper body strength.

Ethical dilemmas: He has forbidden the nurse to contact his children even though they could provide needed support.

Nurse–client process: Client argues with the nurse about each suggestion made and prefers to see himself as the expert.

TREATMENT PLANNING: SETTING JOINTLY AGREED-UPON GOALS

In the case of the client discussed above, the following goals were agreed upon:

1. Practice wheelchair exercises.
2. Change eating patterns.

TREATMENT

Acceptance of condition/attitude change: The client chose the following affirmation to use to replace the upset he feels: "I can make loving choices about my life." Client agreed to write the affirmation on 3 x 5 cards and say the words at least 20 times each day.

Facilitating the healing process/healing intention formulation: From a list of meditative statements, client chose the following one to assist in the healing process: "I am safe and free." Asked client to meditate on the words while in a relaxed state. Nurse will use caring nonverbal and verbal communication, centering, and a meditative state to enhance client healing, will verbalize observed patterns that may be holding the client back and offer alternate approaches.

Creating a sacred space: During client sessions, a soft lamp light will burn in the room and Beethoven tapes will play in the background.

Encouraging re-storying: Encouraged client to recall an upsetting situation with his children and choose an ending that inspires him.

Integrative practices planned: Will use therapeutic touch and guided imagery to assist client in the healing process.

Role model strategies: Nurse showed client how to role play problematic interchanges with his children.

Protection plan: Client pictures martial arts experts surrounding him.

Family strategies: Encouraged client to invite his children to a session with nurse to practice more open communication between them.

Life issues/life purpose work: Client has agreed to think about meditating on his life purpose.

Treatment possibilities/considerations: Other suggested treatments appear below. Most are evidence-based.

ADDITIONAL INFORMATION AND TREATMENTS TO SHARE WITH CLIENTS

NUTRITIONAL APPROACHES

1. *Switch to a vegan or quasi-vegan diet* (McCarty, 2001), eliminating meat and poultry, milk, eggs, and cheese.

2. *Eat flavonoids.* They have been shown to protect the myelin (Hendriks et al., 2003). Foods to focus on are fruits, vegetables, and tea.

3. *Eat plenty of foods rich in omega-3 fatty acids to reduce inflammatory processes* (Bowling & Stewart, 2003; Shapiro, 2003) including sardines, Atlantic mackerel, Atlantic salmon, Pacific herring, Atlantic herring, lake trout, bluefin tuna, scallops, lemon sole, haddock, sturgeon, anchovies, olive oil, sunflower oil, spinach (Salem, 1999), and flaxseeds.

4. *Take extra B-vitamins to help form and maintain the myelin around nerves* (Bowling & Stewart, 2003). Foods that contain B12 are especially important, including sardines, herring, nutritional yeast,

mackerel, trout, sea vegetables (kombu, dulse, kelp, wakame), and fermented soyfoods (tempeh, natto, and miso).

5. *Drink fresh juices every day.* Buy a juicer if necessary. Start with a pint (2 glasses) of fresh carrot juice or 9 ounces of carrot juice with 5 ounces of celery juice and 2 ounces of parsley juice, or 12 ounces of carrot juice mixed with 4 ounces of parsley juice. Dilute half and half with filtered water. Work up to several quarts of fresh juice a day.

6. *Drink 8–10 glasses of water each day.* Much pain is due to dehydration (Williams, 1992).

7. *Put turmeric (curcumin) in and on foods.* Decorate baked potatoes, salads, soups, fish, and other foods with this spice. It has profound anti-inflammatory activity and MS is a cell-mediated inflammatory disease (Natarajan & Bright, 2002).

8. *Obtain additional magnesium and zinc.* Both minerals have been shown to be decreased in central nervous system tissues in MS. A magnesium deficit may induce dysfunction of the nerve cells or lymphocytes and may be a causative factor in the development of the condition. Magnesium interacts with other minerals and/or metals such as calcium, zinc, and aluminum in biological systems, affecting the immune system and influencing the content of these elements in CNS tissues. Zinc helps prevent virus infections and may also be implicated in the etiology of MS (Yasui & Ota, 1992). Food sources of magnesium include whole grain breads and cereals, fresh peas, brown rice, soy products, wheat germ, nuts, Swiss chard, figs, green leafy vegetables, and citrus fruits. Food sources of zinc include oysters, herring, eggs, nuts, wheat germ, and red meats.

SUPPLEMENTS AND HERBS

Gingko, vitamin D (Bowling & Stewart, 2003), fish oil capsules, (McCarty, 2001), the Ayurvedic tonic herb ashwagandha, methylsulfonymethane or MSM (Parcell, 2002), vitamin C, vitamin B12, bromelain from pineapple (Ghadirjan, Jain, Ducic, Shatenstein, & Morisset, 1998), evening primrose oil, or black currant oil capsules may also prove helpful (Weil, 2000).

EXERCISE

1. *T'ai chi.* One study found that walking speed, hamstring flexibility and psychosocial well-being improved after taking t'ai chi (Husted, Pham, Hekking, & Niederman, 1999).

2. *Exercise class* can improve bowel and bladder function and significantly increase upper and lower extremity strength and aerobic capacity. It can also lower triglycerides and reduce depression, anger, and fatigue (Petajan, Gappmaier, & White, 1996).

3. *Look into aquatic exercise.* Aquatic therapy with a pool temperature of 94 degrees F. can improve mobility (Peterson, 2001).

PROTECTION FROM ALUMINUM TOXICITY

Aluminum toxicity is associated with mitochondrial dysfunction and the inhibition of cell growth (Yamamoto, Kobayashi, Devi, Rikiishi, & Matsumoto, 2002). Active oxygen is key to the damage in neuromuscular disorders (Davison, Tibbits, Shi, & Moon, 1988). Avoid multiple vaccinations over a short period of time. Several reviews of the literature, at least one study, and the World Health Organization have linked aluminum-containing vaccines as a possible cause of multiple sclerosis (Authier et al., 2001; Gherardi, 2003; Piyasirisilp & Hemachudha, 2002). Multiple vaccinations performed over a short period of time in the Persian gulf area have been recognized as the main risk factor for Gulf War syndrome (Gherardi, 2003).

COUNSELING/MINDFULNESS OF MOVEMENT

1. *Obtain psychological counseling.* It can improve depression, anxiety, and self-esteem (Huntley & Ernst, 2000).

2. *Participate in a mindfulness of movement short course.* The approach can improve balance and a broad range of symptoms (Mills & Allen, 2000).

MUSIC THERAPY

Join a music therapy group. Clients who received music therapy showed more expiratory muscle strength than individuals who attended music appreciation class (Wiens, Reimer, & Guy, 1999).

BIOFEEDBACK

Beneficial effects were noted after biofeedback sessions for patients whose bowel symptoms were having a major impact on their life. It worked well for constipation and fecal incontinence (Wiesel et al., 2000).

Yoga with Breathing

Gentle stretches can help maintain strength, flexibility, and balance. Focused breathing exercises can reduce stress and symptoms (Gosselink, Kovacs, Ketelaer, Carton, & Decramer, 2000).

Hypnosis

A study showed that hypnosis helped patients get out of wheel chairs, walk with better balance, and experience reduced pain. A secondary effect of hypnosis was an increased sense of hopefulness (Sutcher, 1997).

Homeopathy

Problems of urinary incontinence, sexual dysfunction, cramps and spasms, tremor and trigeminal neuralgia, fatigue, and emotional lability may respond to various homeopathic remedies (Whitmarsh, 2003).

Affirmations

Affirmations that may prove useful include

- I choose loving, joyous thoughts.
- I am safe.
- I am free.
- I create love and joy.

EVALUATING TREATMENT

The client described above rated his progress as follows: "I've been practicing my exercises in the pool and in my wheelchair. My trainer says I have more strength and I believe I have. I've also stopped eating meat and cheese. I think it's helping."

REFERENCES

Authier, F. J., Cherin, P., Creange, A., Bonnotte, B., Ferrer, X., & Abdelmoumni, A. (2001). Central nervous system disease in patients with macrophagic myofascitis. *Brain, 124*(Pt. 5), 974–983.

Bowling, A. C., & Stewart, T. M. (2003). Current complementary and alternative therapies for multiple sclerosis. *Current Treatment Options in Neurology, 5*(1), 55–68.

Chang, S. T. (1986). *The complete system of self-healing exercises.* San Francisco: Tao.

Davison, A., Tibbits, G., Shi, Z. G., & Moon, J. (1988). Active oxygen in neuromuscular disorders. *Muscular and Cell Biochemistry, 84,* 199–216.

Ghadirian, P., Jain, M., Ducic, S., Shatenstein, B., & Morisset, R. (1998). Nutritional factors in the etiology of multiple sclerosis: A case control study. *International Journal of Epidemiology, 27,* 842–852.

Gosselink, R., Kovacs, L., Ketelaer, P., Carton, H., & Decramer, M. (2000). Respiratory muscle weakness and respiratory muscle training in severely disabled multiple sclerosis patients. *Archives of Physical and Medical Rehabilitation, 81,* 747–751.

Hendriks, J. J., de Vries, H. E., van der Pol, S. M., van den Berg, T. K., van Tol, E. A., & Dijkstra, C. D. (2003). Flavonoids inhibit myelin phagocytosis by macrophages: A structure-activity relationship study. *Biochemistry and Pharmacology, 65,* 877–885.

Huntley, A., & Ernst, E. (2000). Complementary and alternative therapies for treating multiple sclerosis symptoms: A systematic review. *Complementary Therapies in Medicine, 8,* 97–105.

Husted, C., Pham, L., Hekking, A., & Niederman, R. (1999). Improving quality of life for people with chronic conditions: The example of t'ai chi and multiple sclerosis. *Alternative Therapies in Health and Medicine, 5*(5), 70–74.

McCarty, M. F. (2001). Upregulation of lymphocyte apoptosis as a strategy for preventing and treating autoimmune disorders: A role for whole-food vegan diets, fish oil and dopamine agonists. *Medical Hypotheses, 57,* 258–275.

Mills, N., & Allen, J. (2000). Mindfulness of movement as a coping strategy in multiple sclerosis: A pilot study. *General Hospital Psychiatry, 22,* 425–431.

Natarajan, C., & Bright, J. J. (2002). Curcumin inhibits experimental allergic encephalomyelitis by blocking IL-12 signaling through Janus kinase-STAT pathway in T lymphocytes. *Journal of Immunology, 168,* 6506–6513.

Nordvik, I., Myhr, K. M., Nyland, H., & Bjerve, K. S. (2000). Effect of dietary advice and n-3 supplementation in newly diagnosed MS patients. *Acta Neurology Scandinavia, 102,* 143–149.

Parcell, S. (2002). Sulfur in human nutrition and applications in medicine. *Alternative Medicine Review, 7,* 22–44.

Petajan, J. H., Gappmaier, E., & White, A. T. (1996). Impact of aerobic training on fitness and quality of life in multiple sclerosis. *Annals of Neurology, 39,* 432–441.

Peterson, C. (2001). Exercise in 94 degrees F water for a patient with multiple sclerosis. *Physical Therapy, 81,* 1049–1058.

Piyasirisilp, S., & Hemachudha, T. (2002). Neurological adverse events associated with vaccination. *Current Opinion in Neurology, 15,* 333–338.

Salem, N. (1999). Introduction to polyunsaturated fatty acids. *PUFA Backgrounder, 3*(1), 1–8.

Shapiro, H. (2003). Could n-3 polyunsaturated fatty acids reduce pathological pain by direct actions on the nervous system? *Prostaglandins Leukot Essential Fatty Acids, 68,* 219–234.

Sutcher, H. (1997). Hypnosis as adjunctive therapy for multiple sclerosis: A progress report. *American Journal of Clinical Hypnosis, 39,* 283–290.

Weil, A. (2000, June). Natural help for multiple sclerosis. *Integrative Medicine, 8.*

Whitmarsh, T. E. (2003). Homeopathy in multiple sclerosis. *Complementary Therapy and Nurse Midwifery, 9*(1), 5–9.

Wiens, M. E., Reimer, M. A., & Guy, H. L. (1999). Music therapy as a treatment method for improving respiratory muscle strength in patients with advanced multiple sclerosis: A pilot study. *Rehabilitation Nursing, 24*(2), 74–80.

Wiesel, P. H., Norton, C., Roy, A. J., Storrie, J. B., Bowers, J., & Kamm, M. A. (2000). Gut focused behavioral treatment (biofeedback) for constipation and fecal incontinence in multiple sclerosis. *Journal of Neurosurgical Psychiatry, 69,* 240–243.

Williams, D. G. (1992). Dehydration and pain. *Alternatives, 3*(2), 12.

Yamamoto, Y., Kobayashi, Y., Devi, S. R., Rikiishi, S., & Matsumoto, H. (2002). Aluminum toxicity is associated with mitochondrial dysfunction and the production of reactive oxygen species in plant cells. *Plant Physiology, 128*(1), 63–72.

Yasui, M., & Ota, K. (1992). Experimental and clinical studies on dysregulation of magnesium metabolism and the aetiopathogenesis of multiple sclerosis. *Magnesium Research, 5,* 295–302.

CHAPTER 17

Osteoporosis

Osteoporosis is a progressive condition with deterioration of bone tissue that results in loss of bone mass and the resultant increased risk of fractures from minimal trauma. Medical treatment includes hormone replacement therapy (which increases the risk of heart attack, cancer, stroke, breast cancer, blood clots, and vaginal bleeding), biphosphonates, Calcitonin, selected estrogen receptor modulators, and Raloxifene.

HOLISTIC NURSING ASSESSMENT

Study the holistic nursing assessment for Mrs. M., a 70-year-old woman diagnosed with osteoporosis. Working in collaboration with clients diagnosed with osteoporosis, adapt the following holistic nursing assessment format.

Client learning needs: "I've lost an inch in height and I have a lot of back pain."

Indicants of readiness to learn: "The doctor told me I could have another compression fracture and I don't want that to happen."

Soul/spirituality symbol(s): "I think of my soul as the core of me, the part that will survive long after I die."

Meaning of the condition to client: "I guess I'm just getting old and falling apart."

Relationship needs/effects as perceived by the client: "My husband doesn't understand why I lie in bed. He doesn't know how much pain I have."

Patterns/attitudes that may create dis-ease for this client: Client uses negative affirmations (e.g., "I'm always in pain" and "Maybe I'll just shrink away to nothing").

Life purpose: "I want to live long enough to see my great-granddaughter."

Client strengths: Has a good sense of humor and wants to learn what she can do to feel better.

Ability to participate in care: Client looks fragile and is underweight, but verbalizes the wish to change.

Ethical dilemmas: None identified.

Nurse–client process: Client denies her feelings and tries to please.

TREATMENT PLANNING: SETTING JOINTLY AGREED-UPON GOALS

In the case of the client discussed above, the following goals were agreed upon:

1. Start a meal plan that builds bone.
2. Begin an exercise program to strengthen bone.
3. Share her feelings with her husband.

TREATMENT

Acceptance of condition/attitude change: The client chose the following affirmation to use to replace the upset she feels: "I stand up for myself." Client agreed to write the affirmation on 3 x 5 cards and say the words at least 20 times each day.

Facilitating the healing process/healing intention formulation: From a list of meditative statements, client chose the following one to assist in the healing process: "Life protects and supports me." Nurse asked client to meditate on the words while in a relaxed state. Nurse will use caring nonverbal and verbal communication, centering, and a meditative state to enhance client healing, will verbalize observed patterns that may be holding the client back and offer alternate approaches.

Creating a sacred space: Client asked to start sessions with a prayer and to play her favorite hymn in the background.

Encouraging re-storying: Encouraged client to recall an upsetting situation with her husband and choose an ending that inspires her.

Integrative practices planned: Nurse will use healing touch and guided imagery to assist client in the healing process.

Role model strategies: Nurse showed client how to role play problematic interchanges with her husband.

Protection plan: Client plans to use a circle of angels around her for protection.

Family strategies: Nurse encouraged client to invite her husband to a session with nurse to practice more open communication between them.

Life issues/life purpose work: Client wants to die. "I've done my work on earth. My children are grown and my husband doesn't need me any more."

Treatment possibilities/considerations: Other suggested treatments appear below. Most are evidence-based.

ADDITIONAL INFORMATION AND TREATMENTS TO SHARE WITH CLIENTS

1. *Eat more foods high in calcium,* including tofu, broccoli, kale, raw spinach, turnip greens, okra, beet greens, collards, sardines, perch, salmon, dried beans (pinto, black), chickpeas, sesame seeds or tahini, almonds, Brazil nuts, hazelnuts, peanuts, some mineral waters (check the label), miso, soy flour, and nonfat yogurt.

2. *Avoid high-fiber foods while eating calcium-rich foods.* Although fiber has a positive effect on digestion and cholesterol, eating too many fiber-rich foods (popcorn, whole grains, fruits and vegetables that don't contain calcium) at the same time can interfere with the body's ability to absorb calcium.

3. *Avoid too much salt.* It can lead to calcium excretion in the urine (Matkovic, Ilich, Andon, Hsieh, Tzagournis, Lagger, et al., 1995).

4. *Stay away from carbonated beverages.* The phosphate in the drinks bind with calcium, reducing its absorbability (Wyshak & Frisch, 1994).

5. *Obtain sufficient essential fatty acids.* Their lack can also lead to osteoporosis (Kruger & Horrobin, 1997). Some of the best sources are fish and fish oils, flax oil, olive oil, borage oil, and evening primrose oil (Curtis et al., 2002; Kruger, Coetzer, deWinter, Gericke, & van Papendorp, 1998).

6. *Avoid taking drugs that interfere with calcium metabolism.* Benzodiazepines (Dalmane, Doral, Halcion) increase risk for osteoporosis (Cummings et al., 1995).

7. *Eliminate animal proteins (meat, cheese, eggs, milk), which increase the elimination of calcium.* When the diet consists of more than 15% protein, the kidneys require much more water than usual to excrete it. As a result, calcium is flushed out. At the very least, reduce intake of animal protein to 3–6 ounces a day (Allolio, 1996).

8. *Drink 3 glasses of carrot, parsley, and spinach juice a day.* That will exceed the U.S. RDA for calcium, build bone strength, strengthen eyes, and aid digestion. Eat lots of fruits, vegetables, and (dried) beans. Prunes are especially good. They contain boron, which has a positive effect on calcium absorption, reduces excretion of calcium, and lowers blood phosphorus levels, another factor associated with osteoporosis (Stacewicz-Sapuntzakis, Bowen, Hussain, Damayanti-Wood, & Farnsworth, 2001).

9. *Take 1,500 milligrams of calcium citrate daily* to maintain bone strength. Take it in divided doses every other day (1,500 mg at night first day, 750 mg morning and evening the second day) to increase bone resorption and protect against osteoporosis (Scopacasa et al., 2000). If not out in the sun daily, take a vitamin D supplement to further prevent postmenopausal bone loss (Hunter et al., 2000).

10. *Eat more soy products.* A study showed that eating whole soy foods resulted in significant reductions in clinical risk factors for osteoporosis (Arjmandi et al., 2003; Scheiber, Liu, Subbiah, Rebar, & Setchell, 2001) and reduced fracture rate (Greendale et al., 2002). Another study found that soy protein stops bone loss in the lumbar spine in women who are around menopausal age (Alekel et al., 2000). Consider using soy as a main source of protein. According to a report, most people eat too much protein and it increases calcium excretion (Lewis & Modlesky, 1998).

11. *Eat more onions, vegetables, and salads.* They can prevent low bone mass and reduce the incidence of osteoporotic fractures. Their base buffers metabolic acid thought to dissolve bone. (Muhlbauer, Lozano, & Reinli, 2002). In one study, dried onion taken daily prevented the bone loss that would normally occur due to the decrease in estrogen levels. It also reversed bone loss seen in osteoporosis, and the effect was greater than that of the prescription drug Calcitonin (Morselli, Neuenschwander, Perrelet, & Pippuner, 2000).

12. *Exercise.* Men who used moderate to vigorous levels of physical activity were protected from future hip fractures (Kujala et al., 2000). Women who folk-danced or participated in gymnastics

showed improved muscular performance and body balance, in addition to increased bone mass (Uusi-Rasi et al., 1999). The Rehabilitation Institute of Chicago recommends weight-bearing exercise to help develop bone mass and strength, 20–30 minutes 3–4 times a week or 3 minutes 10 times a day. Even walking, as long as it is performed briskly, can enhance bone minerals (Lewis & Modlesky, 1998). Back-strengthening exercises are also beneficial. Even standing up can enhance bone health. According to a study, spending less than four hours standing increased risk for hip fracture (Cummings et al., 1995). Weight lifting can maintain bone mineral density and ward off osteoporosis (Dohn, 1996). Combining weight training with exercise, 1,000 mg of calcium citrate malate and 400 IU of vitamin D works well for strengthening bone in postmenopausal women (Brown, 2003). Even gardening once a week can prevent osteoporosis. Women over the age of 50 who did yard work at least once a week had stronger bones than women who jogged and did aerobics. Weight training was the only other activity that significantly strengthened bones (Turner, Bass, Ting, & Brown, 2002).

13. *Avoid antacids as a regular source of calcium.* They can interrupt the effect of other drugs and are especially damaging for individuals with kidney disease (Maton & Burton, 1999).

14. *Don't smoke.* Smoking reduces bone mass and increases risk of fractures (Brander, 1995).

15. *Avoid heavy alcohol use.* Heavy drinking results in decreased bone mass and increased risk for falls and fractures. A maximum of 2 drinks a day is a good rule (Brander, 1995).

16. *Eliminate caffeine* (coffee, caffeinated tea, colas, chocolate, and cocoa) from your meal plan. High caffeine intake is associated with increased risk for hip fracture (Cummings et al., 1995) and with risk of lower bone density in lean elderly women (Korpelainen, Korpelainen, Heikkinen, Vaananen, & Keinanen-Kiiukaanniemi, 2003). Avoid carbonated drinks, even non-colas, because they make calcium less absorbable.

17. *Eat lettuce and green leafy vegetables at least once a day.* Women who ate lettuce once a day had half the risk of hip fractures of women who didn't. Vitamin K was thought to play a key role in allowing certain proteins to be taken up by the bones (Anderson, 1999). Other foods that are rich in this vitamin are broccoli, Brussels sprouts, cabbage, kale, and spinach.

18. *Eat more prunes.* They are a source of boron, which is believed to play a role in the prevention of osteoporosis (Stacewicz-Sapuntzakis, Bowen, Hussain, Damayanti-Wood, & Farnsworth, 2001).

19. *Move toward a plant-based diet.* It is beneficial to bone health (Anderson, 1999).

20. *Maintain body weight.* Older women who weighed less than they had at age 25 had two times the risk of hip fracture (Cummings et al., 1995).

21. *Encourage children to take part in sports.* A study revealed that sports participation during adolescence resulted in less osteoporosis later in life (Puntila et al., 1997).

22. *Avoid taking steroids* (prescribed for asthma, rheumatoid arthritis, glaucoma, and other conditions). Corticosteroids are linked to bone loss, according to the American College of Rheumatology (Saag, 2003).

23. *Get plenty of vitamin C.* It is a cofactor in collagen formation, the glue that holds bones in place (Weber, 1999) and is related to bone mineral density (Ilich, Brownbill, & Tamborini, 2003). Eat plenty of foods high in vitamin C, including green peppers, honeydew melon, cooked broccoli or Brussels sprouts, cooked kale, cantaloupe, strawberries, papaya, cooked cauliflower, oranges, watercress, raspberries, parsley, raw cabbage, grapefruit, blackberries, lemons, onions, sprouts, raw spinach, and tomatoes.

24. *Limit intake of foods high in oxalic acid, which inhibits calcium absorption:* almonds, cashews, chard, rhubarb, asparagus, and spinach.

25. *Obtain daily vitamin B6.* It can function as a cofactor to build up cross-links, which stabilize the collagen chains of the bone. In one study, participants who had low vitamin B6 blood levels were more likely to sustain hip fracture (Reynolds, Marshall, & Brain, 1992; Weber, 1999). Foods rich in this vitamin include brewer's yeast, sunflower seeds, toasted wheat germ, brown rice, soybeans, white beans, liver, chicken, mackerel, salmon, tuna, bananas, walnuts, peanuts, sweet potatoes, and cooked cabbage.

26. *Increase intake of silicon.* Increasing evidence suggests that silicon is important in bone formation (Seaborn & Nielsen, 2002). Major sources of silicon include bananas, string beans (Jugdaohsingh et al., 2002) and the herbs oatstraw and horsetail (Paul et al., 1994).

27. *Eat foods high in manganese, magnesium, copper, and zinc to build bone* (Branca, Valtuena, & Vatuena, 2001), including nuts (except cashews and almonds), seeds, whole grains, fruits and vegetables, dry beans and peas, oatmeal, fresh peas, brown rice, soy flour, wheat germ, figs, citrus fruits, oysters, herring, liver, eggs, red meat, avocados, dandelion greens, and lentils.

28. *Say or write one of the following affirmations 20 times a day.*

- I stand strong and healthy.
- Life itself supports me.
- I walk forward in love.

29. *Complete a bone breathing exercise* at least once a day: Lie prone in a comfortable place or sit in a chair once the process has been mastered. Keep arms next to the body and feet slightly apart. Keep eyes closed and take a few easy breaths, letting breathing move toward the center of the body. When exhaling, let go of everything it's time to let go of, letting it flow down the body and out the toes. When inhaling, let energy come in the toes and flow up through the bones of the legs, up through the spine and neck and out the top of the head. On the next inhale, let energy flow through the bones of the chest, down the arm bones and out each fingertip. Repeat the whole sequence 3–4 times.

EVALUATION OF TREATMENT

Client described above self-evaluated her treatment this way: "I eat a big salad every day and I'm taking a weight-lifting class they have on TV. I still can't talk to my husband, but I'm working on it."

REFERENCES

Alekel, D. D. L., Germain, A. S., Peterson, C. T., Hanson, K. B., Stewart, J. W., & Toda, T. (2000). Isoflavone-rich soy protein isolate attenuates bone loss in the lumbar spine of perimenopausal women. *American Journal of Clinical Nutrition, 72,* 844–852.

Allolio, B. (1996). Osteoporosis and nutrition. *Zeitschrift für Arztliche Fortbild ung, 90*(1), 19–24.

Anderson, J. J. (1999). Plant-based diets and bone health: Nutritional implications. *American Journal of Clinical Nutrition, 70*(3, Suppl.), 539S–542S.

Arjmandi, B. H., Khalil, D. A., Smith, B. J., Lucas, E. A., Juma, S., Payton, M. E., et al. (2003). Soy protein has a greater effect on bone in postmenopausal women not on hormone replacement therapy, as evidenced by reducing bone resorption and urinary calcium excretion. *Journal of Clinical Endocrinology and Metabolism, 88,* 1048–1054.

Baeksgaard, L., Andersen, K. P., & Hyldstrup, L. (1998). Calcium and vitamin supplementation increases spinal BMD in healthy, postmenopausal women. *Osteoporosis International, 8,* 255–260.

Branca, F., Valtuena, S., & Vatuena, S. (2001). Calcium, physical activity and bone health—building bones for a stronger future. *Public Health Nutrition, 4*(1A), 177–223.

Brander, V. (1995, October). Prevent or slow down osteoporosis. *Let's Live,* 10.

Brown, T. (2003). UF researcher finds vitamins, regular exercise and weight training may improve bone density without hormone therapy. Press release. University of Florida, Health Science Center, Office of News & Communications, Gainesville, FL 32610-0253; www.news.health.ufl.edu

Cummings, S. R., Nevitt, M. C., Browner, W. S., Stone, K., Fox, K. M., Ensrud, K. E., et al. (1995). Risk factors for hip fracture in white women. *New England Journal of Medicine, 332,* 767–773.

Curtis, C. L., Rees, S. G., Cramp, J., Flannery, C. R., Hughes, C. E., Little, C. B., et al. (2002). Effects of n-3 fatty acids on cartilage metabolism. *Proceedings of Nutrition Society, 61,* 381–389.

Dohn, N. E. (1996). Lifting weight shown to reverse effects of osteoporosis in heart transplant patients. Media release: University of Florida, Health Science Center Communications, PO Box 100253, Gainesville, FL 32610-0253.

Feskanich, D., Willett, W. C., & Colditz, G. A. (2003). Calcium, vitamin D, milk consumption, and hip fractures: A prospective study among postmenopausal women. *American Journal of Clinical Nutrition, 77,* 504–511.

Greendale, G. A., Fitzgerald, G., Huang, M.-H., Sternfeld, B., Gold, E., Seeman, T., et al. (2002). Dietary soy isolated and bone mineral density: Results from the Study of Women's Health Across the Nation. *American Journal of Epidemiology, 155,* 746–754.

Hunter, D., Major, P., Arden, N., Swaminathan, R., Andrew, T., MacGregor, A. J., et al. (2000). A randomized controlled trial of vitamin D supplementation on preventing postmenopausal bone loss and modifying bone metabolism using identical twin pairs. *Journal of Bone Mineral Research, 15,* 2276–2283.

Ilich, J. Z., Brownbill, R. A., & Tamborini, L. (2003). Bone and nutrition in elderly women: Protein, energy, and calcium as main determinants of bone mineral density. *European Journal of Clinical Nutrition, 57,* 554–565.

Jugdaohsingh, R., Anderson, S. H., Tucker, K. L., Elliott, H., Kiel, D. P., Thompson, R. P., et al. (2002). Dietary silicon intake and absorption. *American Journal of Clinical Nutrition, 75,* 887–893.

Korpelainen, R., Korpelainen, J., Heikkinen, J., Vaananen, K., & Keinanen-Kiukaanniemi, S. (2003). Lifestyle factors are associated with osteoporosis in lean women but not in normal and overweight women: A population-based cohort study of 1222 women. *Osteoporosis International, 14*(1), 34–43.

Kroger, H., Lakka, T., Honkanen, R., & Tuppurainen, M. (1997). Physical activity in adolescence and bone density in peri-and postmenopausal women: A population-based study. *Bone, 21,* 363–367.

Kruger, M., & Horrobin, D. (1997). Calcium metabolism, osteoporosis and essential fatty acids: A review. *Progress in Lipid Research, 36,* 131–151.

Kruger, M. C., Coetzer, H., deWinter, R., Gericke, G., & van Papendorp, D. H. (1998). Calcium, gamma-linolenic acid and eicosapentaenoic acid supplementation in senile osteoporosis. *Aging, 10,* 385–394.

Kujala, U. M., Kaprio, J., Kannus, P., Sarna, S., & Koskenvuo, M. (2000). Physical activity and osteoporotic hip fracture risk in men. *Archives of Internal Medicine, 160,* 705–708.

Lewis, R. D., & Modlesky, C. M. (1998). Nutrition, physical activity and bone health in women. *International Journal of Sport Nutrition, 8,* 250–284.

Matkovic, T., Ilich, J. Z., Andon, M. B., Hsieh, L. C., Tzagournis, M. A., Lagger, B. J., et al., (1995). Urinary calcium, sodium and bone mass of young females. *American Journal of Clinical Nutrition, 62,* 417–425.

Maton, P. N., & Burton, M. E. (1999). Antacids revisited: A review of their clinical pharmacology and recommended therapeutic use. *Drugs, 57,* 855–870.

Morselli, B., Neuenschwander, B., Perrelet, R., & Lippuner, K. (2000). Osteoporosis diet. *Therapeutische Umschau, 57,* 152–160.

Muhlbauer, R. C., Lozano, A., & Reinli, A. (2002). Onion and a mixture of vegetables, salads, and herbs affect bone resorption in the rat by a mechanism independent of their base excess. *Journal of Bone and Mineral Research, 17,* 1230–1236.

Paul, S. M., Doell, W., MacKenzie, G., Schauss, A., Heller, L., Benedict, M., & Puntila, E. (1994). Which nutrients are most important to healing? *Nutritional Research News, 10,* 4.

Reynolds, T. M., Marshall, P. D., & Brain, A. M. (1992). Hip fracture patients may be vitamin B6 deficient. *Acta Orthop Scandinavia, 83,* 635–638.

Saag, K. G. (2003). Glucocorticoid-induced osteoporosis. *Endocrinology Metabolic Clinics of North America, 32*(1), vii, 135–157.

Scheiber, M. D., Liu, J. H., Subbiah, M. T., Rebar, R. W., & Setchell, K. D. (2001). Dietary inclusion of whole soy foods results in significant reductions in clinical risk factors for osteoporosis and cardiovascular disease in normal postmenopausal women. *Menopause, 8,* 384–392.

Scopacasa, F., Need, A. G., Horowitz, M., Wishart, J. M., Morris, H. A., & Nordin, B. E. (2000). Inhibition of bone resorption by divided-dose calcium supplementation in early postmenopausal women. *Calcification Tissue International, 67,* 440–442.

Seaborn, C. D., & Nielsen, F. H. (2002). Silicon deprivation decreases collagen formation in wounds and bone, and ornithine transamine enzyme activity in liver. *Biological Trace Elements Research, 89,* 251–261.

Stacewicz-Sapuntzakis, M., Bowen, P. E., Hussain, E. A., Damayanti-Wood, B. I., & Farnsworth, N. R. (2001). Chemical composition and potential health effects of prunes: A functional food. *Critical Review of Food Science Nutrition, 41,* 251–286.

Turner, L. W., Bass, M. A., Ting, L., & Brown, B. (2002). Influence of yard work and weight training on bone mineral density among older U.S. women. *Journal of Women and Aging, 14*(3–4), 139–148.

Uusi-Rasi, K., Sievanen, H., Vuori, I., Heinonen, A., Kannus, P., Pasanen, M., et al. (1999). Long-term recreational gymnastics, estrogen use, and selected risk factors for osteoporotic fractures. *Journal of Bone Mineral Research, 14,* 1231–1238.

Weber, P. (1999). The role of vitamins in the prevention of osteoporosis—a brief status report. *International Journal of Vitamins and Nutrition Research, 69,* 194–197.

Wyshak, G., & Frisch, R. E. (1994). Carbonated beverages, dietary calcium, the dietary calcium/phosphorus ratio, and bone fractures in girls and boys. *Journal of Adolescent Health, 15,* 210–215.

CHAPTER 18

Overweight/Obesity

Recent research has found that frequent dieters show significantly more weight regain than less frequent dieters (Pasman, Saris, & Westerterp-Plantenga, 1999). Weight-reducing efforts led to dysregulation of the normal appetite system, resulting in weight gain and decreased efficiency in metabolism (Stice & Hayward, 1999).

HOLISTIC NURSING ASSESSMENT

Study the holistic nursing assessment for Ms. T., a 20-year-old woman diagnosed with obesity. Working in collaboration with clients diagnosed with obesity, use the holistic nursing assessment format to understand their needs.

Client learning needs: "The doctor says I'm a risk for gallstones and a heart attack. I don't see how a few extra pounds can do that."

Indicants of readiness to learn: "It's either lose weight or buy a new set of clothes again."

Soul/spirituality symbol(s): "I pray a lot, but I've never gotten an answer."

Meaning of the condition to client: "Ever since I gained weight, my husband stays away from me. That's fine with me because I don't want to get pregnant again anyway."

Relationship needs/effects as perceived by the client: "I think my husband is having an affair with his secretary."

Patterns/attitudes that may create dis-ease for this client: Client uses negative affirmations (e.g., "I'm just a big fat blob," and "No wonder he doesn't love me anymore").

Life purpose: Expresses no life purpose.

Client strengths: Is well-educated and has been reading about obesity on the Internet.

Ability to participate in care: Client has difficulty exercising because of her weight.

Ethical dilemmas: None identified.

Nurse–client process: Client denies angry feelings, but indicates anger by coming late to sessions and making snide comments about the nurse.

TREATMENT PLANNING: SETTING JOINTLY AGREED-UPON GOALS

In the case of the client discussed above, the following goals were agreed upon:

1. Stop eating after 7 p.m.
2. Take a class toward a master's degree to enhance self-esteem.
3. Eat one portion of a forbidden food each day.
4. Start a walking program.

TREATMENT

Acceptance of condition/attitude change: The client chose the following affirmation to use to replace the shame she feels: "I take responsibility for my life." Client agreed to write the affirmation on 3 x 5 cards and say the words at least 20 times each day.

Facilitating the healing process/healing intention formulation: From a list of meditative statements, client chose the following one to assist in the healing process: "I am safe and secure." Client was asked to meditate on the words while in a relaxed state. Nurse will use caring nonverbal and verbal communication, centering, and a meditative state to enhance client healing, will verbalize observed patterns that may be holding the client back and offer alternate approaches.

Creating a sacred space: Client brought in water color drawings that she found soothing.

Encouraging re-storying: Nurse encouraged client to recall an upsetting situation with her husband and choose an ending that inspires her.

Integrative practices planned: Nurse will use relaxation therapy, hypnosis, and guided imagery to assist client in the healing process.

Role model strategies: Nurse showed client how to role play problematic interchanges with her husband.

Protection plan: Client plans to imagine pictures of herself thin and strong surrounding her.

Family strategies: Nurse encouraged client to invite her husband to a session with nurse to practice more open communication between them.

Life issues/life purpose work: Client has agreed to meditate on the perfect job.

Treatment possibilities/considerations: Other suggested treatments appear below. Most are evidence-based.

ADDITIONAL INFORMATION AND TREATMENTS TO SHARE WITH CLIENTS

1. *Develop a self-contract or sign one with a trusted significant other to lose weight.* The person must be someone who will provide support, not nag or tease, but will reinforce the goal. Identify a specific goal (e.g., "Lose one pound a week").

2. *Chart food and mood.* Keep a food/stress diary for at least a week. Write down each item ingested, and thoughts and feelings while eating and afterwards. After several days, note patterns of how stress leads to eating too much or too little and plan ways to prevent stress eating. Finding patterns is the first step on the path to controlling weight.

3. *Eliminate sugary foods that can aggravate tension, increase stress, and add unwanted pounds.* The mood enhancement that sugar brings lasts only for a brief time. After one or two hours, fatigue and decreased energy resume (Christensen, 1991, 1993; Christensen & Burrows, 1993). With this dip in mood, the urge to eat more sugar recurs. This cycle is reinforced and weight gain is not far behind (Miller, Niederpruem, Wallace, & Lindeman, 1994). A study showed that eliminating sugar from the diet reduced symptoms of depression, and returning it to the diet brought the depression back (Christensen & Burrows, 1990). In a group of men and women who ate the same number of calories, the ones who ate refined sugars gained more weight (Miller et al., 1994). The same was found for children (Ludwig, Peterson, & Gortmaker, 2001). Eating sugary foods

that are also high in fat puts on even more weight because the foods taste good, yet are not satisfying for long because they're not nutritious. This leads to eating more and more cookies, candy bars, doughnuts, cakes, pies, ice cream, Danish or sweet rolls, and other baked goods.

4. *Eliminate artificially sweetened foods.* Some are linked with cancer. Aspartame is methanol or wood alcohol and contributes to the formation of formaldehyde in the body. Reported reactions to Aspartame (NutraSweet and Equal) include mood swings, headaches, changes in vision, sleep disorders, memory loss and confusion, nausea and diarrhea, and even convulsions (Trocho et al., 1998; Van den Eeden et al., 1994; Walton, Hudak, & Green-Waite, 1993).

5. *Eat more whole foods and avoid processed foods.* Canned and processed foods don't have enough fiber in them to keep blood glucose levels low. Consuming too many processed foods can produce insulin resistance and send blood glucose to fat depositories on the body (Liu, 2002; Liu & Willett, 2002).

6. *Eliminate the stress of caffeine* (coffee, tea, colas, chocolate, cocoa, some prescription and over-the-counter drugs) that can raise your blood pressure, contribute to adrenal exhaustion, create hormonal imbalances, and has even been linked to cancer (Olney, Farber, Spitznagel, & Robins, 1996). *The Merck Manual of Diagnosis and Therapy,* a medical text that has been relied on by physicians for 100 years, lists caffeine as a poison. Homocysteine, a risk factor for heart disease, is correlated with coffee drinking (El-Khairy, Ueland, & Nygard, 1999). Caffeine creates more stress by leaching calming B-vitamins and bone-strengthening calcium and relaxing magnesium from the body (Kynast-Gales & Massey, 1994; Rude et al., 1999; Tucker et al., 1999), elevating blood pressure (Pincomb et al., 1996), increasing the risk for cancer (Singh & Fraser, 1998), and can reduce chances of becoming pregnant (Bolumar, Olsen, Rebagliato, & Bisani, 1997; Curtis, Savitz, & Arbuckle, 1997).

7. *Eliminate oxidized trans-fats from the diet and use olive oil instead.* Trans-fats transform vegetable oils into solid substances during the process called hydrogenation, which can alter the composition, size, and number of fat cells, promoting weight gain (Miller et al., 1994). Trans-fats are found in almost all commercially made doughnuts, crackers, cookies, pastries, fried foods, potato and corn chips, baked goods, frosting, candy products, and most margarines, and are associated with overweight (Caius & Benefice, 2002; Liu, 2002; Liu & Willett, 2002; Rodriguez-Artalejo et al., 2003).

8. *Stay away from meat and animal products* that not only stress kidneys and liver, but leave less room for vegetables and soy protein that enhance fat oxidation (McCarty, 2000).

9. *When eating, always sit down at a table and concentrate only on chewing, tasting, and enjoying.* Avoid thinking or talking about upsetting topics while eating. Eat slowly enough to tune into "fullness" signals and stop eating. Wait at least five minutes before taking seconds. Let digestive processes catch up with the brain.

10. *Don't drink alcohol.* Drinking more than half a glass of wine may short-circuit fullness signals and lead to eating beyond nutritional needs.

11. *Drink a glass of water before eating* and at least 10 glasses of water a day to help digest food and move toxins and wastes through the body. Dehydration can lead to headaches, fatigue, poor physical performance, and bad food choices.

12. *Never eat after 7 p.m. and always eat breakfast.* Examine eating patterns if not hungry in the morning. Go to bed hungry. Drink a glass of water and go to sleep. Get up and eat a big breakfast. Eat the main meal for lunch to give the body time to metabolize the calories. Eating light all day but having a large evening meal made participants in one study store more fat. Even when they reduced their daily calories and exercised vigorously, they could not lose weight. Some even gained weight (Bernadot, Deutz, Martin, & Cody, 2000).

13. *Eat 5 or 6 meals a day.* This is an especially good tactic when suffering from low blood sugar (experience sugar craving, headache, palpitations, jitteriness, weakness, or fatigue). In this case, eat 5 or 6 small meals high in protein (tofu, fish, and skinless chicken are good bets) and low in carbohydrates (especially fruits, cereal, pasta, bread, and rice) at spaced intervals. Don't eliminate vegetables, because they provide vitamins and minerals and protect against illness.

14. *Eat high-satisfaction foods.* Some foods are more filling than other foods. Focus on eating them instead of reaching for a sugary sweet or a non-nutritious snack. The following foods are ranked in order from most satisfying to least satisfying: potatoes, fish, oatmeal, oranges, apples, whole-wheat pasta, baked beans, grapes, whole-grain bread, popcorn, bran cereal, eggs, cheese, white rice, lentils, brown rice, rice crackers. Lose more weight and keep it off by eating foods high in starchy carbohydrates like potatoes and rice because they weigh more than high-fat foods but contain fewer calories (Rolls & Miller, 1997).

15. *Eat foods high in fiber* to reduce stress to the digestive system and lose weight. Eating a moderate amount of high-fiber foods helps

you lose weight because they are filling and take longer to eat. (It takes longer to eat an apple than to drink a glass of apple juice, and crunching is more satisfying than drinking.) Eating more digestible fibers (cereals, fruits, vegetables, beans, whole-grain breads, nuts and seeds) will not only regulate blood sugar and increase satisfaction, but will also reduce risk of heart disease and high cholesterol (Sprecher & Pearce, 2002).

16. *Use psyllium husks* for elimination problems, abdominal discomfort, or heartburn (Maciejko, Braz, Shah, Patil, & Rubenfire, 1994). This indigestible fiber is available at health food stores. It will coat and soothe the digestive tract. Put a teaspoonful in a glass of water, stir, and drink before it gels.

17. *Take tryptophan* (an amino acid found in all protein-rich foods) to reduce premenstrual cravings and enhance sleep. Have some tuna or a piece of chicken on half a slice of bread or eat fish for dinner and have a piece of fruit an hour before bedtime. Vegetarians can eat cooked dried beans or peas for dinner and a little bread or rice about an hour before bedtime. Tryptophan also promotes weight loss by decreasing appetite (Bell & Goodrick, 2002).

18. *Use monounsaturated oil to reduce afternoon cravings.* Drizzle olive oil on luncheon salad or baked potato or cook with it (Maciejko et al., 1994).

19. *Eat high-zinc foods to lose weight and keep it off.* This mineral may influence leptin, a hormone that plays a key role in maintaining energy balance, giving the illusion of fullness that curbs food cravings. A study demonstrated that men fed zinc-deficient diets produced less leptin. The researchers concluded that when fat is lost, leptin production decreases, which may explain why dieters regain weight (Tallman & Taylor, 2003). Foods high in zinc include oysters, herring, eggs, nuts, wheat germ, liver, and red meat. Dietary fiber, calcium, and foods that contain phytate (dried beans, whole grains, peanut butter) can interfere with the body's ability to absorb zinc, so eat them when not eating zinc-rich foods.

20. *Eat foods high in magnesium to reduce chocolate cravings.* Chocolate can be used as a self-medication for dietary deficiency, especially magnesium (Bruinsma & Taren, 1999). Eat healthier foods instead. Foods high in magnesium to focus on include whole-grain breads and cereals, brown rice, fresh peas, wheat germ, nuts, soy products, Swiss chard, figs, green leafy vegetables, and citrus fruits.

21. *Increase intake of B-vitamins* to help metabolize fatty foods (and lose weight) and raise mood (Harnroongroj et al., 2002;

Mason, 2003; Reitman, Friedrich, Ben-Amotz, & Levy, 2002). Foods to concentrate on include sunflower seeds, rolled oats, lima beans, soybeans, raisins, wheat germ, peas, whole grain foods (cereals, breads, pasta), asparagus, brown rice, chicken, peanuts, raw spinach, kale, eggs, tuna, turkey, salmon, mackerel, sweet potatoes, cooked cabbage, bananas, sardines, trout, sea vegetables (dulse, kombu, kelp, wakame), fermented soy foods (tempeh, natto, miso), fresh green uncooked vegetables, lobster, broccoli, cauliflower, sesame seeds, mushrooms, yogurt (plain, low-fat), oranges, grapefruits, peaches, lettuce, and molasses.

22. *Don't diet. It leads to binge eating.* Restricting what is eaten leads to binge eating and weight gain, not permanent weight loss (Adami, Meneghelli, & Scopinaro, 1999; Hart & Chiovari, 1998; Polivy & Herman, 1999; Ponto, 1995; Popkess-Vawter, Wendel, Schmoll, & O'Connell, 1998; Stein & Hedger, 1997).

A. *Eat "feel good" foods.* Serotonin is a feel-good brain chemical that helps to maintain calm. Eating carbohydrates increases serotonin levels, whereas eating protein reduces them. This could be why a high-protein, high-fat diet leads to stressful feelings and binge eating, while chocolate, pasta, and bread may lead to relaxation. When stressed, take a bite of bread or a mouthful of pasta or rice. (Chocolate is not recommended because of its high fat and sugar content and its lack of nutrients.)

B. *Start a binge journal.* Write down when bingeing occurs, the trigger experiences that precede binge eating, and thoughts and feelings before, during, and after a binge. After recording several episodes, patterns will emerge and situations that set up bingeing will become apparent.

C. *Use distraction when the urge to binge strikes.* Count to ten, read a favorite book, exercise, get a hug or massage, or get involved in an enjoyable activity.

D. *Don't get overly hungry, fatigued, hung-over, lonely or stressed.* Any of these situations can lead to binge eating (Oliver & Wardel, 1999; Stein & Hedger, 1997). Carry a handful of unsalted and non-oiled nuts for snacks. Before eating them, ask, "Am I really hungry or am I angry or hurt?" If angry or hurt, listen to a relaxation tape (buy one in advance for moments like these). Take a relaxation break instead of a coffee break every day as a preventive action. Find a quiet spot, kick shoes off, sit in a comfortable spot, and place one hand over the abdomen. With eyes closed, gently let abdomen expand at inhale to breathe in at navel level. As breathing relaxes and moves lower in the body, let it gradually push out the hand. Sit quietly, breathing. Combine this with a meditation to stop bingeing. Breathe in and say, "I am in control of what I eat," and breathe out and say, "I eat only what I need to stay healthy." Alternative statements are, inhale and say, "I breathe in calm and control," and exhale and say, "I breathe out all fear (worry, anger, hurt)."

E. *Eat 1 portion of a "forbidden food" every day.* Restricting pleasing foods and then bingeing on them, then feeling guilty and restricting foods again is a common cycle that can be stopped by eating 1 portion (only) of a food that's been restricted (Hart & Chiovari, 1998).

F. *Eat enough protein to help eliminate cravings.* Some good snacks to carry are a couple of crackers with cheese or peanut butter on them, a hard-boiled egg, a couple of slices of chicken or turkey.

G. *Drink a cup of decaffeinated green tea when cravings develop.* Green tea decreases appetite (Bell & Goodrick, 2002).

H. *Try a tablespoon of flaxseed oil or several flaxseed capsules for an urge to eat fatty foods* such as French fries, burgers, or chips. Walnuts are also a good source of fatty acids. Eat a handful (only).

I. *Take a chromium capsule.* This mineral promotes the composition of the weight lost to be fat rather than lean tissue (Bell & Goodrick, 2002).

J. *Exercise.* Brisk walking can help use insulin more effectively so that bingeing will be less apt to occur and can also elevate mood (Fox, 1999; Hassmen, Koivula, & Uutela, 2000).

K. *Avoid bringing binge foods into the house and don't plan for a time to eat them.* Ask family not to bring binge foods home. During any free time or when bored, plan a noneating activity with someone else.

L. *Use imagery* to picture fitting into desired clothes, meeting eating goals, and letting go of any failures or angers.

M. *Do at least one active thing after eating dinner:* walk, dance, clean. Choose something that engages the mind so eating is not focused on (Heatherton & Baumeister, 1991).

N. *Use affirmations to counter negative ideas* (Lehman & Rodin, 1989). Choose one of the statements below and say or write it 20 times a day.

- I am safe.
- I love myself and approve of my actions.
- I create my own peace and security.

23. *If sexually abused, obtain counseling* (Fonseca, Ireland, & Resnick, 2002). The only significant risk factor for extreme weight control behaviors among adolescents was sexual abuse history.

24. *Prevent obesity in children* by respecting their appetite (they don't need to finish every meal); provide at least five fresh fruits and vegetables every day; avoid prepackaged, processed, and sugared foods; avoid bringing high-calorie snack foods and drinks into the home; limit trips to fast-food restaurants, ice cream parlors, and other high-calorie eating establishments; discourage frequent consumption of high-calorie beverages such as soft drinks and juices; avoid providing food for comfort or reward; don't offer sweets in exchange for finishing a meal; avoid eating in front of the television set; limit time spent viewing television and playing video games to less than two hours a day; encourage active play; establish regular family activities such as walks, swimming in a pool, ball games, and other outdoor activities (Moran, 1999).

For a complete weight loss plan, including ways to implement it, see P. J. Rosch and C. C. Clark, *De-Stress, Weigh Less: A Six-Step No-Diet Plan for Relaxing Your Way to Permanent Weight Loss.*

EVALUATION OF TREATMENT

The client described above provided the following self-evaluation: "I haven't eaten anything after seven at night for a week and I've started to walk every morning. I've been trying to eat a slice of pizza or a piece of chocolate once a day. I haven't been up for an all-night binge in over a month."

REFERENCES

Adami, G., Meneghelli, A., & Scopinaro, N. (1999). Night eating and binge eating disorder in obese patients. *International Journal of Eating Disorders, 25,* 335–338.

Bell, S. J., & Goodrick, G. K. (2002). A functional food product for the management of weight. *Critical Review of Food Science and Nutrition, 42,* 163–178.

Bernadot, D., Deutz, R. C., Martin, D. E., & Cody, M. M. (2000). Relationship between energy deficits and body composition in elite female gymnasts and runners. *Medicine and Science in Sports and Exercise, 32,* 659–668.

Bolumar, F., Olsen, J., Rebagliato, M., & Bisani, L. (1997). Caffeine intake and delayed conception: A European multi-center study on infertility and subfecundity. *American Journal of Epidemiology, 145,* 324–334.

Bruinsma, K., & Taren, D. L. (1999). Chocolate: Food or drug? *Journal of the American Dietetic Association, 99,* 1249–1256.

Caius, N., & Benefice, E. (2002). Food habits, physical activity and over-weight among adolescents. *Review of Epidemiology Sante Publicque, 50,* 531–542.

Christensen, L. (1991). The role of caffeine and sugar in depression. *Nutrition Reports, 9*(3), 17–24.

Christensen, L. (1993). Effects of eating behavior on mood: A review of the literature. *International Journal of Eating Disorders, 14,* 171–183.

Christensen, L., & Burrows, R. (1990). Dietary treatment of depression. *Behavior Therapy, 21,* 183–194.

Curtis, K. M., Savitz, D. A., & Arbuckle, T. E. (1997). Effects of cigarette smoking, caffeine consumption, and alcohol intake on fecundability. *American Journal of Epidemiology, 146*(1), 32–41.

El-Khairy, L., Ueland, P. M., Nyard, D., Refaum, H., & Vollset, S. E. (1999). Lifestyle and cardiovascular disease risk factors as determinants of total cysteine in plasma: The Hordaland Homocysteine Study. *American Journal of Clinical Nutrition, 70,* 1016–1024.

Fonseca, H., Ireland, M., & Resnick, M. D. (2002). Familial correlates of extreme weight control behaviors among adolescents. *International Journal of Eating Disorders, 32,* 441–48.

Fox, K. R. (1999). The influence of physical activity on mental well-being. *Public Health Nutrition, 2*(3A), 411–418.

Harnroongroj, T., Jintaridhi, P., Vudhivai, N., Pongpaew, P., Tungtrongchitr, R., Phonrat, B., et al. (2002). B vitamins, vitamin C, and hematological measurements in overweight and obese Thais in Bangkok. *Journal of the Medical Association of Thailand, 85,* 17–25.

Hart, K. E., & Chiovari, P. (1998). Inhibition of eating behavior: Negative cognitive effects of dieting. *Journal of Clinical Psychology, 54,* 427–430.

Hassmen, P., Koivula, N., & Uutela, A. (2000). Physical exercise and psychological well-being: A population study in Finland. *Preventive Medicine, 30*(1), 17–25.

Heatherton, T. F., & Baumeister, R. F. (1991). Binge eating as escape from self-awareness. *Psychological Bulletin, 110,* 86–108.

Kynast-Gales, S. A., & Massey, L. K. (1994). Effect of caffeine on circadian excretion of urinary calcium and magnesium. *Journal of the American College of Nutrition, 13,* 467–472.

Lehman, A. K., & Rodin, J. (1989). Styles of self-nurturance and disordered eating. *Journal of Consulting and Clinical Psychology, 57,* 117–122.

Liu, S. (2002). Intake of refined carbohydrates and whole grain foods in relation to risk of type 2 diabetes mellitus and coronary heart disease. *Journal of the American College of Nutrition, 21,* 298–306.

Liu, S., & Willett, W. C. (2002). Dietary glycemic load and atherothrombotic risk. *Current Atherosclerosis Reports, 4,* 454–461.

Ludwig, D. S., Peterson, K. E., & Gortmaker, S. L. (2001). Relation between consumption of sugar-sweetened drinks and childhood obesity: A prospective, observational analysis. *Lancet, 357,* 505–508.

Maciejko, J. J., Braz, A., Shah, A., Patil, S., & Rubenfire, M. (1994). Psyllium for the reduction of cholestyramine-associated gastrointestinal symptoms in the treatment of primary hypercholesterolemia. *Archives of Family Medicine, 3,* 955–960.

Mason, J. B. (2003). Biomarkers of nutrient exposure and status in one-carbon (methyl) metabolism. *Journal of Nutrition, 133*(Suppl. 3), 941S–947S.

McCarthy, M. F. (2000). The origins of western obesity: A role for animal protein? *Medical Hypotheses, 54,* 488–494.

Miller, W. C., Niederpruem, M. G., Wallace, J. P., & Lindeman, A. K. (1994). Dietary fat, sugar and fiber predict body fat content. *Journal of the American Dietary Association, 94,* 612–615.

Moran, R. (1999). Evaluation and treatment of childhood obesity. *American Family Physician, 59,* 861.

Oliver, G., & Wardel, J. (1999). Perceived effects of stress on food choice. *Physiological Behavior, 66,* 511–513.

Olney, J. W., Farber, N. B., Spitznagel, E., & Robins, L. N. (1996). Increasing brain tumor rates: Is there a link to aspartame? *Journal of Neuropathology and Experimental Neurology, 55,* 1115–1123.

Pasman, W. J., Saris, W. H., & Westerterp-Plantenga, M. S. (1999). Predictors of weight maintenance. *Obesity Research, 7,* 43–50.

Pincomb, A., Lovallo, W. R., McKey, B. S., Hee Sung, B., Passey, R. B., Everson, A., & Wilson, M. F. (1996). Acute blood pressure elevations with caffeine in men with borderline systemic hypertension. *American Journal of Cardiology, 77,* 270–274.

Polivy, J., & Herman, C. P. (1999). The effects of resolving to diet on restrained and unrestrained eaters: The "false hope syndrome." *International Journal of Eating Disorders, 26,* 434–437.

Ponto, M. (1995). The relationship between obesity, dieting and eating disorders. *Professional Nurse, 10,* 422–425.

Popkess-Vawter, S., Wendel, S., Schmoll, S., & O'Connell, K. (1998). Overeating, reversal theory, and weight cycling. *Western Journal of Nursing Research, 20,* 67–83.

Reitman, A., Friedrich, I., Ben-Amotz, A., & Levy, Y. (2002). Low plasma antioxidants and normal plasma B vitamins and homocysteine in patients with severe obesity. *Israeli Medical Association Journal, 4,* 590–593.

Rodriguez-Artalejo, F., Garcia, E. L., Gorgojo, L O., Garces, C., Royo, M. A., Martin Moreno, J. M., et al. (2003). Consumption of bakery products, sweetened soft drinks and yogurt among children aged 6–7 years: Association with nutrient intake and overall diet quality. *British Journal of Nutrition, 89,* 419–429.

Rolls, B. J., & Miller, D. L. (1997). Is the low-fat message giving people a license to eat more? *Journal of the American College of Nutrition, 16,* 535–543.

Rosch, P. J., & Clark, C. C. (2001). *De-stress, weigh less: A six-step no-diet plan for relaxing your way to permanent weight loss.* New York: St. Martin's Press.

Rude, R. K., Kirschen, M. E., Gruber, H. E., Meyer, M. H., & Luck, D. L. (1999). Magnesium deficiency-induced osteoporosis in the uncoupling of bone formation and bone resorption. *Magnesium Research, 12,* 257–267.

Singh, P. H., & Fraser, G. E. (1998). Dietary risk factors in colon cancer in a low-risk population. *American Journal of Epidemiology, 148,* 761–774.

Sprecher, D. L., & Pearce, G. L. (2002). Fiber-multivitamin combination therapy: A beneficial influence on low-density lipoprotein and homocysteine. *Metabolism, 51,* 1166–1170.

Stein, K. F., & Hedger, K. M. (1997). Body weight and shape self-cognitions, emotional distress, and disordered eating in middle adolescent girls. *Archives of Psychiatric Nursing, 11,* 264–275.

Stice, W. P., & Hayward, C. (1999). Naturalistic weight reduction efforts prospectively predict growth in relative weight and onset of obesity among female adolescents. *Journal of Consulting and Clinical Psychology, 67,* 967–974.

Tallman, D. L., & Taylor, C. G. (2003). Effects of dietary fat and zinc on adiposity, serum leptin and adipose fatty acid composition in C57BL/6J mice. *Journal of Nutrition and Biochemistry, 14*(1), 17–23.

Trocho, C., Pardo, R., Rafecas, I., Virgili, J., Remesar, X, Fernandes-Lopez, J. A, et al. (1998). Formaldehyde derived from dietary aspartame binds to tissue components in vivo. *Life Science, 63,* 337–339.

Tucker, K. L., Hannan, M. T., Chen, H., Cupples, L. A., & Wilson, R. (1999). Potassium, magnesium and fruit and vegetables associated with greater bone mineral density in elderly men and women. *American Journal of Clinical Nutrition, 69,* 727–736.

Van den Eeden, S. K., Koepsell, T. D., Longstreth, W. T., van Belle, G., Daling, J. R., & McKnight, B. (1994). Aspartame ingestion and headaches: A randomized crossover trial. *Neurology, 44,* 1787–1793.

Walton, R., Hudak, R., & Green-Waite, R. J. (1993). Adverse reactions to aspartame: Double-blind challenge in patients from a vulnerable population. *Biological Psychiatry, 34*(1–2),13–17.

CHAPTER 19

Pain

Pain is an unpleasant emotional and sensory experience associated with potential or actual tissue damage. Pain medications, especially nonsteroidal anti-inflammatory drugs (NSAIDs) are usually prescribed. Clients 60 years and older are most apt to experience side effects such as peptic ulcer disease and gastrointestinal bleeding that can lead to death.

HOLISTIC NURSING ASSESSMENT

Study the holistic nursing assessment for Mrs. Y., a 61-year-old client suffering from pain. Working in collaboration with other clients complaining of pain, use the format presented to conduct a holistic nursing assessment.

Client learning needs: Says her pain medication won't work anymore.

Indicants of readiness to learn: "I want to get rid of all this pain, but I'm not sure how to go about it."

Soul/spirituality symbol(s): "I just pray to the Lord."

Meaning of the condition to client: "I think I'm being punished."

Relationship needs/effects as perceived by the client: "I spend all my time trying to get pain free. I don't have time for my family anymore."

Patterns/attitudes that may create dis-ease for this client: Client uses negative affirmations (e.g., "I feel like this pain has me," and "This pain is ruling me. I can't think of anything else").

Life purpose: "It's time for me to die now. My husband is more interested in his work than he is in me, and my children are grown up
and don't need me."

Client strengths: Is lucid when not in pain. Has a college education
and has looked up pain measures on the Internet.

Ability to participate in care: Client is malnourished and weak.

Ethical dilemmas: Client denies suicidal thoughts, but has tried to
stockpile pain meds twice, according to the hospital chart.

Nurse–client process: Client talks little about herself. When she
does, she focuses on dying and "leaving this world. I'm waiting
for the Lord to take me home."

TREATMENT PLANNING: SETTING JOINTLY AGREED-UPON GOALS

In the case of the client discussed above, the following goals were
agreed upon:

1. Use a pain diary to detect patterns.
2. Listen to a relaxation tape twice a day.
3. Start an exercise program.

TREATMENT

Acceptance of condition/attitude change: The client chose the following affirmation to use to replace the pain she feels: "I release
the past." Client agreed to write the affirmation on 3 x 5 cards and
say the words at least 20 times each day.

Facilitating the healing process/healing intention formulation:
From a list of meditative statements, client chose the following
one to assist in the healing process: "All is well in my world."
Client was asked to meditate on the words while in a relaxed
state. Nurse will use caring nonverbal and verbal communication,
centering, and a meditative state to enhance client healing, will
verbalize observed patterns that may be holding the client back
and offer alternate approaches.

Creating a sacred space: During client sessions, relaxing music chosen by the client will play.

Encouraging re-storying: Nurse encouraged client to recall an upsetting situation with someone in her family and choose an ending that inspires her.

Integrative practices planned: Nurse will use therapeutic touch and guided imagery to assist client in the healing process.

Role model strategies: Nurse showed client how to role play problematic interchanges with her children.

Protection plan: Client plans to use an "image of the Lord" around her for protection.

Family strategies: Nurse encouraged client to invite her son or daughter to a session with nurse to practice more open communication between them.

Life issues/life purpose work: Client has agreed to meditate on her life purpose.

Treatment possibilities/considerations: Other suggested treatments appear below. Most are evidence-based.

ADDITIONAL INFORMATION AND TREATMENTS TO SHARE WITH CLIENTS

FOR ALL TYPES OF PAIN

1. *Avoid NSAIDs.* Pain medications, especially nonsteroidal anti-inflammatory drugs (NSAIDs), are usually prescribed, but clients over 60 years of age are more likely to experience side effects. Older adults are more apt to develop peptic ulcer disease and are five times as likely to die from gastrointestinal bleeding as those who do not take NSAIDs (Loeb, 1999).

The NSAID most likely to irritate stomach and intestines is aspirin. Clients who have a history of stomach or intestinal irritation, are taking steroids, smoke, have abnormal kidney function, drink alcohol, or take high doses of NSAIDs, are at greater risk for developing adverse effects. According to the American Geriatrics Society Panel on Chronic Pain in Older Persons (1998), other side effects to watch out for are liver damage (Tylenol), abnormal kidney function, constipation, confusion, damaged cartilage, increased blood pressure, internal bleeding, ulcers, pain, and headaches (Motrin, Advil, Nuprin, Naprosyn, Trilisate, Midol IB, Bayer Select Pain Relief, and IBU). Even one or two ibuprofen (Motrin) capsules taken two or three days a week can cause kidney damage.

Sometimes opiates are prescribed. One opiate that has many problems is Norpropoxyphene. It's associated with fluid in the lungs, heart toxicity, difficulty breathing, cardiac arrest, and even death. If this drug is prescribed with diazepam (Valium), the occurrence of adverse effects is increased, including falls, an already serious problem among older adults (Perin, 2000).

2. *Think of pain as a message the body provides.* Help unravel what message pain is giving and examine in depth the cost of pain to life. How does it decrease the ability to enjoy beloved activities, family, friends, peace of mind? Gently explore what hidden benefits pain has brought you. This is called secondary gain. It could be that the only time anyone pays any attention to you is when you are in pain. Studies have shown that people who get support from their pain usually have high levels of it and are more disabled than those who don't. Pain can also be used as an excuse for not dealing with other problems in life like a bad marriage or fear about discussing important issues. It's not easy to talk about some of these topics, but a good therapist can help you do it and keep you feeling safe. A major goal of this kind of approach is to find a way for you to meet life goals in a healthy way rather than relying on being in pain to achieve them.

Mind/body strategies have been known to work even when all else failed. People who have been through a therapeutic experience that addressed their pain report significant reductions in pain severity, depression, anxiety, and feeling out of control. They even report that pain interferes less in their activities of daily life. Even if the pain continues, the negative emotions, which make the pain worse, are reduced and participants can take an active role in life again (Astin, Shapiro, Eisenberg, & Forys, 2003).

3. *Start a pain diary.* Record level of pain every hour and see how it is related to time of day, mood, fatigue, stress, activities, and other people.

4. *Try a psychotherapeutic approach.* If drugs, local anesthetics, surgical procedures, ice, heat, electrical stimulation, and massage don't work, consider a referral to a mental health nurse practitioner with pain management skills.

5. *Embrace pain.* Avoid thinking of it as the enemy. Take ownership of the pain to try to understand how it fits into the whole of life experience. Listen to the message of pain deep within. It is a valuable gift that can be understood. Once the basis of pain is understood, control over the pain and life can be regained.

6. *Express feelings.* Keeping pain unexpressed will only increase it. This does not mean complaining more; it means saying, "I feel angry when . . ." or "I'm afraid of . . ." and then being very specific about what evokes anger or fear. This kind of assertive communication may require assertiveness training or counseling with a mental health nurse practitioner who has assertiveness skills.

7. *Use relaxation therapy.* Evidence is strong for the effectiveness of relaxation as a class of techniques to reduce chronic pain (National Institutes of Health, Technology Assessment Panel, 1996). At minimum, listen to a relaxation tape in the morning and before bed. For quicker results, leave it playing at a low volume all day long, except when driving or using heavy machinery.

8. *Learn massage techniques.* Purchase a book on self- or couple massage and practice the techniques with a partner. Even rubbing someone else's feet and having that person return the favor can bring many benefits. A 20-minute massage once daily just before the morning debridement of skin in burn patients provided a measurable decrease of anxiety after the massage session and significant lower pain ratings after a week of treatment (Field, 1998). A University of Florida in Gainesville report revealed that massage and relaxation therapy both reduced pain. The researcher believed it was because both treatments caused blood vessels to dilate, improving blood flow (Ross, 2000).

9. *Exercise.* Movement is a distractor that can help the body release endorphins, natural body painkillers. Exercise also strengthens muscles, improves joint mobility, promotes comfort, restores coordination and balance, and improves sleep. There is no evidence that one type of exercise is better than another, but slow movement such as walking or t'ai chi is less stressful than other exercises. Fitness walking reduced pain more than a pain education program (instruction and demonstration of the use of heat, cold, massage, relaxation, and distraction) or usual medical care (Ferrell, Josephson, Pollan, Loy, & Ferrell, 1997). Purchasing a book, joining a health club, or finding a personal trainer are ways to get into an exercise program. Whichever method is selected, an exercise schedule should be gentle, regular, and gradual to avoid introducing additional pain.

10. *Meditate.* One technique called "mindfulness" encourages passive focus on pain by just observing it (Bonadonna, 2003). This can help distinguish between pain and its experience. Once arriving at this point, it will be self-evident that pain can be controlled. Practicing the procedure and developing a meditation audiotape can help.

11. *Try guided imagery;* for example, picturing the areas where pain is located in the body, turning those areas a color, then a liquid, and then imagining the liquid leaving the body and flowing away to a place where it can no longer influence often helps.

12. *Engage in at least one pleasurable activity a day.* To stop feeling guilty about comfort and pleasure, spending at least half an hour a day engaged in an activity that gives pleasure is mandatory (Hooker, 1996). Put that activity on the calendar and then follow through, taking a walk, listening to music, soaking in a bubble bath, reading a book, seeing a play or television show or doing whatever brings enjoyment.

13. *Use affirmations.* Catastrophic and negative thoughts increase pain (Van Damme, Cromley, & Eccleston, 2004). Write or say one of the following positive statements at least 20 times a day and stop yourself when you hear yourself saying words that are in opposition to it:

- release the past and let it go.
- I am free and everyone is free.
- I forgive myself and everyone else.
- I deserve to be free and pain-free.

14. *Try Feldenkrais for headaches or musculoskeletal problems.* In one study, a group that used the Feldenkrais Method reported mobility and decreased pain up to a year after treatment, compared to other groups (Bearman & Shafarman, 1999).

15. *Use Reiki* (Olson & Hanson, 1997).

16. *Investigate herbs and supplements that reduce pain.* Gingko biloba has been found to reduce leg pain and increase walking distance (Pittler & Ernst, 2000). Other herbs that have shown promise for pain treatment include garlic and feverfew (especially for headaches because it either prevents blood vessel spasm or blocks prostaglandins that increase inflammation). Cayenne has been shown to reduce arthritis pain (Mills, Jacoby, Chacksfield, & Willoughby, 1996). Blue-green algae may help treat pain (Gerwick, 2000). A useful topical agent, cajeput oil, which is usually combined with peppermint, clove, menthol, eucalyptus, cayenne, or arnica oil, can relieve musculoskeletal pain, headache, hemorrhoid pain, neuralgia, rheumatic pain, and pain resulting from sports injuries.

17. *Learn self-hypnosis.* The evidence supporting the effectiveness of hypnosis in alleviating chronic pain, especially with cancer, is strong. It is also effective for reducing pain in irritable bowel syndrome, post-surgical pain, TMJ, and tension headaches (Montgomery,

David, Winkel, Silverstein, & Bovbjerg, 2002; Palsson, Turner, Johnson, Burnelt, & Whitehead, 2002), reducing the pain perceived by patients on mechanical ventilation (Thomas, 2003), those suffering from rectal pain (Palsson et al., 2002), and pediatric pain (Zeltzer et al., 2002). A meta-analysis of studies using hypnosis postsurgery revealed that participants in hypnosis treatment groups had better clinical outcomes than 89% of participants in control groups (Montgomery et al., 2002).

18. *Massage the ileocecal valve points* to relieve low back pain, chest pain, or headaches (see Digestive Problems).

19. *Drink 6 to 8 glasses of water every day.* Much pain is due to dehydration (Williams, 1995).

20. *Eat foods high in sulfur or take methysulfonylemethane (MSM).* Sulfur compounds have been shown to reduce pain (Parcell, 2002). Food high in sulfur include cabbage, peas, beans, eggs, cauliflower, horseradish, shrimp, chestnuts, mustard greens, onions, and asparagus.

21. *Eat pineapple or take bromelain* (Rowan, Buttle, & Barrett, 1990).

22. *Try healing touch.* A study found that after healing touch treatment, relief was reported by 6 of 11 clients (55%) experiencing pain (Wilkinson et al., 2002).

23. *Explore therapeutic touch.* People with chronic pain who were about to participate in a cognitive-behavioral pain treatment program were randomized to either relaxation training or therapeutic touch (TT) plus relaxation (experimental group). Participation in the TT group was found to be associated with less distress and disability. Participants also exhibited greater self-efficacy and unitary power as well as lower attrition rates (Smith, Arnstein, Rosa, & Wells-Federman, 2002).

24. *Look into a wellness intervention.* A wellness two-phase program consisting of lifestyle-change classes for 8 weeks, then telephone follow-up for 3 months, produced significant effects on self-efficacy for health behaviors, health-promoting behaviors, and mental health and pain scales (Stuifbergen et al., 2003).

ARTHRITIS PAIN

In a repeated-measures investigation, 30 women diagnosed with rheumatoid arthritis responded to the McGill Pain Questionnaire prior to listening to music of their choice, during music, and 1 to 2 hours after completing the intervention. The results of the study supported the use of music as a transformative intervention (Schorr, 1993).

BACK PAIN

The majority of clients with back pain, even those with radiculopathy, improve with conservative management. Surgery is unnecessary (Wipf & Deyo, 1995).

1. *Rate pain pre- and post-treatment* (also a good idea for other types of pain). The best measures for chronic low back pain are the 101-point Numeric Rating Scale or NRS and the Box scale or BS (Strong, Ashton, & Chant, 1991). The NRS asks clients to "Please indicate on the line below the number between 0 and 100 that best describes your pain." A zero (0) would mean "no pain" and a one hundred (100) would mean "pain as bad as it could be." The BS has boxes with 1 to 10 and the words, "If a zero (0) means 'no pain,' and a ten (10) means 'pain as bad as it could be,' on this scale of 0 to 10, what is your level of pain? Put an 'x' through that number."

2. *Examine beliefs.* Participants in a study who had low back pain had more catastrophizing thoughts ("It only feels bad. I cannot think or do anything.") and higher levels of psychological distress than those without such pain and can benefit from active behavioral coping procedures (Harkapaa, 1991).

3. *Try manual therapy and exercise.* A multicenter, randomized, controlled trial with 1-year follow-up found improvement for back pain from both manual therapy and exercise therapy, but manual therapy showed significantly greater improvement in low back pain (Aure, Nilsen, & Vasseljen, 2003).

4. *Take willow bark extract.* It is the natural form of salicylic acid (aspirin), has comparable anti-inflammatory activities, and has no adverse effects on the stomach mucosa (Marz & Kemper, 2002).

BREAST PAIN

Fish oil, evening primrose oil, corn oil with wheatgerm oil, and even plain corn oil decreased breast pain in premenopausal women with severe chronic mastalgia who took part in a randomized, double-blind, factorial clinical trial, although evening primrose oil and fish oil resulted in a greater decrease in breast pain than the other oils (Blommers, de Lange-DeKlerk, Kuik, Bezemer, & Meijer, 2002). Restriction of dairy products and foods high in saturated fats can relieve mild to moderate breast pain, but not severe pain (Berry, 2001).

Burns

Massage therapy can help reduce pain of burn debridement (Field, 1998). Vitamin E and castor oil are soothing and healing topical agents for burns (Williams, 1995).

Chemotherapy Distress

A study indicated that relaxation training and cognitive distraction resulted in less distress and nausea prior to chemotherapy for treatment groups, but not controls (Vasterling, Jenkins, Tope, & Burish, 1993).

Chest Pain

Some chest pain may be due to a stuck ileocecal valve. Massage of points right below the bony ridge at the back of the right side of the head, on an angle from the chest to the right arm, up and down the sides of both legs and the outer calf of the right leg for 10 to 20 seconds (but no longer) can help (Williams, 1992a, 1992b).

Gynecologic and Obstetrical Pain

Foot reflexology used after gynecological surgery resulted in study participants needing less pain medication than a control group (Kesselring, 1994). Pure lavender oil in a sitz bath reduced perineal discomfort more effectively than synthetic lavender oil or an inert bath additive between the third and fifth days postpartum (Dale & Cornwell, 1994). Prophylactic use of acupressure bands bilaterally on the P-6 acupoint significantly reduced the incidence of nausea and vomiting after epidural morphine for post-Cesarean section pain relief (Ho, Hseu, Tsai, & Lee, 1996). Relaxation and music reduced pain after gynecologic surgery in a randomized controlled trial (Good, Anderson, Stanton-Hicks, Grass, & Makii, 2002).

Headache

1. *Start a food/mood/stress diary.* Identify and eliminate substances and situations that trigger headaches. Factors that can precipitate a headache include food allergies, emotional changes, low magnesium levels, intense emotions such as anger, hormonal changes (menstruation, ovulation, birth control pills), exhaustion, poor posture, eyestrain, withdrawal from caffeine, smoking or second-hand

smoke (Hannerz, 1997), or muscle tension. The most common allergens are milk, aged cheeses, chocolate, food additives, wheat, citrus fruits, overripe bananas, sauerkraut, smoked or pickled meats and fish, cold cuts, hot dogs, sausage, liver, beans (lima, soy, and fava), lentils and peas, sourdough and yeast breads, bouillon cubes, soy sauce (and other foods containing MSG), nuts, peanut butter, colas, coffee, tea, artificial sweeteners like Aspartame (Nutrasweet), fish, tomatoes, cheese, wheat gluten (Hadjivassiliou et al., 2001), beer, and wine (Savi et al., 2002).

Tension-type headaches usually occur in the context of stress, either environmental (loud noise, heat, bright or flickering fluorescent lights, perfumes, strong odors, second-hand cigarette smoke), motion (travel, athletic activities, complex moving visual patterns, weather changes), smoking, drugs (nitroglycerin, hydralazine, reserpine, diuretics, anti-asthma medications, overuse of pain medications), head trauma, medical tests, excess exertion (sports, sexual orgasm), neck disorders (arthritis, disk narrowing), or interpersonal events (arguments, anger, guilt, etc.). Food can also bring on a tension headache (Savi et al., 2002).

2. *Rest* in a darkened room. Fatigue can bring on headaches and so can too much sleep. Keep a regular sleep/wake regime.

3. *Eat foods and drink beverages that are room temperature.*

4. *Take magnesium.* Low magnesium levels can also lead to daily headaches in adults (Ramadan et al., 1989; Swanson, 1988) and adolescents (Aloisi, Marrelli, Porto, Tozzi, & Cerone, 1997). Having a mitral valve prolapse doubles the risk for migraines because of low magnesium blood levels. Participants in one study who took 600 mg of magnesium (trimagnesium dicitrate) daily for 12 weeks had 41.6% fewer headaches than those in the placebo group (Matthew, 1993). Adverse events were diarrhea (18.6%) and stomach irritation (4.7%). Start with 600 mg of magnesium citrate, aspartate, or chelate in divided doses to treat both headaches and mitral valve prolapse (Gallai, Baker, & McLellan, 1986).

5. *Avoid drugs correlated with headaches.* According to a review of clinical studies, 70% of chronic daily headaches may be drug-induced (Murray, 1994). There are two kinds of headaches of this type: analgesic rebound and ergotamine rebound. Withdrawing the medication in one study resulted in decreased frequency and severity of headaches, increased well-being, enhanced sleep patterns, and a reduction in irritability, depression, and lethargy (Ramadan et al., 1989). In another study patients with daily headaches were told to stop taking pain medication. A month later 66% were

improved and by the end of the second month 81% were improved (Peikert, Wilimzig, & Kohne-Volland, 1996). Taking a large number of analgesics for migraine headaches (more than 8 pills a day or 50 in a week) may cause more headaches (Selman, 2000). Many headache medicines also contain caffeine or a sedative. Eliminating these drugs can lead to withdrawal symptoms (nausea, abdominal cramps, diarrhea, restlessness, sleeplessness, and anxiety) for 24 to 48 hours. Withdrawal of ergotamine can also produce rebound headaches. As most migraine headaches do not occur more frequently than every few days, daily headaches are probably due to an ergotamine rebound effect.

6. *Use herbs.* One study found that feverfew was associated with a reduction in the number and severity of migraines and in the degree of vomiting, and there were no serious side effects (Murphy, Heptinstall, & Mitchell, 1988; Pettit, 2001). Applying a topical ointment with cayenne in and around the nostril several times a day may help. Use a small amount and expect it to burn a little at first. Try a couple of sprinkles of ginger or a ginger extract. Repeat every two hours as needed. Gingko, 50 mg, three times a day with water or as a tincture might help because it increases circulation to the brain, but check with a pharmacist first to make sure it won't interact with any other medications you're taking. Try skullcap tea, available at health food stores. Drink room temperature valerian tea, take 200 mg valerian capsules or take as a tincture. Take 750 mg willow bark up to three times daily. It can also be taken as a tincture or tea. It contains the same active ingredients as aspirin but has none of its adverse effects. Try massaging the affected area with a 10 percent solution of peppermint oil.

7. *Try complete breaths.* Place one hand at navel level and gently try to push that hand out with each exhalation. Put reminders around the house to "breathe in your abdomen." If that doesn't help, take a yoga or meditation class to help slow down and breathe right.

8. *Obtain time management counseling.* Feeling overstressed can tighten up muscles, cut off blood supply to neck and shoulders, and bring on a headache. Consider professional time management or counseling help when activities or responsibilities feel overwhelming.

9. *Use ice.* Wrap an ice cube in a thin scarf and slowly stroke along painful areas.

10. *Rotate the neck.* Headaches can result from neck and shoulder tension. Prevent them by gently rotating the neck from side to side and shrugging shoulders at least hourly to break the tension held in

muscles and more often when sitting at a monitor or holding the head still.

11. *Learn self-hypnosis.* Hypnosis has been shown to be effective for adults, but it can help children, too (Holden, Deichmann, & Levy, 1999). Check for elevated anxiety and depression in youngsters, as the rate of chronic headaches in children and teens age 9 to 15 years is 25% higher than other children ("Are Headaches a Warning Sign?," 1998).

12. *Try massage.* It can decrease the incidence of chronic tension headache (Quinn, Chandler, & Moraska, 2002) and tension-type headache in children (Sarioglu et al., 2003). Reflexology was shown to be as helpful as medication in one study (Kesselring, 1994). For self-massage, follow these directions:

A. Stretch the muscles on, above, and below the bony ridge across the back of the head. When those muscles go into spasm (from stress or lack of magnesium), histamine is released, stimulating the sinus linings to overproduce fluid. The membranes swell shut and pressure builds up. Massaging these muscles gently can relieve spasms and reduce swelling, thereby reducing headache. Use 6 strokes across the muscle, then tap the muscle 6 times. Repeat until muscle relaxes.

B. Massage the point between the outer corner of your eye and the outer end of your eyebrow. Let the finger rest on a ridge of bone, the outer edge of the eye socket. Move only a finger's width toward the ear and find a small hollow. Massage there.

C. Massage big toes. Twirl them, pinch them, and use the fingernails to press into the top of the toes. In reflexology, the head is represented on the big toe, so massage well in the spot where the headache would be.

13. *Take a vitamin B* complex supplement at the first hint of pain (Schoenen, Jacquy, & Lenaerts, 1998). Riboflavin alone works as well as beta blockers in the treatment of migraine (Sandor, Afra, Ambrosini, & Schoenen, 2000).

14. *Try fatty acids* or EFAs, including salmon and evening primrose oil, which are anti-inflammatory substances that can relieve headache (Harel et al., 2002; Tapiero, Ba, Couvreur, & Tew, 2002). Find EPO at health food stores. Use fish as a protein source, especially the oily varieties like salmon, tuna, sardines, and mackerel.

15. *Try olive oil.* One study found it worked as well as fish oil (Harel et al., 2002).

16. *Rule out sleep disorders.* According to one study, sleep disturbances were often related to headaches occurring during the night
or early morning. (Paiva et al., 1997). When the sleep disturbance
was treated, the headaches disappeared.

17. *Try biofeedback.* Participants who had biofeedback before
cognitive therapy had better results than those who did not. The
biofeedback helped them recognize the influence of their thoughts
and emotions on their headaches and prepared them for successful cognitive treatment (Kropp, Gerber, Keinath-Specht, Kopal, &
Niederberger, 1997). Biofeedback worked as well as guided imagery
training in two studies (Arena, Bruno, Hannah, & Meador, 1995;
Ilacqua, 1994).

18. *For menstrual migraines,* try a combination of 60 mg soy
isoflavones, 100 mg dong quai, and 50 mg black cohosh (Burke,
Olson, & Cusack, 2002).

19. *Explore chiropractic.* Treatment by a chiropractor reduced the
number of headache hours per day by 69% and headache intensity
by 36%, compared to a group that received soft tissue massage for
their headaches (Nilsson, Christensen, & Hartvigsen, 1997).

20. *Use oil of peppermint.* Peppermint oil applied topically on the
temples and forehead treats headaches (Williams, 1995).

21. *Relaxation therapy* works better for tension headaches, and
autogenic training works better for migraines (Janssen & Neutgens,
1986).

22. *Multidisciplinary intervention:* A low-cost, group, multidisciplinary migraine headache intervention in a community-based nonclin-
ical setting included 18 group-supervised exercise therapy sessions,
2 group stress management and relaxation therapy lectures, 1 group
dietary lecture, and 2 massage therapy sessions. The treatment
group experienced statistically significant changes in self-perceived
pain frequency, pain intensity, health status, pain-related disability,
and depression (as compared to a standard care group), and the
effects were still apparent at the 3-month follow-up (Lemstra, Stewart,
& Olszynski, 2002).

23. *Drink 6 to 8 glasses of water a day* (Williams, 1992a).

24. *Try guided imagery* (Mannix, Chandurkar, Rybicki, Tusek, &
Solomon, 1999).

25. *Investigate acupuncture.* In one study, a group using acupuncture resulted in a significantly greater positive results than a group
undergoing conventional drug therapy (Gao, Zhao, & Xie, 1999).

26. *Exercise aerobically.* Walking, jogging, running, swimming, or
bike riding may help (Mauskop, 2001).

HEART PAIN

Try oral L-arginine. This semi-essential amino acid that stimulates nitric oxide, a key component of endothelial-derived relaxing factor, can be utilized in therapeutic regimens for angina (Appleton, 2002).

INTERSTITIAL CYSTITIS

A randomized, double-blind, placebo-controlled study showed that the treatment group (who took L-arginine) had a decrease in pain intensity and frequency of pain and showed greater globe improvement than the control (placebo) group (Korting, Smith, Wheeler, Weiss, & Foster, 1999).

LEG PAIN

Gingko biloba can reduce pain and increase walking distance for intermittent claudication (Pittler & Ernst, 2000).

MENSTRUAL PAIN

Acupressure was as effective as ibuprofen for 216 female high school students who complained of dysmenorrhea, and was recommended as the treatment of choice because it has no side effects (Pouresmail & Ibrahimzadeh, 2002).

MUSCLE SORENESS

Massage has been shown to reduce muscle soreness (Hilberg, Sforzo, & Swensen, 2003).

1. *Rub any sore, cold, or inflexible body parts* with gentle compassion, bringing fresh blood and energy to those spots. Obtain a massage if unable to self-massage.

2. *Lie prone on one side* with a hand over head and the other resting on a soft mat, rug, or mattress. Bend the knee of the top leg, but keep the bottom leg straight. Breathe in and out very slowly while tightening the muscles of the anus. Hold the muscles tight for as long as possible, then relax. Repeat until feeling weary or strained, then stop and relax (Chang, 1986).

NERVE PAIN

Apply peppermint oil (Williams, 1995), staying away from eyes and washing hands carefully after touching the oil.

PEDIATRIC PROCEDURE PAIN

Distraction and imagery were found to decrease pain in children during painful procedures (Broome, Lillis, McGahee, & Bates, 1992). Other cognitive-behavioral pain reduction strategies that may work include parent-caregiver participation; minimizing environmental stimulation; discussing the procedure in advance and/or providing a sensory demonstration of how the procedure will feel and sound; offering choice of injection site or adhesive bandage to enhance client control; holding or rocking; teaching progressive muscle relaxation, therapeutic touch, or massage; "blowing" the pain away by using forced exhalation at the first sensation of pain; teaching rhythmic deep breathing (in through the nose, out through pursed lips); looking at toys or books; counting clouds; counting ceiling tiles; singing; reciting a rhyme or story; listening to music with headphones; watching a video; playing a game; calling upon a fantasy character or superhero to help fight pain; saying coping statements ("I'll be OK," "This is almost over"); and using a "magic" glove or blanket to touch the painful area (Schlag, 1996).

PEDIATRIC STOMACH PAIN

Children with recurrent abdominal pain reported complete elimination of pain and lower levels of relapse after participating in cognitive-behavioral family therapy (Sanders, Shepherd, Cleghorn, & Woolford, 1994). In another study, four out of five children resolved their recurrent abdominal pain without an identifiable physical cause within three weeks after a single session of instruction in self-hypnosis (Anbar, 2001).

SICKLE CELL PAIN

Results from a small University of Florida pilot study that compared massage and relaxation therapy showed both procedures safely and effectively reduced sickle cell pain (Ross, 2000).

SURGICAL PAIN

Using pleasant imagery resulted in significantly less post-surgical pain and significantly less pain medication for elective surgeries (Daake & Gueldner, 1989). A topical capsaicin cream decreased postsurgical neuropathic pain and was preferred by participants over a placebo by a three-to-one margin (Ellison et al., 1997). Acupuncture during epidural anesthesia in appendectomy reduced the amount of intestinal gas excreted, the analgesics and antibiotics administered, and the rate of wound infection post surgery (Sun, Li, & Si, 1992). Firm pressure on 15 classical acupoints (as compared to light pressure in the same areas) decreased postoperative pain (Felhendler & Lisander, 1996). Music can decrease sedative requirements during spinal anesthesia (Lepage, Drolet, Girard, Grenier, & DeGagne, 2001). An experimental study examined the effects of second- and third-day postoperative music interventions (music, music video) on pain and sleep in 96 postoperative participants having coronary artery bypass graft. Those in the music group had significantly lower scores on postoperative day 2 than the rest period control group (Zimmerman, Nieveen, Barnason, & Schmaderer, 1996). A review of the effects of relaxation and music on postoperative pain found them to be helpful (Good, 1996).

TRAUMA PAIN

Acupressure resulted in significantly less pain and anxiety, lower heart rate, and a greater satisfaction in a double-blinded trial that included 60 victims of trauma riding in an ambulance (Kober et al., 2002).

TREATMENT EVALUATION

Using the Numeric Rating Scale, the client described above rated herself an average of 8 prior to therapeutic touch and guided imagery and an average of 10 after treatment. She reported that her pain increased before dinner every evening when she felt the most stressed. Using the nurse's suggestion, the client paid a neighborhood teenager to make dinner two nights a week so she could rest, and negotiated dinner out once a week with her husband.

REFERENCES

American Geriatric Society Panel on Chronic Pain in Older Persons. (1998). The management of chronic pain in older persons: New guides from the American Geriatrics Society. *Clinician Reviews, 8*(9), 69–106.
Aloisi, P., Marrelli, A., Porto, C., Tozzi, E., & Cerone, G. (1997). Visual evoked

potentials and serum magnesium levels in juvenile migraine patients. *Headache, 37,* 383–385.

Anbar, R. D. (2001). Self-hypnosis for the treatment of functional abdominal pain in childhood. *Clinical Pediatrics, 40,* 447–451.

Appleton, J. (2002). Arginine: Clinical potential of a semi-essential amino. *Alternative Medicine Review, 7,* 512–522.

Are headaches a warning sign? (1998). *Clinician Reviews, 8*(10), 38.

Arena, J. G., Bruno, G. M., Hannah, S. L., & Meador, K. J. (1995). A comparison of frontal electromyographic biofeedback training, trapezius electromyographic biofeedback training, and progressive muscle relaxation therapy in the treatment of tension headache. *Headache, 35,* 411–419.

Astin, J. A., Shapiro, S. L., Eisenberg, D. M., & Forys, K. L. (2003). Mind–body medicine: State of the science, implications for practice. *Journal of the American Board of Family Practice, 16,* 131–147.

Aure, O. F., Nilsen, J. H., & Vasseljen, O. (2003). Manual therapy and exercise therapy in patients with chronic low back pain: A randomized, controlled trial with 1-year follow-up. *Spine, 28,* 525–531.

Bearman, D., & Shafarman, S. (1999). The Feldenkrais Method in the treatment of chronic pain: A study of efficacy and cost effectiveness. *American Journal of Pain Management, 9,* 22–27.

Berry, J. A. (2001). Breast pain: All that hurts is not cancer. *American Journal for Nurse Practitioners, April,* 9–10, 15–18.

Blommers, J., de Lange-DeKlerk, E. S., Kuik, D. J., Bezemer, P. D., & Meijer, S. (2002). Evening primrose oil and fish oil for severe chronic astalgia: A randomized, double-blind, controlled trial. *American Journal of Obstetrics and Gynecology, 187,* 1389–1394.

Bonadonna, R. (2003). Medication's impact on chronic illness. *Holistic Nurse Practitioner, 17,* 309–319.

Broome, M. E., Lillis, P. P., McGahee, T. W., & Bates, T. (1992). The use of distraction and imagery with children during painful procedures. *Oncology Nursing Forum, 19,* 499–502.

Burke, B. E., Olson, R. D., & Cusack, B. J. (2002). Randomized, controlled trial of phytoestrogen in the prophylactic treatment of menstrual migraine. *Biomedical Pharmacotherapy, 56,* 283–288.

Daake, D. R., & Gueldner, S. H. (1989). Imagery instruction and the control of postsurgical pain. *Applied Nursing Research, 2,* 114–120.

Dale, A., & Cornwell, S. (1994). The role of lavender oil in relieving perineal discomfort following childbirth: A blind randomized clinical trial. *Journal of Advanced Nursing, 19*(1), 89–96.

Ellison, N., Loprinzi, C. L., Kugler, J., Hatfield, A. K., Miser, A., Sloan, J. A., et al. (1997). Phase III placebo-controlled trial of capsaicin cream in the management of surgical neuropathic pain in cancer patients. *Journal of Clinical Oncology, 15,* 2974–2980.

Felhendler, D., & Lisander, B. (1996). Pressure on acupoints decreases postoperative pain. *Clinical Journal of Pain, 12,* 326–329.

Ferrell, B. A., Josephson, K. R., Pollan, A. M., Loy, S., & Ferrell, B. R. (1997). A randomized trial of walking versus physical methods for chronic pain management. *Aging, 9*(1–2), 99–105.

Field, T. (1998). Massage therapy and burn debridement. *Journal of Burn Care Rehabilitation, 10,* 241–244.

Gallai, L. D., Baker, S. M., & McLellan, R. K. (1986). Magnesium deficiency in the pathogenesis of mitral valve prolapse. *Magnesium, 5,* 165–174.

Gao, S. Y., Zhao, D. L. & Zie, Y. G. (1999). A comparative study on the treatment of migraine headache with combined distant and local acupuncture points versus conventional drug therapy. *American Journal of Acupuncture, 27* (1–2), 27–30.

Gerwick, W. (2000, December). *Potent new compound from blue-green algae may help treat, elucidate nerve disorders.* Presented at the 2000 International Chemical Congress of Pacific Basin Societies, Honolulu, HI.

Good, M. (1996). Effects of relaxation and music on postoperative pain: A review. *Journal of Advanced Nursing, 24,* 905–914.

Good, M., Anderson, G. C., Stanton-Hicks, M., Grass, J. A., & Makii, M. (2002). Relaxation and music reduce pain after gynecologic surgery. *Pain Management in Nursing, 3,* 61–70.

Hadjivassiliou, M., Grunewald, R. A., Lawden, M., Davies-Jones, G. A., Powell, T., & Smith, C. M. (2001). Headache and CNS white matter abnormalities associated with gluten sensitivity. *Neurology, 56,* 385–388.

Hannerz, J. (1997). Symptoms and diseases and smoking habits in female episodic cluster headache in migraine patients. *Cephalgia, 17,* 499–500.

Harel, Z., Gascon, G., Riggs, S., Vaz, R., Brown, W., & Exil, G. (2002). Supplementation with omega-3 polyunsaturated fatty acids in the management of recurrent migraines in adolescents. *Journal of Adolescent Health, 31,* 154–161.

Harkapaa, K. (1991). Relationships of psychological distress and health locus of control beliefs with the use of cognitive and behavioral coping strategies in low back pain patients. *Clinical Journal of Pain, 7,* 175–180.

Hilberg, J. E., Sforzo, G. A., & Swensen, T. (2003). The effects of massage on delayed onset muscle soreness. *British Journal of Sports Medicine, 37,* 72–75.

Ho, C. M., Hseu, S. S., Tsai, S. K., & Lee, T. Y. (1996). Effect of P-6 acupressure on prevention of nausea and vomiting after epidural morphine for post-cesarean section pain relief. *Acta Anaesthesiology Scandinavia, 40,* 372–375.

Holden, E. W., Deichmann, M. M., & Levy, J. D. (1999). Empirically supported treatments in pediatric psychology: Recurrent pediatric headache. *Journal of Pediatric Psychology, 24,* 91–109.

Hooker, G. A. (1996, May/June) Chronic pain can be managed. *Emotional Wellness Matters,* 1–3.

Ilacqua, G. E. (1994). Migraine headaches: Coping efficacy of guided imagery training. *Headache, 34*(3), 99–102.

Janssen, K., & Neutgens, J. (1986). Autogenic training and progressive relaxation in the treatment of three kinds of headache. *Behavioral Research Therapy, 24,* 199–208.

Kesselring, A. (1994). Foot reflex zone massage. *Schweizerische Medizinische Wochenschrift, 62,* 88–93.

Kober, A., Scheck, T., Greher, M., Lieba, F., Fleischhackl, R., Fleischhackl, S., et al. (2002). Prehospital analgesia with acupressure in victims of minor trauma: A prospective, randomized, double-blinded trial. *Anesthesia and Analgesia, 95,* 723–727.

Korting, G. E., Smith, S. D., Wheeler, M. A., Weiss, R. M., & Foster, H. E., Jr. (1999). A randomized double-blind trial of oral L-arginine for treatment of interstititial cystitis. *Journal of Urology, 161,* 558–565.

Kropp, P., Gerber, W. D., Keinath-Specht, A., Kopal, T., & Niederberger, U. (1997). Behavioral treatment in migraine. Cognitive-behavioral therapy and blood-volume-pulse biofeedback: A crossover study with a two-year follow-up. *Functional Neurology, 12*(1),17–24.

Lemstra, M., Stewart, B., & Olszynski, W. P. (2002). Effectiveness of multidisciplinary intervention in the treatment of migraine: A randomized clinical trial. *Headache, 42,* 845–854.

Lepage, C., Drolet, P., Girard, M., Grenier, Y., & DeGagne, R. (2001). Music decreases sedative requirements during spinal anesthesia. *Anesthesia and Analgesia, 93,* 912–916.

Loeb, J. L. (1999). Pain management in long-term care. *American Journal of Nursing, 99*(2), 48–52.

Mannix, L. K., Chandurkar, R. S., Rybicki, L. A., Tusek, D. L., & Solomon, G. D. (1999). Effect of guided imagery on quality of life for patients with chronic tension-type headache. *Headache, 39,* 326–334.

Marz, R. W., & Kemper, F. (2002). Willow bark extract—effects and effectiveness. Status of current knowledge regarding pharmacology, toxicology and clinical aspects. *Wien Medili Wochenschrift, 152,* 354–359.

Matthew, N. T. (1993). Transformed migraine. *Cephalgia, 13*(Suppl. 12), 78–83.

Mauskop, A. (2001). Alternate therapies in headache. Is there a role? *Medical Clinics of North America, 85,* 1077–1084.

Mills, S. Y., Jacoby, R. K., Chacksfield, M., & Willoughby, M. (1996). Effect of a proprietary herbal medicine on the relief of chronic arthritic pain: A double-blind study. *British Journal of Rheumatology, 35,* 874–878.

Montgomery, G. H., David, D., Winkel, G., Silverstein, J. H., & Bovbjerg, D. H. (2002). The effectiveness of adjunctive hypnosis with surgical patients: A meta-analysis. *Anesthesia and Analgesia, 94,* 1639–1645.

Murphy, J. J., Heptinstall, S., & Mitchell, J. R. (1988). Randomized double-blind placebo-controlled trial of feverfew in migraine prevention. *Lancet, 2,* 189–192.

Murray, M. T. (1994). Do headache medicines cause chronic headaches? *American Journal of Natural Medicine, 1*(2), 5–7.

National Institutes of Health, Technology Assessment Panel. (1996). Integration of behavioral and relaxation approaches into the treatment of chronic pain and insomnia. *Journal of the American Medical Association, 276,* 313–318.

Nilsson, N., Christensen, H. W., & Hartvigsen, J. (1997). The effect of spinal manipulation in the treatment of cervicogenic headache. *Journal of Manipulative Physiological Therapy, 20,* 326–330.

Olson, K., & Hanson, J. (1997). Using Reiki to manage pain: A preliminary report. *Cancer Prevention and Control, 1,* 108–113.

Paiva, T., Farinha, A., Martins, A., Batista, A., & Guilleminault, C. (1997). Chronic headaches and sleep disorders. *Archives of Internal Medicine, 157,* 1701–1705.

Palsson, O. S., Turner, M. J., Johnson, D. A., Burnelt, C. K., & Whitehead, W. E. (2002). Hypnosis treatment for severe irritable bowel syndrome: Investigation of mechanism and effects on symptoms. *Digestive Diseases and Science, 47,* 2605–2614.

Parcell, S. (2002). Sulfur in human nutrition and applications in medicine. *Alternative Medicine Review, 7*(11), 22–44.

Peikert, A., Wilimzig, C., & Kohne-Volland, R. (1996). Prophylaxis of migraine with oral magnesium: Results from a prospective, multi-center, placebo-controlled and double-blind randomized study. *Cephalalgia, 16,* 257–263.

Perin, M. L. (2000). Problems with propoxyphene. *American Journal of Nursing, 100*(6), 22.

Pettit, J. L. (2001). Feverfew. *Clinician Reviews, 11,* 113–114.

Pittler, M. H., & Ernst, E. (2000). Gingko biloba extract for the treatment of intermittent claudication: A meta-analysis of randomized trials. *American Journal of Medicine, 108,* 276–281.

Pouresmail, Z., & Ibrahimzadeh, R. (2002). Effects of acupressure and ibuprofen on the severity of primary dysmenorrhea. *Journal of Traditional Chinese Medicine, 22,* 205–210.

Quinn, C., Chandler, C., & Moraska, A. (2002). Massage therapy and frequency of chronic tension headaches. *American Journal of Public Health, 92,* 1657–1661.

Ramadan, N. M., Halvorson, H., Vande-Linde, A., Levine, S. R., Helpern, J. A., & Welsh, K. M. (1989). Magnesium deficiency in migraine patients. *Headache, 34,* 160–165.

Rappoport, A. M. (1985). Analgesic-rebound headache: Theoretical and practical implications. *Cephalgia, 5*(Suppl. 3), 448–449.

Ross, M. F. (2000). UF pilot study shows massage, relaxation reduce sickle cell anemia pain. Media release, University of Florida Health Science Center. Gainesville, FL. Accessed September 25, 2000, at www.health.ufl.edu/hscc

Rowan, A., Buttle, D., & Barrett, A. (1990). The cysteine proteinases of the pineapple plant. *Biochemistry Journal, 266,* 869–875.

Sanders, M. R., Shepherd, R. W., Cleghorn, G., & Woolford, H. (1994). The treatment of recurrent abdominal pain in children: A controlled comparison of cognitive-behavioral family intervention and standard pediatric care. *Journal of Clinical Psychology, 62,* 306–314.

Sandor, P. S., Afra, J., Ambrosini, A., & Schoenen, J. (2000). Prophylactic treatment of migraine with beta-blockers and riboflavin: Differential effects on the intensity dependence of auditory evoked cortical potentials. *Headache, 40*(1), 30–35.

Sarioglu, B., Erhan, E., Serdaroglu, G., Doering, B. G., Eremis, S., & Tutuncuoglu, S. (2003). Tension-type headache in children: A clinical evaluation. *Pediatrics International, 45,* 186–189.

Savi, L., Rainero, I., Valfre, W., Gentile, S., Lo Giudice, R., & Pinessi, L. (2002). Food and headache attacks: A comparison of patients with migraine and tension-type headache. *Panminerva Medicine, 44*(1), 27–31.

Schlag, K. A. (1996, April). Pint-sized pain. *Advance for Nurse Practitioners,* pp. 22–29.

Schoenen, J., Jacquy, J., & Lenaerts, M. (1998). Effectiveness of high-dose riboflavin in migraine prophylaxis: A randomized controlled trial. *Neurology, 50,* 466–470.

Schorr, J. A. (1993). Music and pattern change in chronic pain. *Advances in Nursing Science, 15*(4), 27–36.

Selman, J. E. (2000). Contemporary diagnosis and management of headache. *Clinical Advisor, June,* 37–46.

Smith, D. W., Arnstein, P., Rosa, K. C., & Wells-Federman, C. (2002). Effects of integrating therapeutic touch into a cognitive behavioral pain treatment program: Report of a pilot clinical trial. *Journal of Holistic Nursing, 20,* 267–287.

Strong, J., Ashton, R., & Chant, D. (1991). Pain intensity measurement in chronic low back pain. *Clinical Journal of Pain, 7,* 209–218.

Stuifbergen, A. K., Becker, H., Timmerman, G., & Kullberg, V. (2003). A randomized clinical trial of a wellness intervention for women with multiple sclerosis. *Archives of Physical Medicine and Rehabilitation, 84,* 467–476.

Sun, P., Li, L., & Si, M. (1992). Comparison between acupuncture and epidural anesthesia in appendectomy. *Chen Tzu Yen Chiu, 17*(2), 87–89.

Tapiero, H., Ba, G. N., Couvreur, P., & Tew, K. D. (2002). Polyunsaturated fatty acids (PUFA) and eicosanoids in human health and pathologies. *Biomedical Pharmacotherapy, 56,* 215–222.

Thomas, L. A. (2003). Clinical management of stressors perceived by patients on mechanical ventilation. *AACN Clinical Issues, 14,* 73–81.

Van Damme, S., Cromley, G., & Eccleston, C. (2004). Disengagement from pain: The role of catastrophic thinking about pain. *Pain, 107*(1–2), 70–76.

Vasterling, J., Jenkins, R. A., Tope, D. M., & Burish, T. G. (1993). Cognitive distraction and relaxation training for the control of side effects due to cancer chemotherapy. *Journal of Behavioral Medicine 16,* 65–79.

Wilkinson, D. W., Knox, P. L., Chatman, J. E., Johnson, T. L., Barbour, N., Myles, Y., et al. (2002). The clinical effectiveness of healing touch. *Journal of Alternative and Complementary Medicine, 8,* 33–47.

Williams, D. G. (1992a). Ileocecal valve. *Alternatives, 1*(14), 1.

Williams, D. G. (1992b). How to work with the ileocecal valve. *Alternatives, 1*(3), 1–4.

Williams, D. G. (1995). Three common methods of using castor oil. *Alternatives, 5,* 161–165.

Wipf, J. E., & Deyo, R. A. (1995). Low back pain. *Medical Clinics of North America, 79,* 231–246.

Zeltzer, L. K., Tsao, J. C., Stelling, C., Powers, M., Levy, S., & Waterhous, M. (2002). A phase I study on the feasibility and acceptability of an acupuncture/hypnosis intervention for chronic pediatric pain. *Journal of Pain Symptom Management, 24,* 437–446.

Zimmerman, L., Nieveen, J., Barnason, S., & Schmaderer, M. (1996). The effects of music interventions on postoperative pain and sleep in coronary artery bypass graft (CABG) patients. *Scholarly Inquiry in Nursing Practice, 10,* 153–157.

CHAPTER 20

Parkinson's Disease

Tremor is the classic symptom of Parkinson's disease (PD). Stress and fatigue can intensify tremors, but they disappear during concentrated effort or sleep. Cramps in the legs, neck, or trunk are also common. Shuffling, stooped posture, and imbalance occur in later phases of the condition as do loss of control over some functions (facial expression, blinking, swallowing), sleeping problems, and difficulty adjusting posture when seated. Levodopa (L-dopa) is the standard treatment. Its effect decreases over time and it has many adverse effects, from vomiting to heart irregularities and confusion to uncontrollable grimacing and foot tapping. Sinemet (carbidopa) is usually given to counteract the annoying effects of L-dopa. Unfortunately, it has its own set of adverse reactions from hallucinations to dizziness, headache, back pain, eyelid spasms, kidney and liver disorders, seizures, drooling, and more. Some forms of exercise can help for a few years and surgery can relieve some symptoms, but is only used for young, otherwise healthy individuals. Even when successful, vision loss due to damage to the optic nerve is always a danger.

HOLISTIC NURSING ASSESSMENT

Study the holistic nursing assessment for one client, Mr. F., a 52-year-old man diagnosed with Parkinson's disease. Working in collaboration with clients diagnosed with Parkinson's disease, use the format presented to conduct a holistic nursing assessment.

Client learning needs: "I have to be able to stop this trembling."

Indicants of readiness to learn: "I'm going to my son's graduation and I have to stop shaking so much."

Soul/spirituality symbol(s): "I haven't been to church in years, but I was raised Catholic."

Meaning of the condition to client: "I had a pesticide business for many years. The doctor says that's probably why I shake."

Relationship needs/effects as perceived by the client: "My son and I never got along very well. Now he's graduating and moving away."

Patterns/attitudes that may create dis-ease for this client: Client uses negative affirmations (e.g., "I shake all the time" and "You can't trust anyone").

Life purpose: Expresses no life purpose except to stop trembling.

Client strengths: Has articulated two goals.

Ability to participate in care: Client verbalizes the wish to change.

Ethical dilemmas: None identified.

Nurse–client process: Client directs the nurse's every action.

TREATMENT PLANNING: SETTING JOINTLY AGREED-UPON GOALS

In the case of the client discussed above, the following goals were agreed upon:

1. Eat foods and take supplements that protect the nervous system.
2. Start an exercise program.
3. Start singing in the community choir.

TREATMENT

Acceptance of condition/attitude change: The client chose the following affirmations to use to counter negative thoughts and feelings: "I relax." "I am safe." "I trust my life processes." Client agreed to write the affirmations on 3 x 5 cards and say the words at least 20 times each day.

Facilitating the healing process/healing intention formulation: From a list of meditative statements, client chose the following one to assist in the healing process: "I trust the processes of life." Asked client to meditate on the words while in a relaxed state. Nurse will use caring nonverbal and verbal communication, centering, and a meditative state to enhance client healing, will verbalize observed patterns that may be holding the client back and offer alternate approaches.

Creating a sacred space: During client sessions, soft lighting, client-chosen music, and aromatherapy will be used to facilitate healing.

Encouraging re-storying: Encouraged client to recall an upsetting situation with his son and choose an ending that satisfied him.

Integrative practices planned: Nurse will use therapeutic touch and guided imagery to assist client in the healing process.

Role model strategies: Showed client how to role play problematic interchanges with his son.

Protection plan: Client plans to picture the light of God surrounding him.

Family strategies: Encouraged client to invite his son to a session with nurse to practice more open communication between them.

Life issues/life purpose work: Client has agreed to write in his journal about his life purpose.

Treatment possibilities/considerations: Other suggested treatments appear below. Most are evidence-based.

ADDITIONAL INFORMATION AND TREATMENTS TO SHARE WITH CLIENTS

1. *Avoid drugs and other chemicals that evoke the condition.* The following situations are correlated with an increased risk for PD: exposure to neurotoxic drugs (Compazine, Trilafon, Mellaril, Prolixin, Stelazine, Thorazine, Trilafon, Haldol, Reglan, Clozaril, Risperdal, Zyprexa and other tranquilizers, tetrabenazine, cinnarizine, flunarizine, amiodarone, bethanechol, pyridostigmine, lithium, Valium, Prozac, Nardil, Demerol, amphotericin B, caphaloridine, 5-fluorouracil, vincristine-doxorubicin, and the synthetic heroin compound MPTP), poisoning by chemicals (manganese dust, carbon disulfide, copper or carbon monoxide) and/or pesticides (Broussole & Thobosi, 2002; Reis, 1995; Tuchsen & Jensen, 2000; Vanacore et al., 2002).

2. *Switch to a vegetarian eating plan.* Diets high in animal fat or cholesterol are associated with substantial increase in risk for PD. In contrast, fat of plant origin (olive oil, sesame oil) does not appear to increase risk. There is a possibility that vegetarian diets are beneficial in PD because they slow the loss of surviving dopaminergic neurons, retarding the progress of the syndrome (McCarty, 2001). Fruits and vegetables will also help clear toxins and rebuild tissue.

3. *Avoid wheat.* Gluten sensitivity is an important consideration in gait and balance dysfunction in Parkinsonism (Manek & Lew, 2003). Wheat is found in breads, cereals, pastas, pie crust, cakes, cookies, some soy sauces, candies, and other processed foods. Avoid them completely. Alternative flours include soy, spelt, corn, and rice, but check labels carefully as wheat is often included.

4. *Eat at least one sour apple a day.* Apples and other fruits contain malic acid, which is neuroprotective (Mazzio & Soliman, 2003).

5. *Avoid using herbicides and pesticides.* Use natural substances such as garlic, soap and water, and oil to spray outdoor plants and protect them from insects. Learn to live with the balance of nature, and accept that insects provide a valuable service. Eliminate lawn and xeriscape yard with native plants and flowers that are insect resistant.

6. *Cleanse the liver.* Take silymarin (milk thistle) to cleanse the liver and take large doses of vitamin C if exposed to toxins.

7. *Learn relaxation procedures.* Tremors can be reduced significantly after biofeedback training (Chung, Poppen, & Lundervold, 1995).

8. *Find an Alexander Technique therapist.* Clients with Parkinson's disease who used the Alexander Technique showed reduced depression and improved capacity to manage their disability (Stallibrass, 1997).

9. *Work with an Ayurvedic practitioner.* An Ayurvedic approach showed statistically significant reductions in symptoms of sixty persons with Parkinson's disease (Parkinson's Disease Study Group, 1995).

10. *Start an exercise program.* A 10-week exercise program improved spinal flexibility and function in people with Parkinson's disease who were in the early and mid-stages of PD. Swimming, stationary bike, or walking (if balance is good), might be appropriate choices, but consult with a personal trainer or find a special exercise program for people with PD (Schenkman et al., 1998).

11. *Consider osteopathic manipulation.* Standard osteopathic manipulative treatment improved the gait in patients diagnosed with PD (Wells et al., 1999).

12. *Eat more foods high in zinc and consider taking a supplement.* Individuals with PD show a significantly decreased zinc status (Kunikowska & Jenner, 2003). Foods high in zinc include eggs, nuts, herring, and oysters. Zinc supplementation has been shown to significantly increase superoxide dismutase, which aids in the protection of neurons from free radicals (Forsleff, Schauss, Bier, & Stuart, 1999), so also consider investing in a good multimineral that includes no more than 15 mg/day of zinc.

13. *Investigate music.* Choral singing, voice exercise, rhythmic and free body movements can have a significant overall effect, increasing happiness and the ability to control walking patterns (Pacchetti et al., 2000).

14. *Try Chinese herbs.* One study showed that Chinese traditional medicine, Banxia Heup Tang (BHT) significantly improved the swallowing reflex in PD (Iwasaki et al., 2000).

15. *Take butcher's broom for low blood pressure.* Butcher's broom (*Ruscus aculeatus*), an herb, may be of benefit in treating chronic low blood pressure (orthostatic hypotension), which can accompany this condition (Redman, 2000).

16. *Acupuncture may help.* Acupuncture reduces PD symptoms, delays the disease's progression, and decreases the dosage needed for anti-parkinsonian drugs (Zhuang & Wang, 2000).

17. *Take coenzyme Q-10 and sesame oil.* There is considerable evidence that mitochondrial dysfunction and oxidative damage play a role in the development of PD (Beal, 2003). Several agents are available that can modulate cellular energy metabolism and exert antioxidative effects. Coenzyme Q-10 and N-acetylcysteine are two substances that provide protection against toxicity (Mazzio, Huber, Darling, Harris, & Soliman, 2001). In one study, the enzyme was tolerated well and had no side effects in dosages up to 1200 mg/d. Less disability developed in participants assigned to coenzyme Q-10 than in those assigned to placebo, and the benefit was greatest in subjects receiving the highest dosage (Shults et al., 2002). Coenzyme Q-10 is found in mackerel, salmon, sardines, peanuts and spinach. Purchase the enzyme as a capsule in the health food store. Look for a liquid or oil form that contains a small amount of vitamin E to preserve the coenzyme. N-acetylcysteine helps detoxify harmful toxins and protect the body, but can inactivate insulin.

18. *Drink green tea.* Green tea has neuroprotective properties and has been shown to guard against neurotoxins (Levites, Amit, Mandel, & Youdim, 2003).

19. *Take vitamins C and E.* These vitamins are antioxidants that offer protection against the free radicals produced by L-dopa. Taking these vitamins before symptoms appear may protect against developing the condition (de Rijk et al. 1997). Take 1,000 to 3,000 mg a day of vitamin C and 800 IU a day of vitamin E.

20. *Eat foods high in lycopene.* Recent interest has focused on antioxidants such as lycopene (Rao & Balachandran, 2002). At least one study found an association between lycopene, found in tomatoes and tomato products, and protecting against PD risks (Scheider et al., 1997).

21. *Maintain bone strength.* Individuals with PD tend to have lower bone mineral density, more severe osteoporosis, and more falls and fractures. Take at least 1200 mg a day of calcium citrate (the most absorbable form) and eat calcium-rich foods that are easy to absorb including broccoli, kale, green leafy vegetables, tomatoes, whole wheat bread, yogurt, canned sardines, molasses, almonds, soy milk, buttermilk, and tofu.

22. *Eat foods rich in B vitamins.* B vitamins can elevate mood, reduce tingling or burning sensations in the feet or legs, and take away fatigue (Wade, Young, Chaudhuri, & Davidson, 2002). Both folate and vitamin B12 can help remyelinate in neurologica disorders such as PD; a deficiency can cause depression, dementia, myelopathy, and peripheral neuropathy (Bottiglieri, Hyland, & Reynolds, 1994). Eat more sunflower seeds, rolled oats, lima beans, soybeans, raisins, wheat germ, peas, whole-wheat-flour foods, asparagus, brown rice, chicken, peanuts, spinach (raw), kale, eggs, tuna, turkey, salmon, mackerel, sweet potatoes, cooked cabbage, bananas, sardines, trout, sea vegetables (dulse, kombu, kelp, wakame), fermented soy foods (tempeh, natto, miso), fresh green uncooked vegetables, lobster, broccoli, cauliflower, sesame seeds, mushrooms, yogurt (plain, low-fat), oranges, grapefruits, peaches, lettuce, and molasses.

23. *Take SAMe.* S-adenosylmethionine (SAMe) is required in numerous transmethylation reactions involving nucleic acids, proteins, phospholipids, amines, and other neurotransmitters. It is also linked with folate and vitamin B12. When these B vitamins are deficient, neurologic and psychological disturbances, including depression, dementia, myelopathy, and peripheral neuropathy, develop (Bottiglieri et al., 1994). SAMe can be found in the supplement section of health food stores and may be available at some pharmacies.

24. *Eat foods rich in copper.* In PD, copper is significantly decreased (Kunikowska & Jenner, 2003). Foods to concentrate on are almonds, avocados, barley, beans, dandelion greens, and lentils.

25. *Reduce or eliminate dairy foods.* In two large prospective cohort studies, a positive association was found between dairy intake and PD risk, especially in men (Chen, Zhang, Hernan, Willett, & Acherio, 2002).

26. *Take a selenium supplement.* Most of the soil in America is depleted of selenium, yet the trace element is important to elevating mood. Oxidative injury plays a role in neurodegenerative conditions such as Parkinson's, and selenium is an antioxidant that could help (Benton, 2002).

27. *Try massage therapy* (Manyam & Sanchez-Ramos, 1999).

TREATMENT EVALUATION

Client reported he had decreased the amount of meat eaten to 4 meals a week, started t'ai chi class, and signed up for choir practice.

REFERENCES

Beal, M. F. (2003). Bioenergetic approaches for neuroprotection in Parkinson's disease. *Annals of Neurology, 53*(Suppl. 3), S47–S48.

Benton, D. (2002). Selenium intake, mood and other aspects of psychological functioning. *Nutrition and Neuroscience, 5,* 363–374.

Bottiglieri, T., Hyland, K., & Reynolds, E. H. (1994). The clinical potential of ademetionine (S-adenosylmethionine) in neurological disorders. *Drugs, 48,* 137–152.

Broussole, E., & Thobois, S. (2002). Genetic and environmental factors of Parkinson's disease. *Review of Neurology, 158*(Spec. no. 1), S11–S23.

Chen, H., Zhang, S. M., Hernan, M. A., Willett, W. C., & Ascherio, A. (2002). Diet and Parkinson's disease: A potential role of dairy products in men. *Annals of Neurology, 52,* 793–801.

Chung, W., Poppen, R., & Lundervold, D. A. (1995). Behavioral relaxation training for tremor disorders in older adults. *Biofeedback and Self-Regulation, 20,* 123–135.

de Rijk, M. C., Breteler, M. M., den Breeijen, J. H., Launer, L. J., Grobbee, D. E., van der Meche, F. G., & Hofman, A. (1997). Dietary antioxidants and Parkinson's disease: The Rotterdam Study. *Archives of Neurology, 54,* 762–765.

Esposito, E., Rotilio, D., Di Matteo, V., Di Giulio, C., Cacchio, M., & Algeri, S. (2002). A review of specific dietary antioxidants and the effects on biochemical mechanisms related to neurodegenerative processes. *Neurobiology and Aging, 23,* 719–735.

Forsleff, L., Schauss, A. G., Bier, I. D., & Stuart, S. (1999). Evidence of functional zinc deficiency in Parkinson's disease. *Journal of Alternative and Complementary Medicine, 5,* 57–64.

Iwasaki, K., Wang, Q., Seki, H., Satch, K., Takeda, A., Arai, H., & Sasaki, H. (2000). The effects of the traditional Chinese medicine, "Banxia Houpo Tang (Hange-Kobku T)" on the swallowing reflex in Parkinson's disease. *Phytomedicine, 7,* 259–263.

Kunikowska, G., & Jenner, P. (2003). Alterations in m-RNA expression for Cu,Zn-superoxide dismutase and glutathione peroxidase in the basal ganglia of MPTP-treated marmosets and patients with Parkinson's disease. *Brain Research, 968,* 206–218.

Levites, Y., Amit, T., Mandel, S., & Youdim, M. B. (2003). Neuroprotection and neurorescue against Abetatoxicity and PKC-dependent release of non-amyloidogenic soluble precursor protein by green tea polyphenol-epigallocatechin-3-gallate. *Federation of American Societies for Experimental Biology, 17,* 952–954.

Manek, S., & Lew, M. F. (2003). Gait and balance dysfunction in adults. *Current Treatment Options, 5,* 177–185.

Manyam, B. V., & Sanchez-Ramos, J. R. (1999). Traditional and complementary therapies in Parkinson's disease. *Advances in Neurology, 80,* 565–574.

Mazzio, E., Huber, J., Darling, S., Harris, N., & Soliman, K. F. (2001). Effect of antioxidants on L-glutamate and N-methyl-4-phenylpyridinium ion induced-neurotoxicity in PC12 cells. *Neurotoxicology, 22,* 283–286.

Mazzio, E., & Soliman, K. F. (2003). The role of glycolysis and gluconeogenesis in the cytoprotection of neuroblastoma cells against 1-methyl 4-phenylpyridinium ion toxicity. *Neurotoxicology, 24*(1), 137–147.

McCarty, M. F. (2001). Does a vegan diet reduce risk for Parkinson's disease? *Medical Hypotheses, 57,* 318–323.

Pacchetti, C., Mancini, F., Aglieri, R., Fundaro, C., Martignoni, E., & Nappi, G. (2000). Active music therapy in Parkinson's disease: An integrative method for motor and emotional rehabilitation. *Psychosomatic Medicine, 62,* 386–393.

Parkinson's Disease Study Group. (1995). An alternative medicine treatment for Parkinson's disease: Results of a multi-center clinical trial. *Journal of Alternative and Complementary Medicine, 1,* 249–255.

Rao, A. V., & Balachandran, B. (2002). Role of oxidative stress and antioxidants in neurogenerative diseases. *Nutrition and Neuroscience, 5,* 291–309.

Redman, D. A. (2000). Ruscus aculeatus (butcher's broom) as a potential treatment for orthostatic hypotension, with a case report. *Journal of Alternative and Complementary Medicine, 6,* 539–549.

Reis, J. G. (1995). A Parkinson's primer. *Nursing Spectrum,* June 26, pp. 12–14.

Scheider, W. L., Hershey, L.A., Vena, J. E., Holmlund, T., Marshall, J. R., & Freudenheim, J. L. (1997). Dietary antioxidants and other dietary factors in the etiology of Parkinson's disease. *Movement Disorders, 12,* 190–196.

Schenkman, M., Cutson, T. M., Kuchibhatia, M., Chandler, J., Pieper, C. F., & Laub, K. C. (1998). Exercise to improve spinal flexibility and function for people with Parkinson's disease: A randomized, controlled trial. *Journal of the American Geriatric Society, 46*(1d), 1207–1216.

Shults, C. W., Oakes, D., Kieburtz, K., Beal, M. F., Haas, R., Plumb, S., et al. (2002). Effects of coenzyme Q10 in early Parkinson disease: Evidence of slowing of the functional decline. *Archives of Neurology, 59,* 1541–1550.

Stallibrass, C. (1997). An evaluation of the Alexander Technique for the management of disability in Parkinson's disease—a preliminary study. *Clinical Rehabilitation, 11,* 8–12.

Tuchsen, F., & Jensen, A. A. (2000). Agricultural work and the risk of Parkinson's disease in Denmark 1981–1993. *Scandinavian Journal of Work and Environmental Health, 26,* 359–362.

Vanacore, N., Nappo, A., Gentile, M., Brustolin, A., Palange, S., Liberati A., et al. (2002). Evaluation of risk of Parkinson's disease in a cohort of licensed pesticide users. *Neurology and Science, 23*(Suppl. 2), S1119–S1120.

Wade, D. T., Young, C. A., Chaudhuri, K. R., & Davidson, D. L. (2002). A randomized placebo controlled exploratory study of vitamin B-12, lofepramine, and L-phenylalanine (the "Cari Loder regime") in the treatment of multiple sclerosis. *Journal of Neurology and Neurosurgical Psychiatry, 73,* 246–249.

Wells, M. R., Giantinoto, S., D'Agate, D., Areman, R. D., Fazzini, E. A., & Dowling Bosak, A. (1999). Standard osteopathic manipulative treatment acutely improves gait performance in patients with Parkinson's disease. *Journal of the American Osteopathic Association, 99,* 92–98.

Zhuang, X., & Wang, L. (2000). Acupuncture treatment of Parkinson's disease—a report of 29 cases. *Journal of Traditional Chinese Medicine, 20,* 265–267.

CHAPTER 21

Sleep Disorders

Approximately 35% of the American population has insomnia, often due to prescription medications. Lack of restful sleep can affect the ability to heal from other conditions so it's an important condition to bring under control. Medical treatment includes short-term use of sleeping pills, but there are no safe and effective medications for the routine treatment of sleep apnea (long, frequent pauses in breathing during sleep). A common treatment for this type of apnea is continuous positive airway pressure or CPAP. A small blower is attached with a flexible tube onto a snug-fitting mask and placed over the nose. Air pressure delivered through the device keeps the airway open during the night. This treatment is difficult to tolerate, but can rapidly reverse daytime sleepiness caused by apnea. Oral or dental appliances may help with mild to moderate sleep apnea. Surgery may help, but none of the procedures are 100 percent effective.

HOLISTIC NURSING ASSESSMENT

Study the holistic nursing assessment for Ms. U., a 34-year-old client diagnosed with a sleep disorder. Working in collaboration with clients diagnosed with sleep disorders, use the format presented to conduct a holistic nursing assessment.

Client learning needs: "I can't sleep."

Indicants of readiness to learn: "Feels like I haven't slept for weeks. This has got to stop."

Soul/spirituality symbol(s): "I gave up church when my grandfather started sexually abusing me."

Meaning of the condition to client: "I don't trust anybody."

Relationship needs/effects as perceived by the client: "I have to confront my grandfather."

Patterns/attitudes that may create dis-ease for this client: Client uses negative affirmations (e.g., "I keep getting hooked up with men who abuse me").

Life purpose: Expresses no life purpose except to sleep.

Client strengths: Has articulated two goals.

Ability to participate in care: Client verbalizes the wish to change.

Ethical dilemmas: None identified. Client vacillates between wanting to confront her grandfather and the pain such an action may cause her family.

Nurse–client process: Client cancels sessions, comes late, and refuses to discuss the meaning of her behavior.

TREATMENT PLANNING: SETTING JOINTLY AGREED-UPON GOALS

In the case of the client discussed above, the following goals were agreed upon:

1. Decide whether to confront her grandfather or not.
2. Stop smoking.
3. Try different sleep disorder treatments until one works.

TREATMENT

Acceptance of condition/attitude change: The client chose the following affirmation to use to replace the negative affirmations she repeats to herself: "I release the day and slip into peaceful sleep." Client agreed to write the affirmation on 3 x 5 cards and say the words at least 20 times each day.

Facilitating the healing process/healing intention formulation: From a list of meditative statements, client chose the following one to assist in the healing process: "I am safe knowing tomorrow will take care of itself." Nurse asked client to meditate on the words while in a relaxed state. Nurse will use caring nonverbal and verbal communication, centering, and a meditative state to enhance client healing, will verbalize observed patterns that may be holding the client back and offer alternate approaches.

Creating a sacred space: During client sessions, soft lighting and comfortable room temperature will be used to facilitate healing.

Encouraging re-storying: Nurse encouraged client to recall an upsetting situation with her grandfather and choose an ending that satisfied her.

Integrative practices planned: Nurse will teach self-hypnosis and guided imagery to assist client in the healing process.

Role model strategies: Nurse showed client how to role play problematic interchanges with her grandfather and boyfriend.

Protection plan: Client plans to picture a white light surrounding her.

Family strategies: Nurse encouraged client to invite her boyfriend to a session with nurse to practice more open communication between them.

Life issues/life purpose work: Client has agreed to write in her journal about the abuse in her life.

Treatment possibilities/considerations: Other suggested treatments appear below. Most are evidence-based.

ADDITIONAL INFORMATION AND TREATMENTS TO SHARE WITH CLIENTS

Natural remedies usually take longer than pharmaceuticals, but they have fewer side effects, and once a healthy sleep pattern is established, medications can slowly be phased out. Prior to choosing treatments, collect the following information: consult with bed partner or if living alone, tape record a night's sleep. This will provide a baseline and permanent record of nighttime difficulties and a basis for problem solving and choosing from the available treatments below. Also keep a sleep diary for 1–2 weeks. Record bedtime, total sleep time, time to sleep onset, number of awakenings, use of sleep medications, time out of bed in the morning, and a rating of subjective quality of sleep and daytime symptoms. This diary can serve as a baseline for assessing what works to help you sleep and what doesn't. Some questions to be answered include

- When did the sleep problem begin?
- Do I have any psychiatric, medical, or female-related condition that may cause insomnia?
- Am I trying to sleep in a quiet room with the correct temperature and lighting?
- Do I have creeping, crawling, or uncomfortable feelings in my legs that are relieved by moving them?
- Does my bed partner report that I jerk my arms or legs in sleep?
- Am I a shift worker or do I fly a lot?
- What time do I go to bed and get up on the weekdays? Weekends?
- Do I use caffeine, tobacco, alcohol, over-the-counter, or prescription drugs?
- What daytime consequences does using these substances have?
- Do I doze off or stay awake during routine tasks, especially while driving?

Once a baseline is gathered, choose from the following treatments:

1. *Lose weight if overweight.* This can cure sleeping disorders (Tiihonen, Partinen, & Narvanen, 1993). (See Overweight/Obesity chapter for ideas.)

2. *Avoid drinking alcohol in the evening* (Brown, 1999).

3. *Avoid caffeine in the evening* (Brown, 1999). Don't drink coffee, tea, colas, or hot chocolate, or eat chocolate. Some drugs to avoid are Anacin, Aqua-Ban Plus, Caffedrine, NoDoz, Quick Pep, Tirend, Midol, Vanquish, Vivarin, Extra Strength Excedrin, and Bayer Select Maximum. Herbal products that contain ephedra, caffeine, or guarana also can keep you awake.

4. *Exercise every day, but not at night.* Walking is a good choice. Do some gentle stretches, but nothing too strenuous before bedtime because it is stimulating (Montgomery & Dennis, 2002; Nadolski, 2003).

5. *Try hypnosis.* It may help with sleep (Stradling, Robers, Wilson, & Lovelock, 1998).

6. *Take a B-complex capsule every day.* The B vitamins are known to calm and reduce nightmares and restless sleep, especially vitamin B12 ("Methylcobalamin," 1998). Pantothenic acid is particularly good for drying the sinuses and easing breathing.

7. *Maintain a consistent bedtime routine.* Changes in usual patterns can disturb sleep (Bernardo, 1999; Nadolski, 2003).

8. *Eat a light meal no less than 3 hours before retiring* (Nadolski, 2003). If the body is still digesting food, it will be difficult to sleep well. This effort will also assist with weight loss.

9. *Keep bedroom quiet and dark.* Avoid any situation that distracts from sleeping (Nadolski, 2003).

10. *Participate in a relaxing activity prior to sleeping.* Read a boring book, take a short walk, or enjoy a warm bath to relax. If these activities are insufficient, purchase a relaxation tape and listen to it while in bed.

11. *To reduce worrying at night, write down concerns about upcoming or past events.* If necessary, write down a plan for dealing with the concern the next day (Azar, 1996; Brown, 1999).

12. *Have a small evening snack of foods containing tryptophan.* This substance is known to bring on drowsiness and induce sleep. It is found in milk, turkey, and potatoes.

13. *Look into taking melatonin.* This supplement lessens jet lag and can induce sleep in some people although there have been no long-term trials (Chase & Gidal, 1997; Hughes, Sack, & Lewy, 1998). It works best for older adults. A better method is to increase the production of melatonin by shining a light on the back of the knee. Researchers at Cornell University (1998) showed that body temperature and melatonin levels were altered when light was shined on the back of the knee. This may reset the body's circadian clock and should work to reduce jet lag, the effects of shift work, and changes in usual sleep behavior (Williams, 1998).

14. *Take valerian.* This herb has been validated in Europe for its effectiveness in relieving insomnia. Germany's Commission E has approved it for sleep disorders and as a minor tranquilizer. No side effects have been reported. Valerian was just as good as an anti-anxiety insomnia (benzodiazepine) preparation but has no withdrawal symptoms (Schmitz & Jackal, 1998). Whereas medications for insomnia have a "morning hangover" effect, valerian doesn't (Gerhard, Linnenbrink, Georghiadou, & Hobi, 1996). Follow directions on the bottle.

15. *Try kava root.* Since 1869, European herbal medicine has recommended kava root in many forms as a treatment for anxiety. Several studies comparing kava to tranquilizers have shown that it's very effective for insomnia when 150–210 milligrams are taken as a single dose 1 hour before going to bed (Gyllenhaal, Merritt, Peterson, Block, & Gochenour, 2000). *Caution:* do not take kava with alcohol or prescription anti-anxiety medicines, such as Valium.

16. *Use better sleep posture.* Elevate the head with a pillow while sleeping on the back or use a cervical support pillow.

17. *Get out of bed if not asleep after 20 minutes.* Avoid eating, studying, watching TV, or reading in bed. Any of these behaviors can create negative cues and provide conditioning for insomnia (Bernardo, 1999).

18. *Avoid nicotine* (Nadolski, 2003). Take a smoking cessation course or hire a hypnotist to quit smoking. Until smoke free, at least avoid nicotine near bedtime and upon night awakenings. It is a stimulant.

19. *Take folate for restless leg syndrome.* Women who had unpleasant sensations in their legs and difficulty falling asleep had lower blood levels of folate (Lee, 2001). Foods to eat to increase intake of folic acid include asparagus, fresh liver, fresh dark green uncooked vegetables, turnips, potatoes, orange juice, black-eyed peas, lima beans, watermelon, oysters, and cantaloupe.

20. *Take additional magnesium or eat magnesium-rich foods,* including whole grain breads and cereals, fresh peas, brown rice, soy flour, wheat germ, nuts, Swiss chard, figs, green leafy vegetables, and citrus fruits. Magnesium depletion has been associated with dysregulating biorhythms including delayed and advanced sleep phase syndrome, night work disorders, and age-related insomnia (Durlach et al., 2002).

21. *Investigate acupressure.* Acupressure was found to produce a significant effect in reducing nighttime awakening and improving the quality of sleep (Chen, Lin, Wu, & Lin, 1999). Try the following, holding each spot with the index, third, and fourth fingers of the hand until a smooth, quiet pulsation is felt in all three fingers (Dayton, 1994):

A. One thumb. Repeat with other thumb.
B. The fatty area above the thumb on the palm. Repeat with other thumb.
C. Outside of heel on both feet.
D. Right above the wrist right below the little finger on both hands.
E. Inside of elbow on both arms.
F. Middle top of hip bone on both sides.
G. Middle bottom of buttocks on both sides.
H. At the back of the head along the occipital ridge on both sides.
I. Along bottom of rib cage on both sides.

22. *Avoid salt.* Using salt for dinner can aggravate sleep disorders, acting as a stimulant to adrenal glands (Williams, 1995).

23. *Rebalance blood sugar.* Falling asleep easily but waking in the middle of the night could be due to low blood sugar level. Change your meal plan to include more nutritious foods. In the meantime, a

quick fix is to consume a teaspoon of unsweetened juice, cottage cheese, or peanut butter (Williams, 1995).

24. *Change beds and/or pillows* if unable to sleep.

25. *Try sex.* Graedon (1994) recommends sex as a wonderful way to help fall asleep.

26. *Investigate the sleep-robbing effects of every drug taken.* Look up every over-the-counter, prescription, or recreational drug taken and avoid the ones that affect sleep. Common drugs that affect sleep are Norpramine, Prozac, Sarafem, Effexor, Wellbutrin, Tofranil, Nardil, Zoloft, and narcotics (Mindell & Hopkins, 1998). Additional drugs that may cause insomnia include other antidepressants, antihypertensives, antineoplastics, bronchodilators, central nervous system stimulants, corticosteroids, decongestants, diuretics, anticholinergics, histamines, smoking cessation aids (Nadolski, 2003), beta blockers, and recreational drugs (Members of the National Heart, Lung, and Blood Institute Working Group on Insomnia, 1998).

27. *For children who don't sleep, try a bedtime pass* (allows child to leave the bedroom for 10 minutes instead of receiving a lecture or scolding), *a snack, discussion of concerns, and the avoidance of stimulating television shows* (Frimen et al., 1999).

28. *Avoid fatigue and extreme temperature changes* (Schutte & Doghramji, 2003).

29. *Use affirmations* to replace negative thoughts (Hay, 2000). Say or write at least one of the following statements 20 times a day to balance negative thinking patterns:

- I release the day.
- I slip into peaceful sleep.
- Tomorrow will take care of itself.

30. *Identify and elaborate on an interesting and engaging imagery task during the pre-sleep period.* One study revealed that this kind of imagery task was associated with shorter sleep onset and less frequent and distressing pre-sleep thought than general distraction or usual bedtime behavior (Harvey & Payne, 2002).

TREATMENT EVALUATION

Client reported she has decided not to confront her grandfather, who is old and sick. Instead, she plans to write him a letter detailing all her feelings and discuss her words with the nurse rather than mailing the message. Client is in a Stop Smoking class and is using imagery to prepare herself for sleep. She reports good results.

REFERENCES

Azar, B. (1996). Intrusive thoughts proven to undermine our health. *American Psychological Association Monitor, 27,* 10.

Bernardo, M. L. (1999). Disturbances of sleep. *Alternative Health Practitioner, 5*(1), 1–2.

Brown, D. B. (1999). Managing sleep disorders. *Clinician Reviews, 9*(10), 51–70.

Chase, J. E., & Gidal, B. E. (1997). Melatonin: Therapeutic use in sleep disorders. *Annals of Pharmacotherapy, 31,* 1218–1226.

Chen, M. L., Lin, L. C., Wu, S. C., & Lin, J. G. (1999). The effectiveness of acupressure in improving the quality of sleep of institutionalized residents. *Journal of Gerontology and Biological Science and Medical Science, 54,* M389–M394.

Cornell University. (1998). The effect of light exposure on release of melatonin. *Science, 279,* 333–334, 396–399.

Dayton, B. R. (1994). *High touch acupressure workbook II.* Friday Harbor, WA: High Touch Network.

Durlach, J., Pages, N., Bac, P., Bara, M., Guiet-Bara, A., & Agrapart, C. (2002). Chronopathological forms of magnesium depletion with hypofunction or with hyperfunction of the biological clock. *Magnesium Research, 15,* 263–268.

Friman, P. C., Hoff, K. E., Schnoes, C., Freeman, K. A., Woods, D. W., & Blum, N. (1999). The bedtime pass: An approach to bedtime crying and leaving the room. *Archives of Pediatrics & Adolescent Medicine, 153,* 1027–1029.

Gerhard, U., Linnenbrink N., Georghiadou C., & Hobi, V. (1996). Vigilance-decreasing effects of 2 plant-derived sedatives. *Schweizerische Rundschau fur Medez in Praxis, 85,* 473–481.

Graedon, J. (1994). Graedon's guide to getting a good night's sleep. *The people's pharmacy.* King Features, Graedon Enterprises, Inc. (no city).

Gyllenhaal, C., Merritt, S. L., Peterson, S. D., Block, K. I., & Gochenour, T. (2000). Efficacy and safety of herbal stimulants and sedatives in sleep disorders. *Sleep Medicine Research, 4,* 229–251.

Harvey, A. G., & Payne, S. (2002). The management of unwanted pre-sleep thoughts in insomnia: Distraction with imagery versus general distraction. *Behavioral Research, 40,* 267–277.

Hay, L. (2000). *Heal your body.* Carlsbad, CA: Hay House.

Hughes, R. J., Sack, R. L., & Lewy, A. J. (1998). The role of melatonin and circadian phase in age-related sleep-maintenance insomnia: Assessment in a clinical trial of melatonin replacement. *Sleep, 21,* 52–68.

Lee, K. A. (2001). The effect of folate and iron on restless legs syndrome. *Journal of Women's Health and Gender Based Medicine, 10,* 335–341.

Members of the National Heart, Lung, and Blood Institute Working Group on Insomnia. (1998). *Insomnia: Assessment and management in primary care.* Rochester, MN: American Academy of Sleep Medicine.

Methylcobalamin. (1998). *Alternative Medical Reviews, 3,* 461–463.

Mindell, E., & Hopkins, V. (1998). *Prescription alternatives.* New Canaan, CT: Keats.

Montgomery, P., & Dennis, J. (2002). Physical exercise for sleep problems in adults aged 60+. *Cochrane Database System Review, 4,* CD003404.

Nadolski, N. (2003). Getting a good night's sleep: Diagnosing and treating insomnia. *American Journal for Nurse Practitioners,* (Special Supplement), S2–S14.

Schmitz, M., & Jackal, M. (1998). No title available. *Wien Med Wochenschr, 148*(13), 291–298.

Schutte, S., & Doghramji, K. (2003, February). Eyes wide open: Update on sleep disorders. *Clinical Advisor,* pp. 17–27.

Stradling, J., Robers, D., Wilson, A., & Lovelock, F. (1998). Controlled trial of hypnotherapy for weight loss in patients with obstructive sleep apnea. *International Journal of Obesity and Related Metabolic Disorders, 22,* 278–281.

Tiihonen, M., Partinen, M., & Narvanen, S. (1993). The severity of obstructive sleep apnea is associated with insulin resistance. *Journal of Sleep Research, 2,* 56–61.

Williams, D. G. (1995). Safe "shuteye"—natural remedies for insomnia. *Alternatives, 6*(4), 25.

Williams, D. G. (1998). Seven steps to healthy sleep. *Alternatives, 7*(14), 108–109.

CONTACT DR. CLARK

For updated information, a holistic health forum, and a free weekly e-mail newsletter, contact Dr. Clark @ http://HolisticHealth.bellaonline.com.

For information about consultation, workshops, continuing education units or to provide feedback, please contact the author at http://home.earthlink.net/~cccwellness

INDEX

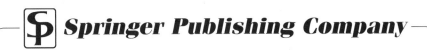

Springer Publishing Company

Spirituality In Nursing
From Traditional to New Age, 2nd Edition
Barbara Stevens Barnum, RN, PhD, FAAN

Praise for second edition:

"Clearly describes historical and current relationships between nursing and spirituality."

"Provides an excellent overview of spirituality."
—American Journal of Nursing

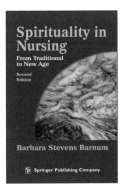

Thoroughly updated, the new edition of this award-winning book looks at spirituality and nursing from many perspectives: theoretical, historical, religious, psychological, and physiological.

Partial Contents:

Part I: Spirituality Today and Yesterday
- Spirituality in Nursing: Past and Present Trends
- Spirituality and Nursing's History

Part II: Spirituality and the Emerging Paradigm
- Spirituality, Physics, Philosophy, and Psychology

Part III: Spirituality and the Individual
- Spirituality and the Mind
- Spirituality, Illness, and Death

Part IV: Spirituality and Nursing's New Paradigm
- Spirituality as a Component in Nursing Theories

Part V: Spiritual Interventions in Health Care
- Spirituality and New Age Therapeutics

Part VI: Spirituality and Ethics
- Spirituality and Ethics: A Contrast in Forms

AJN Book of the Year Award Winner
2003   216pp   0-8261-9181-9   hard

11 West 42nd Street, New York, NY 10036-8002 • Fax: 212-941-7842
Order Toll-Free: 877-687-7476 • Order On-line: www.springerpub.com

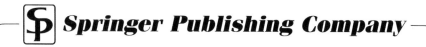

Springer Publishing Company

Nursing as a Spiritual Practice

A Contemporary Application of Florence Nightingale's Views

Janet A. Macrae, PhD, RN

Florence Nightingale is widely regarded as the founder of modern nursing. What is less well known is that she also had well-developed ideas about the spiritual aspects of nursing care. Her views draw from both Eastern and Western spiritual traditions and have a startling relevance to nursing practice today. Janet Macrae, a Nightingale scholar and a nationally recognized expert on therapeutic touch, outlines Nightingale's ideas on spirituality in this book and discusses how a variety of techniques can be used to achieve a more spiritual and humane form of nursing care. The techniques, which include yoga, meditation, and relaxation exercises, can be used by both nurses and patients.

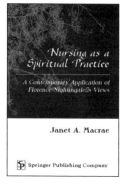

Contents:

PART 1: Nightingale on Spirituality

- Nightingale's Spiritual Vision
- Spirituality, Religion, and Health Care
- Spiritual Development

PART II: Spirituality in Nursing Practice: Using the Nightingale Influence

- Stress Reduction and Relaxation
  Compassion
- Listening and Awareness
- On Prayer
- Spirituality and Conduct
- True Work

2001   144pp   0-8261-1387-7   hard

11 West 42nd Street, New York, NY 10036-8002 • Fax: 212-941-7842
Order Toll-Free: 877-687-7476 • Order On-line: www.springerpub.com